MW00353690

A Practical Approach to Pain Management

Edited by

Mathew Lefkowitz, M.D.

Clinical Associate Professor, Department of
Anesthesiology, State University of New
York Health Science Center at Brooklyn;
Attending Physician, Long Island College
Hospital, Brooklyn, New York

Allen H. Lebovits, Ph.D.

Associate Professor, Department of
Anesthesiology, State University of New
York Health Science Center at Brooklyn;
Co-Director, Pain Management Service,
University Hospital of Brooklyn and Long
Island College Hospital, Brooklyn, New
York

with

David J. Wlody, M.D.

Clinical Associate Professor, Department of
Anesthesiology, State University of New
York Health Science Center at Brooklyn;
Director of Obstetric Anesthesia, Long
Island College Hospital, Brooklyn, New
York

Stuart A. Rubin, M.D.

Visiting Assistant Professor, Department of
Rehabilitation Medicine, Albert Einstein
College of Medicine of Yeshiva University,
Bronx, New York; Private Practice—Pain
Management and Rehabilitation Medicine,
Boca Raton/Boynton Beach, Florida

Little, Brown and Company
Boston   New York   Toronto   London

Copyright © 1996 by Mathew Lefkowitz and Allen H. Lebovits
First Edition

All rights reserved. No part of this
book may be reproduced in any form
or by any electronic or mechanical
means, including information storage
and retrieval systems, without
permission in writing from the
publisher, except by a reviewer who
may quote brief passages in a review.

Library of Congress Cataloging-in-Publication Data

A practical approach to pain management / edited by Mathew Lefkowitz,
    Allen H. Lebovits; with David J. Wlody, Stuart A. Rubin.
        p.   cm.
    Includes bibliographical references and index.
    ISBN 0-316-51958-8
    1. Pain—Treatment. 2. Analgesia. I. Lefkowitz, Mathew.
    II. Lebovits, Allen H.
    [DNLM: 1. Pain—therapy. WL 704 P8948 1996]
    RB127.P72   1996
    616'.0472—dc20
    DNLM/DLC
    for Library of Congress   95-39061
                                                                CIP

Printed in the United States of America

RRD–VA

Editorial: Nancy E. Chorpenning, Richard L. Wilcox
Production Services: Tracey A. Solon
Copyeditor: Genevieve MacLellan
Indexer: Hagerty and Holloway
Production Supervisor: Mike Burggren
Cover Designer: Mike Burggren

To our families and friends, who have always been there for us, but most of all to our patients—we hope we have been there for you

Contents

Preface

Pain is a ubiquitous symptom and, in its chronic form, a syndrome that draws from nearly all medical specialties—anesthesiology, physiatry, psychiatry, neurology, pharmacology, obstetrics and gynecology, pediatrics, otolaryngology, neurosurgery, and dentistry, to name just a few. Thus, nearly all physicians and health care specialists require knowledge about the evaluation and treatment of pain. The field of pain management, as evidenced by the proliferation of journals and books devoted to pain, is growing so rapidly, however, that it is challenging for even the most seasoned pain management practitioner to keep up with all aspects of this multifaceted specialization.

The complexity of acute and chronic pain mandates a comprehensive evaluation and treatment approach. Single-specialty training of health care providers is not adequate where pain management is concerned. Bonica's first introduction of the concept of multidisciplinary pain management over 40 years ago is now the accepted gold standard of practice. Given the current health care crisis and the increasing emphasis on demonstration of short- and long-term outcome effectiveness, there is growing pressure for the specialist to be well versed in all aspects of pain evaluation and treatment. Paradoxically, the trend toward specialization in medicine as well as in private practice promotes a narrow, tunnel-vision framework, when what is needed for optimal pain management is a broad, multifaceted understanding of the field.

This book aims to provide the busy single-specialty provider with a detailed and in-depth review of the significant clinical practice approaches to pain management. Many times the challenge for the clinician is in referring the patient to the right specialist. An understanding of the techniques currently being used by pain specialists will enable practitioners to provide their patients with competent referrals. Educated clinicians can more effectively direct their patient to the appropriate specialist or clinic for definitive diagnosis and treatment. If appropriate, the clinician might also apply some aspects of the techniques himself or herself.

A Practical Approach to Pain Management is not intended as a comprehensive textbook; rather, it is a how-to handbook written in outline format. Practical clinical aspects have been emphasized rather than theory. The reader is encouraged to explore the references or suggested readings at the end of each chapter for further coverage and a more theoretical approach.

This book is divided into two sections. The first section, Therapeutic and Diagnostic Approaches, includes chapters on nearly every major therapeutic and diagnostic approach to pain evaluation and management. Chapters cover acute pain management, pharmacologic management, regional techniques, psychological approaches, physical techniques, and various other approaches and issues. The second section, Pain Syndromes, focuses on the specific pain syndromes most commonly encountered in practice, including the complex issue of pediatric pain. The authors are recognized specialists in their fields, sharing expertise and clinical insight they have accrued over many years of practice.

A book the length and scope of *A Practical Approach to Pain Management* cannot be prepared without the assistance and support of a great many people. We gratefully acknowledge the support of the members of the Department of Anesthesiology, State University of New York Health Science Center at Brooklyn; and Long Island College Hospital. We also thank Ms. Ellen Jackson for her help with manuscript preparation and organization; Ms. Irma Rudnick; and Mr. Tom Eagan for his editorial assistance. Lastly, we thank our contributors for their patience over this long process, and our coeditors, Drs. David J. Wlody and Stuart A. Rubin, whose contributions were invaluable to the production of this book.

A.H.L
M.L.

Contributing Authors

Lynette E. Bassman, Ph.D.

Assistant Professor, University Counseling Center, Shippensburg University, Shippensburg, Pennsylvania

Bennett Blumenkopf, M.D.

Associate Professor, Department of Neurological Surgery, Vanderbilt University School of Medicine, Nashville, Tennessee

Arlene M. Braker, M.D.

Assistant Professor of Physical Medicine and Rehabilitation, Medical College of Wisconsin, Milwaukee

William Breitbart, M.D.

Associate Professor, Department of Psychiatry, Cornell University Medical College; Associate Attending Psychiatrist, Memorial Sloan-Kettering Cancer Center, New York

May L. Chin, M.D.

Associate Professor, Department of Anesthesiology, George Washington University School of Medicine and Health Sciences; Director, Acute Pain Service, Department of Anesthesiology, George Washington University Medical Center, Washington

Mathelyn Claudio-Santiago, R.N., B.S.N.

Senior Clinical Associate, Department of Anesthesiology, Pain Management Program, Montefiore Medical Center, Bronx, New York

Mary M. Conaway, R.N., B.S.N.

Nurse Representative, Pharmacy, Lehigh Valley Hospital, Allentown, Pennsylvania

Barry C. Cooper, D.D.S.

Former Associate Professor of Clinical Otolaryngology, New York Medical College, Valhalla, New York; Attending Physician, Department of Surgery (Dentistry), St. Vincent's Hospital and Medical Center of New York, New York

John P. Dodaro, M.D.

Chief Resident, Department of Otolaryngology, State University of New York Health Science Center at Brooklyn; Chief Resident, Department of Otolaryngology, Long Island College Hospital, Brooklyn, New York

Joseph Dryer, M.D.	Clinical Instructor, Department of Orthopedic Surgery, New York Medical College, Valhalla, New York; Attending Physician, St. Vincent's Hospital and Medical Center of New York, New York
Eric B. Fishman, M.D.	Clinical Assistant Instructor, Department of Anesthesiology, State University of New York at Stony Brook Health Sciences Center, Stony Brook, New York
Mark G. Greenbaum, M.D.	Assistant Professor, Department of Rehabilitation Medicine, Albert Einstein College of Medicine of Yeshiva University; Director, Lubin Rehabilitation Center, Jack D. Weiler Hospital of the Albert Einstein College of Medicine, Bronx, New York
Paul Gusmorino, M.D.	Assistant Clinical Professor of Psychiatry, Albert Einstein College of Medicine of Yeshiva University, Bronx, New York; Medical Director, Pain Center, Department of Behavioral Medicine, Hospital for Joint Diseases, New York
Thomas R. Haher, M.D.	Professor of Orthopedic Surgery, New York Medical College, Valhalla, New York; Chairman, Department of Orthopedic Surgery, St. Vincent's Hospital and Medical Center of New York, New York
Robert Jablonski, Jr., M.D.	Assistant Attending Physician, Department of Plastic and Reconstructive Surgery, New York Eye and Ear Infirmary, New York
Subhash Jain, M.D.	Associate Professor of Anesthesiology, Cornell University Medical College; Director, Pain Management, Department of Anesthesiology and Critical Care Medicine, Memorial Sloan-Kettering Cancer Center, New York
Edith R. Kepes, M.D.	Clinical Professor Emeritus, Department of Anesthesia, Albert Einstein College of Medicine of Yeshiva University; Attending Anesthesiologist, Montefiore Medical Center, Bronx, New York
Yasin N. Khan, M.D.	Clinical Assistant Professor of Anesthesiology, Pennsylvania State University College of Medicine, Hershey, Pennsylvania; Medical Director of Pain Medicine, Sacred Heart Hospital, Allentown, Pennsylvania

Allen H. Lebovits, Ph.D.	Associate Professor, Department of Anesthesiology, State University of New York Health Science Center at Brooklyn; Co-Director, Pain Management Service, University Hospital of Brooklyn and Long Island College Hospital, Brooklyn, New York
Mathew Lefkowitz, M.D.	Clinical Associate Professor, Department of Anesthesiology, State University of New York Health Science Center at Brooklyn; Attending Physician, Long Island College Hospital, Brooklyn, New York
Alan M. Levine, M.D.	Director of Acute Postoperative Pain Service, Palms of Pasadena Hospital, St. Petersburg, Florida
Mark A. Liker, M.D.	Medical Student, Department of Orthopedic Surgery, State University of New York Health Science Center at Brooklyn, Brooklyn, New York
Frank E. Lucente, M.D.	Professor and Chairman, Department of Otolaryngology, State University of New York Health Science Center at Brooklyn; Chairman, Department of Otolaryngology, Long Island College Hospital and University Hospital of Brooklyn, Brooklyn, New York
Douglas R. Lyman, Ph.D.	Clinical Staff Psychologist, Pain Rehabilitation Center, Elmbrook Memorial Hospital, Brookfield, Wisconsin
N. Timothy Lynch, Ph.D.	Assistant Professor of Anesthesiology, Medical College of Wisconsin, Milwaukee
Robert A. Marini, M.D.	Assistant Clinical Professor, Department of Rehabilitation Medicine, Albert Einstein College of Medicine of Yeshiva University; Attending Physician, Department of Rehabilitation Medicine, Jack D. Weiler Hospital of the Albert Einstein College of Medicine, Bronx, New York
Nancy Chiyo Maruyama, M.D.	Instructor, Department of Psychiatry and Human Behavior, Brown University School of Medicine; Staff Psychiatrist, Department of Psychiatry, Roger Williams Medical Center, Providence, Rhode Island
Alexander Mauskop, M.D.	Assistant Professor, Department of Neurology, State University of New York Health Science Center at Brooklyn, Brooklyn, New York; Director, New York Headache Center, New York

John S. McDonald, M.D. — Professor and Chairman of Anesthesiology, Professor of Obstetrics and Gynecology, and Director, Pain Control Center (Anesthesiology), Ohio State University College of Medicine, Columbus, Ohio

Robert C. Nucci, M.D. — Active Staff, Department of Orthopedics, Helen Ellis Hospital, Tarpon Springs, Florida

Jyoti Patel-Silvera, M.D. — Clinical Assistant Professor, Department of Anesthesia, University of Florida College of Medicine, Gainesville, Florida; Director of Pain Management, Department of Anesthesia, Flager Hospital, St. Augustine, Florida

Isaac Pinter, Ph.D. — Assistant Professor, Rehabilitation Medicine, Mount Sinai School of Medicine of the City University of New York; Administrative Director, Pain Center, Department of Behavioral Medicine, Hospital for Joint Diseases, New York

Russell K. Portenoy, M.D. — Associate Professor, Department of Neurology, Cornell University Medical College; Director of Analgesic Studies, Pain Service, Department of Neurology, Memorial Sloan-Kettering Cancer Center, New York

Howard L. Rosner, M.D. — Assistant Professor of Anesthesiology, Cornell University Medical College; Director of Pain Management, The New York Hospital, New York

Stuart A. Rubin, M.D. — Visiting Assistant Professor, Department of Rehabilitation Medicine, Albert Einstein College of Medicine of Yeshiva University, Bronx, New York; Private Practice—Pain Management and Rehabilitation Medicine, Boca Raton/Boynton Beach, Florida

Vincent R. Saladini, Jr., M.D. — Director, Pain Treatment Service, and Attending Physician, Department of Anesthesiology, Hackensack Medical Center, Hackensack, New Jersey

Joseph G. Sankoorikal, M.D. — Medical Director, Rehabilitation Services, St. Francis Hospital, Topeka, Kansas

Alan C. Santos, M.D. — Associate Professor of Anesthesiology and Obstetrics and Gynecology, Albert Einstein College of Medicine of Yeshiva University; Director of Obstetric Anesthesia, Abraham Jacobi Hospital, Bronx, New York

Robert J. Schwartzman, M.D.

Professor and Chairman, Department of Neurology, Medical College of Pennsylvania and Hahnemann University; Clinical Services Chief, Department of Neurology, Medical College of Pennsylvania and Hahnemann University, Philadelphia

Barbara S. Shapiro, M.D.

Assistant Clinical Professor, Department of Pediatrics, University of Pennsylvania School of Medicine; Attending Physician, Division of General Pediatrics, Children's Hospital of Philadelphia, Philadelphia

Barry R. Snow, Ph.D.

Adjunct Assistant Professor, School of Public Health, Columbia University College of Physicians and Surgeons; Clinical Psychologist and Associate Director, Pain Center, Department of Behavioral Medicine, Hospital for Joint Diseases, New York

Rajka Soric, M.D.

Assistant Professor and Director, Division of Physiatry, Department of Medicine, University of Toronto Faculty of Medicine; Physiatrist-in-Chief, Department of Rehabilitation Medicine, Mount Sinai Hospital, Toronto

Ellen S. Steinberg, M.D.

Clinical Assistant Professor of Anesthesiology and Obstetrics and Gynecology, State University of New York at Stony Brook Health Sciences Center; Director of Obstetric Anesthesia, The University Hospital at Stony Brook, Stony Brook, New York

Sridhar V. Vasudevan, M.D.

Clinical Professor, Department of Physical Medicine and Rehabilitation, Medical College of Wisconsin, Milwaukee; Medical Director, Pain Rehabilitation Center, Elmbrook Memorial Hospital, Brookfield, Wisconsin

Ronald E. Wilson, M.D.

Assistant Clinical Professor, Department of Neurology, Vanderbilt University School of Medicine; Neurologist, Centennial Medical Center, Nashville, Tennessee

David J. Wlody, M.D.

Clinical Associate Professor, Department of Anesthesiology, State University of New York Health Science Center at Brooklyn; Director of Obstetric Anesthesia, Long Island College Hospital, Brooklyn, New York

A Practical Approach to Pain Management

Notice. The indications and dosages of all drugs in this book have been recommended in the medical literature and conform to the practices of the general medical community. The medications described do not necessarily have specific approval by the Food and Drug Administration for use in the diseases and dosages for which they are recommended. The package insert for each drug should be consulted for use and dosage as approved by the FDA. Because standards for usage change, it is advisable to keep abreast of revised recommendations, particularly those concerning new drugs.

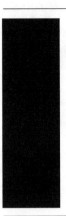

Therapeutic and Diagnostic Approaches

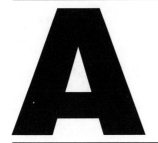

Acute Pain

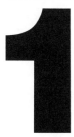

The Pharmacologic Management of Acute Postoperative Pain

Howard L. Rosner

I. Background
A. Definition of acute pain
1. Pain of recent onset
2. Duration of 0 to 7 days
3. Mild to severe in nature
4. Having an etiology that is usually a single "fixable" event or one in which the body will heal itself
5. Having input into the CNS through peripheral nociceptors
6. Its treatment is usually aimed at the cause of the pain

B. Pain classification by duration of symptoms is outlined in Table 1-1.

C. Management.
Although pain is rarely life-threatening, the need for pain reduction can be urgent, requiring prompt attention. Analgesics, both narcotic and nonnarcotic, are indicated for the management of acute pain. Historically, narcotic analgesics have been the mainstays of treatment for acute pain. The most common routes of administration are oral, rectal, subcutaneous, intramuscular, intravenous, and neuraxial. Newer methods of administration are sublingual, transbuccal, intranasal, and transdermal.[1,2]

II. Systemic narcotic administration
effectively manages acute pain by raising the serum opiate concentration into a therapeutic range. The time of onset of analgesia differs with the route of administration. The following methods are effective systemic dosing techniques.

A. Parenteral bolus administration
1. Intramuscular injection
2. Subcutaneous injection
3. Intravenous injection

B. Enteral administration
techniques have the disadvantage of a slower onset of action than parenteral; however, they can successfully maintain a therapeutic serum level as well as parenteral administration can.

C. Patient-controlled analgesia (PCA) pumps
(PCA in general is discussed in greater detail in Chap. 2). One of the most exciting advances in microprocessor technology has been the advent of "smart" pumps to deliver narcotic analgesics to postoperative patients. These modified infusion pumps are able to administer
1. Infusions of narcotics
2. Small preprogrammed bolus doses on patient demand
3. Larger bolus by prescription
4. Taken together, these PCA specifications allow patients to titrate their narcotic doses as needed, while avoiding the toxic side effects that result from high peak serum levels which commonly result from parenteral techniques (e.g., IM prn dosage)[3]

III. Neuraxial narcotic administration.
Narcotics, local anesthetics, and mixtures of narcotics and local anesthetics are routinely administered into the neuraxis (by epidural or subarachnoid injection) for postoperative analgesia. The advantages of this type of analgesia are widely documented, as are many of its associated problems. Neuraxial narcotics can be classified on the basis of their lipid solubility, which indicates the duration of action and the time from injection to effect. In this classification system, a narcotic can be hydrophilic (lipophobic) or lipophilic.

A. Hydrophilic narcotics
such as morphine, when placed in the lumbar epidural space (in doses of 3–5 mg) or the subarachnoid space (in doses of 0.5–1.5 mg), provide excellent analgesia for 12 to 24 hours per dose. Morphine can also be given by epidural infusion (0.1 mg/ml at 3–5 ml/hr) with periodic adjustments

Table 1-1. Pain classification by duration of symptoms

Acute
Duration of 0 to 7 days
Mild to severe
Etiology known or unknown, usually a single, "fixable" event
Input from nociceptors (peripheral pain receptors)
Treatment of causes and pain reduction, often urgent: analgesics are narcotic and nonnarcotic
Mild psychological contribution

Subacute
Duration of 7 days to 6 mo
Mild to severe
Etiology as in acute pain
Input from nociceptors
Treatment of causes and pain reduction, usually not urgent: analgesics are narcotic and nonnarcotic
Mild psychological contribution

Ongoing acute
Any duration of time
Usually severe
Due to ongoing tissue damage from neoplasms

Input from nociceptors
Treatment of causes and pain reduction: analgesics are narcotic and nonnarcotic
Depression and anxiety common

Recurrent acute
Any duration of time
Mild to severe
Due to chronic organic nonmalignant pathology
Input from nociceptors
Treatment of causes and pain reduction: analgesics are nonnarcotic and co-analgesics used as
    first-line treatment; narcotics sometimes indicated
Depression and anxiety common

Chronic intractable benign pain syndrome
Duration of more than 6 mo
Mild to severe
Etiology unknown
No known nociceptive input
Treatment aimed at pain reduction: analgesics are nonnarcotic, and co-analgesics are used; usually
    no indication for narcotics
Psychological factors very important; psychotherapy indicated
Patient may or may not have adequate coping mechanisms

to ensure adequate analgesia. Hydrophilic narcotics remain within the water phase of the cerebrospinal fluid (CSF) for prolonged periods of time and thus can spread throughout the neuraxis, including the ventricles of the brain. Because the CSF acts as the reservoir and the drugs will take up to 24 hours to dissipate from the CSF, these drugs can provide analgesia in areas distant from the injection site. This is also why complications such as respiratory suppression, pruritus, nausea, and vomiting can occur (as opiate receptors in the brain stem are stimulated).[4]

B. **Lipophilic narcotics,** such as fentanyl and sufentanil, are more commonly administered epidurally. Their use is associated with fewer complications because they spend far less free time in the CSF compared with morphine. Rather, they are taken up quickly into the high-lipid-content tissue of the spinal cord. This provides excellent but highly segmental analgesia. These agents can affect areas distant from the injection site only by adding volume to the injectate (e.g., 15–20 ml total volume for thoracic analgesia from a lumbar epidural catheter). Fentanyl (in doses of 100–150 µg) or sufentanil (in doses of 10–15 µg) provide analgesia for 3 to 6 hours in single-bolus doses.[5,6]

Lipophilic narcotics are also commonly used by infusion when the epidural catheter is placed in proximity to the affected segments. A rate of 3–5 ml/hr for thoracic catheters and 5–10 ml/hr for lumbar catheters is most commonly employed. Fentanyl is diluted to a therapeutic concentration of 5–10 µg/ml and sufentanil to 0.5–1 µg/ml for these infusions.

C. The addition of a dilute **local anesthetic** (e.g., 0.05–0.10% bupivacaine) to an infusion increases the depth of analgesia without causing substantial motor, sensory, or sympathetic blockade. Local anesthetic infusions without narcotics can also provide analgesia, but the concentrations required are high enough to cause some impairment of motor, sensory, and sympathetic function. A lower concentration of narcotic is required to produce analgesia when mixed with a local anesthetic.[5–7]

IV. Epidural narcotic analgesia

A. Dosage

1. Although clinicians find it difficult to agree on an absolute dose, most think the optimal dosage for epidural morphine is in the range of 3 to 4 mg every 12 to 24 hours. No added benefit (but a greater incidence of side effects) has been noted by increasing the dose beyond 4 mg, although substantial decreases in benefit are observed below 3 mg. Side effects are also minimized in this dosage range.

2. Fentanyl and other lipophilic drugs have a segmental dosage pattern. They can be administered by bolus dose to begin an analgesic regimen, by intermittent bolus for prolonged analgesia, or as a rescue for inadequate analgesia due to neuraxial morphine. Lipophilic narcotics work exceedingly well when administered by a bolus loading dose followed by an infusion. If the tip of the epidural catheter is juxtaposed to the dermatomes that need to be blocked, then the doses required are quite low (e.g., 50–100 µg loading dose) and a low rate of infusion is needed (up to 50 µg/hr) to maintain analgesia. If the surgical site is more distant (as in thoracic surgery with a lumbar catheter), then a higher rate of infusion (up to 150 µg/hr) may be necessary.

B. Summary of neuraxial narcotics

1. The analgesia produced is intense, segmental, dose related, and effective for postoperative and visceral-type pain.

2. Lipid solubility is an important criterion for the disposition of these agents. Hydrophilic compounds such as morphine, which possess high receptor binding affinity, produce an intense and prolonged analgesic period with a latency of 30 minutes to 1 hour. Lipophilic compounds such as fentanyl produce an intense analgesia with more rapid onset and a shorter duration of action (1–3 hr).

3. Neuraxial narcotics do not produce sympathetic or motor blockade in clinically relevant doses.

4. Respiratory depression of a significant and consistent nature has been found to occur when morphine in large doses (10 mg) is injected into the epidural space of pain-free volunteers.

5. Lipid-soluble agents such as methadone, fentanyl, and hydromorphone cause relatively little respiratory suppression.

6. Pain from abdominal malignancy can be relieved by small doses of morphine (0.5 mg spinal or 2 mg epidural) every 24 hours.
7. The concomitant use of low-dose morphine (2 mg) and fentanyl (50 μg) by bolus injection can provide better analgesia and longer duration of action.
8. Analgesia for labor can be achieved with small doses (0.5 mg) of spinal morphine but requires doses of epidural morphine larger than 8 mg, which would produce sufficiently high blood levels to depress the neonate. Labor analgesia is especially effective with neuraxial sufentanil. Fentanyl is also commonly used.
9. Side effects include nausea, vomiting, pruritus, drowsiness, dizziness, urinary retention, and respiratory depression. Hydrophilic narcotics such as morphine have a greater incidence of side effects than those that are more lipophilic. Higher doses of morphine have a greater incidence of side effects.
10. Naloxone in very small doses (0.01–0.05 mg/hr infusion) can prevent the side effects from occurring and in slightly higher doses (0.05–0.10 mg bolus) can reverse side effects that have occurred. Low-dose naloxone does not usually reverse the analgesia of epidural or intrathecal narcotics.
11. Neuraxial narcotics hasten ambulation and decrease hospital stays in postoperative patients and can make the entire postoperative period less traumatic.

V. Neuraxial narcotic infusions and patient-controlled epidural analgesia (PCEA)

A. **Program parameters** are in milligrams or milliliters. Infusions will typically use milliliters as the program parameter.
B. **Drug concentration.** Fentanyl at a concentration of 5–10 μg/ml is the most common agent used. A mixture of local anesthetic and narcotic may be used if the catheter tip is adjacent to the surgical site, e.g., fentanyl (5 μg/ml) plus 0.05–0.10% bupivacaine (0.5–1.0 mg/ml). Alternative narcotics such as sufentanil (0.5–1.0 μg/ml) or morphine (100 μg/ml) may be substituted.
C. **Initial bolus loading** is the loading dose required to achieve analgesia. Typically this will require 3–5 ml q5–6min until analgesia, with a maximum of 20 ml (before reevaluation).
D. **Demand dose** is the dose that the patient will receive when he or she presses the demand button if a PCA pump is used and the patient is given control of the infusion (patient-controlled epidural analgesia or PCEA).[8]
   Note: For the most part, this technique is not widely practiced; therefore, patients receiving epidural narcotics usually receive infusions with no demand feature. This would be ordered as a demand dose of 0 ml per attempt. (The demand button itself will be detached from the infuser for epidural use.)
E. **Dosage interval** is the interval during which the machine will not deliver any medication. Since the demand dose is set to 0 ml per attempt, the dosage interval is moot (any setting is fine, just specify a number that the machine will accept, e.g., 1 min).
F. **Basal infusion** is the infusion portion of the pump and the major focus of epidural narcotic analgesia. This should be ordered in the range of 3–10 ml/hr depending on the proximity of the catheter to the dermatomal level of the incision.
G. **One-hour limit.** The machine will shut down when this limit is reached. The most convenient way of setting this limitation is for the maximum that the other settings will deliver. The machine will not allow a higher limit than the product of the basal rate and the demand doses, but it will allow a smaller limit than this product. If the machine shuts down, it will sound an alarm until a staff member turns the alarm off. In this setting, the 1-hour limit should equal the hourly rate of infusion.
H. **Sample orders**
   1. **Epidural infusion only**
      a. Drug and concentration: fentanyl 10 μg/ml (alternative mixture: fentanyl 5 μg/ml plus 0.05% bupivacaine)
      b. Demand dose: 0 ml per attempt
      c. Dosage interval: 0 min
      d. Basal infusion: 5 ml/hr
      e. One-hour limit: 5 ml
      f. Typical antiemetic: prochlorperazine (Compazine) 10–25 mg IM, PO, or rectally q4–6h prn (alternative antiemetics: trimethobenzamide [Tigan] 150 mg IM, PO, or rectally; or hydroxyzine [Vistaril] 25 mg IM or PO q4–6h prn; or transdermal scopolamine patch, every 3 days)

g. Typical hypnotic: triazolam (Halcion) 0.125–0.25 mg PO or SL prn at bedtime (alternative hypnotics: diphenhydramine [Benadryl] 25 mg IM or PO; or zolpidem tartrate [Ambien] 10 mg PO prn at bedtime)

2. Epidural PCA (PCEA)

a. Drug and concentration: sufentanil 1 µg/ml (alternative mixture: sufentanil 0.5 µg/ml plus 0.05% bupivacaine)

b. Demand dose: 2 ml per attempt

c. Dosage interval: 20 min

d. Basal infusion: 4 ml/hr

e. One-hour limit: 10 ml

f. Typical antiemetic: prochlorperazine 10–25 mg IM, PO, or rectally q4–6h prn (alternative antiemetics: trimethobenzamide 150 mg IM, PO, or rectally; or hydroxyzine 25 mg IM or PO q4–6h prn; or transdermal scopolamine patch every 3 days)

g. Typical hypnotic: triazolam 0.125–0.250 mg PO or SL prn at bedtime (alternative hypnotics: diphenhydramine 25 mg IM or PO; or zolpidem tartrate 10 mg PO prn at bedtime)

I. Other considerations

1. Following the initial orders, there can be **further orders** for pump increases for continued pain and pump decreases for toxic side effects. Changes should be directed at maintaining analgesia without toxicity. In the event of continued pain, patients should receive another bolus under the original orders (approximately 5–10 ml of analgesic mixture), and the rate should be increased by 2–3 ml/hr.

2. If the patient has **excess pain** relative to what might be suspected and the infuser is not delivering adequate analgesia, consider that there is some other process occurring which can cause pain (e.g., urinary retention, compartment syndrome following cast placement). Also, consider that the catheter may not be in the epidural space or that the distance from the catheter tip to the level of the incision is too great.

VI. Other methods of acute pain control include administration of pharmacologic agents such as nonnarcotic analgesics, nerve block injections (either one-shot or continuous techniques), and transcutaneous electrical nerve stimulation (TENS). Nerve blocks and TENS are beyond the scope of this chapter and are discussed in Chapters 7–10 and 14.

A. Nonnarcotic analgesics include acetaminophen, aspirin, and nonsteroidal anti-inflammatory drugs (NSAIDs)[9] (Table 1-2). Acetaminophen and aspirin possess a centrally acting effect that can enhance the activity of narcotics. Aspirin and NSAIDs also possess a peripheral effect in inhibiting prostaglandin synthesis. Prostaglandins are released from the site of tissue injury (e.g., surgery), which sensitizes peripheral nociceptors to stimulus by bradykinin and substance P, released by tissue damage (which starts the pain cascade). By inhibiting prostaglandins, the activation of peripheral nociceptors is reduced. The major problems with NSAID administration to the postoperative patient are fever suppression and platelet dysfunction. If these are not contraindications in a particular case, then NSAIDs can be useful adjuvants to narcotic analgesics (Tables 1-3 and 1-4).

B. Ketorolac (Toradol). The major limiting feature in the use of NSAIDs for postoperative patients has been the route of administration. Until recently these drugs were available in only a capsule form not suited to most patients in the immediate perioperative period. Only indomethacin is available in a suppository form. Both these routes have the limitations of enteral administration, as previously described. However, ketorolac is the first NSAID available for parenteral administration. This drug is administered in a loading dose and maintenance dose format of 30–60 mg and 15–30 mg IM or IV q4–6h. The total daily dose should not exceed 150 mg for the first day and 120 mg for the subsequent days of use.

C. Acetaminophen (in doses of up to 4 g/day) is a useful treatment for mild pain and a widely used adjuvant to opiates for severe pain. The major considerations in the use of acetaminophen are fever suppression and hepatic toxicity. As with the NSAIDs, acetaminophen will suppress fever activity, which may be contraindicated. Acetaminophen is converted by conjugation and hydroxylation in the liver to inactive metabolites; however, high doses result in the formation of N-acetyl-p-benzoquinone, believed to be responsible for hepatotoxicity.

D. Mixed agonist-antagonist opiates include, among others, the drugs pentazocine, butorphanol, nalbuphine, and dezocine. These drugs lack the efficacy of the

Table 1-2. Nonsteroidal anti-inflammatory drugs

Generic name (trade name)	Usual dosages and routes of administration	Maximum dose/day and major side effects*
Aspirin (many)	650–1000 mg PO or rectally qid	4.0 g/day Tinnitus
Diclofenac (Voltaren)	25–75 mg PO bid-tid	150 mg/day Headache, edema, dizziness, tinnitus
Diflunisal (Dolobid)	500 mg PO bid-tid	1.5 g/day Headache, rash, fatigue, dizziness
Fenoprofen (Nalfon)	200–600 mg PO qid	3.2 g/day Dizziness, headache
Ibuprofen (Advil, Nuprin, Rufen, Motrin)	200–800 mg PO tid-qid	3.2 g/day Dizziness, rash
Indomethacin (Indocin)	25–75 mg PO q8–12h, or 50 mg rectally q6–12h	200mg/day Confusion, headache
Ketorolac (Toradol) (Note: only IM/IV NSAID)	30–60 mg IM or IV loading dose, then 15–30 mg IM q4–6h, or 10–30 mg PO q4–6h	150 mg 1st-day, then 120 mg/day thereafter Edema, drowsiness, sweating, dizziness
Meclofenamate (Meclomen)	100 mg PO qid	50–400 mg/day Diarrhea, rash
Naproxen (Naprosyn, Anaprox, Aleve)	200–500 mg PO bid-tid	1.25 g/day Tinnitus, edema, dizziness, rash
Piroxicam (Feldene)	10 mg PO bid, or 20 mg PO every day	20 mg/day Malaise, dizziness
Sulindac (Clinoril)	150–200 mg PO bid	400 mg/day Headache, edema, dizziness, rash

*Common side effects are gastritis, platelet suppression, bowel disturbances, mild renal suppression. Phenylbutazone has not been included on this list because of the severity of its side effects. Choline magnesium trisalicylate (Trilisate) and salsalate (Disalcid) have not been included because of their poor performance when compared with the above medications.

Table 1-3. Narcotic analgesics for mild to moderate pain

Generic name (trade name)	Starting dose and route of administration	Duration of action	Side effects and comments[a]
Codeine (many)[b,c]	30–60 mg PO q4–6h	4–6 hr	See footnote[c]
Hydrocodone (Vicodin, Lorcet)[b]	5–10 mg PO q4–6h	4–6 hr	Dysphoria
Oxycodone (Percodan, Percocet, Tylox)[b]	2.25–4.50 mg PO q3–6h	3–6 hr	Dysphoria, shorter acting
Pentazocine (Talwin)	25–50 mg PO q3–4h	3–6 hr	Dysphoria, agonist/antagonist type. May precipitate withdrawal symptoms if given to narcotic addict. Can be given by injection for more severe pain. Peak dose per day 600 mg PO, 360 mg IM.
Propoxyphene (Darvon, Darvon-N, Darvocet)[b]	32–65 mg PO q4–6h	4–6 hr	Dysphoria, hepatic dysfunction, convulsions with overdose
Naphsylate preparation	50–100 mg PO q4–6h		

[a]Common side effects are respiratory suppression, constipation, somnolence, nausea and vomiting, tolerance with continued use, urinary retention, and pruritus.
[b]These narcotics are commonly compounded with aspirin or acetaminophen with a wide variety of trade names.
[c]In compounds the dose of codeine is notated by a numeral from 1 to 4: 1 indicates a codeine dose of 7.5 mg, 2 a dose of 15 mg, 3 a dose of 30 mg, and 4 a dose of 60 mg. Other constituents of these compounds may include caffeine, barbiturates, and sympathomimetics.

Table 1-4. Narcotic analgesics for severe pain

Generic name (trade name)	Route and starting dose	Peak effect	Equianalgesic doses[a]	Comments[b]
Hydromorphone (Dilaudid)	**PO:** 4–6 mg q3–4h **IM:** 1–2 mg q3–4h **Rectally:** 3–6 mg q4–8h	1–2 hr ½–1 hr 1–2 hr	7.5 mg 1.5 mg 6 mg	Good GI uptake
Levorphanol (Levo-Dromoran)	**PO:** 2–4 mg q6–8h **IM:** 2mg q4–6h	1–2 hr ½–1 hr	4 mg 2 mg	Can accumulate over 2–3 days; long plasma half-life. Good GI uptake
Meperidine (Demerol)	**PO:** 50–200 mg q2–4h **IM:** 50–100 mg q1½–3h1–4 hr	1–4 hr 2–4 hr	150–200 mg 100 mg	Poor GI uptake. Normeperidine (toxic metabolite) can accumulate, leading to CNS excitation.
Methadone (Dolophine)	**PO:** 5–10 mg q6–12h **IM:** 5–10 mg q4–6h	1–2 hr ½–1 hr	15–20 mg 10 mg	Good GI uptake. Can accumulate with chronic use yielding half-life up to 2 days.
Morphine (Controlled-release)	**PO:** 20–60 mg q3–4h **IM:** 5–10 mg q3–4h **PO:** 20–60 mg q6–12h	1–2 hr ½–1 hr 2–4 hr	20–60 mg 10 mg 2–4 hr	Poor GI uptake, improves with chronic use, from 6:1 ratio to 2:1–3:1 ratio of PO to IM dosing.
Oxymorphone (Numorphan)	**IM:** 1 mg q4h **Rectally:** 5–10 mg q4–6h	½–1 hr 1–3 hr	1 mg 5–10 mg	No oral preparation

[a]Equianalgesic doses stated in comparison with morphine 10 mg IM.
[b]Common side effects are respiratory suppression, constipation, somnolence, nausea and vomiting, pruritus, urinary retention, tolerance with continued use, dysphoria, euphoria. Caution should be used in patients in danger of carbon dioxide retention, increased intracranial pressure.

pure agonists and may precipitate withdrawal in opiate-habituated patients. Dysphoria is a common side effect. Because of their receptor antagonist properties, these drugs may also preclude the effect of pure opiate agonists administered afterward for breakthrough pain. Advantages of medications in this group are analgesia with less respiratory depression than pure agonists and a lower potential for habituation and abuse. However, their use is limited by a ceiling effect whereby progressive increases in dose do not produce increases in effects.

References

1. Ashburn MA, Lind GH, Gillie MH, et al. Oral transmucosal fentanyl citrate (OTFC) for the treatment of postoperative pain. *Anesth Analg* 76:377–381, 1993.
2. Caplan RA, Ready LB, Oden RV, et al. Transdermal fentanyl for postoperative pain management. A double blind placebo study. *JAMA* 261:1036, 1989.
3. Ferrante FM, VadeBoncouer TR. *Postoperative Pain Management.* New York: Churchill-Livingstone, 1993.
4. Benzon HT, Wong HY, Belavic AM Jr, et al. A randomized double-blind comparison of epidural fentanyl infusion versus patient-controlled analgesia with morphine for postthoracotomy pain. *Anesth Analg* 76:316–322, 1993.
5. Tanaka M, Watanabe S, Ashimura H, et al. Minimum effective combination dose of epidural morphine and fentanyl for posthysterectomy analgesia: a randomized, prospective, double-blind study. *Anesth Analg* 77:942–946, 1993.
6. Grass JA. Sufentanil: clinical use as postoperative analgesic—epidural/intrathecal route. *J Pain Symptom Manage* 7:271–286, 1992.
7. Yu PY, Gambling DR. A comparative study of patient controlled epidural fentanyl and single dose epidural morphine for post-cesarean section analgesia. *Can J Anaesth* 40:416–420, 1993.
8. Vercauteren MP. PCA by epidural route (PCEA). *Acta Anaesthesiol Belg* 43:33–39, 1992.
9. Moote C. Efficacy of nonsteroidal anti-inflammatory drugs in the management of postoperative pain. *Drugs* 44 (Suppl 5):14–30, 1992.

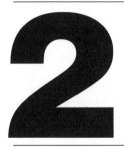

Patient-Controlled Analgesia

Edith R. Kepes
Mathelyn Claudio-Santiago

I. **Background.** Since Sechzer first described in 1968 the use of on-demand intravenous opioid given in small incremental doses,[1] patient-controlled analgesia (PCA) has developed and progressed to the point where it now has a major role in the management of acute and chronic pain.

The goal of continuous medication in small intermittent doses is to achieve an even blood level that produces analgesia and avoids the peaks and valleys of blood levels obtained with conventional intramuscular or oral therapy, which may cause patients to be either oversedated or in pain (Fig. 2-1). The blood concentration of narcotic required to relieve pain varies from patient to patient. There is little correlation between analgesic narcotic requirements and body weight or surface area. Anxiety and abuse of drugs or alcohol, which causes tolerance or cross-tolerance to opioids, increase the amount of drugs needed for adequate pain relief. Endorphin and substance P correlate best with these individual variations.[2] There is also a placebo response for PCA, which at present is poorly understood.

II. **Routes of administration of PCA**

A. **Intravenous administration** is the most frequently used method for pain caused by surgery, trauma, labor, sickle cell crisis, and cancer.

B. **Subcutaneous or intramuscular administration** can be used for patients in whom intravenous access is difficult to maintain. The disadvantage is that larger doses of narcotics are needed to achieve the same level of analgesia because absorption from these sites is less complete.

C. **Oral administration,** long popular in the United Kingdom, is becoming popular on an outpatient basis in the United States. This method results in a high degree of patient satisfaction. Increasing drug usage does not occur, in contrast to the situations in which medication is dispensed by nursing staff in single doses.

D. **Epidural or subarachnoid PCA with local anesthetics and opioids** is popular for use in obstetric, postoperative, and cancer pain. The advantage is the lack of systemic effects such as sedation and nausea, but itching and urinary reduction may be bothersome.

E. **Sublingual PCA with buprenorphine and transnasal PCA with butorphanol** are other effective routes of analgesia and may occupy a place of analgesia control in the future.

F. **Spinal administration.** The favorable spinal-cerebral gradient of opioids depends on the amount injected at the spinal site used, and the drug's water solubility. This technique is most suitable for pain in the pelvis and lower extremities. Even after lumbar administration, redistribution to the brain occurs via blood and CSF, requiring respiratory monitoring in the first 24 hours. Spinal opioids provide a long-lasting CSF reservoir of analgesic drugs, and further doses can be spaced hours apart.

III. **Instrumentation.** The PCA device is activated by patient demand for analgesia, within limits set by the physician. The bolus, incremental and total daily doses, and the lockout interval between doses are preset by the physician. Many PCA devices also are able to provide a continuous infusion of narcotic, which can be used with or without intermittent bolus infusion on demand.

Computer technology permits programming, storage, and retrieval of data by the microprocessor. The number of demands by the patient as well as details of the drug delivered can be recalled. This permits review of analgesic usage, titration of analgesic needs, and also a base for data collection in patient research. Current PCA devices are lightweight, portable, and battery-operated in an effort to aid patient ambulation. Drugs can be put into a disposable reservoir of varying size.

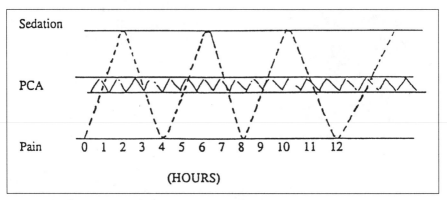

Fig. 2-1. Analgesic pain cycle.

Some PCA devices are well suited to both inpatient and outpatient analgesic usage. Many devices are mounted on an intravenous pole for security, require the use of specific cassettes to that pump, or have a printer built in or a port to attach one. All have some form of security that limits the patient's ability to tamper with the analgesic settings or narcotic store. A mechanical lock and key or electrical access code, or both, are typical security measures. An implantable reservoir for epidural or intrathecal administration of narcotics that works via a hydraulic system is also available.

IV. Choice of patients. PCA is suitable for patients of all ages who can understand the apparatus. Children as young as 5 years of age have successfully managed PCA. Relative contraindications are patients who are abusing illicit drugs or have marked metabolic disorders such as sepsis or severe fluid and electrolyte abnormalities, end-stage renal and hepatic disease, and severe chronic obstructive pulmonary disease or sleep apnea.

V. Indications

A. Postoperative pain and trauma pain. Conventional intramuscular pain medication is administered in a fixed dose at fixed time intervals (hr) by the nurse on request by the patient. Loading bolus doses, which are important to achieve an initial adequate analgesic blood level, are not used. The dose and timing are determined by the physician, and the medication is given or withheld according to the nurse's judgment.

By contrast, in PCA the drug is administered on demand in incremental doses requested by the patient from the PCA machine. The time interval between these incremental doses (lockout period) is in minutes. Only the maximum amount of drug that can be delivered in a fixed time (1- or 4-hr maximum and lockout period) is prescribed by the physician. Loading doses and subsequent bolus doses are commonly utilized to establish or regain analgesia. Studies that examined the efficiency of PCA versus intramuscular medication demonstrated no difference in pain scores.[3-5] These studies, however, were mostly conducted in artificial situations in which a limited number of patients were intensively monitored to permit frequent dosage adjustment to the patients' requirements and nurses were given guidelines of how to administer narcotics. Such intensive scrutiny and attention would be difficult to accomplish on a busy surgical ward with a limited number of nursing staff.

PCA is best initiated in the preoperative period. At this time, the chart is reviewed, the contemplated surgery is evaluated, and the instrument is explained to the patient.

The instrument is programmed in the post-anesthesia care unit (PACU). The setting is determined by the patient's condition, pain scale (0 = no pain; 1 = mild; 2 = moderate; 3 = severe), and sedation scale (1 = wide awake; 2 = drowsy but awake; 3 = drowsy, easily aroused; 4 = sleeping, easily aroused; 5 = sleeping, difficult to arouse; 6 = unarousable).

Unless contraindicated by a history of nausea, hypotension, or confusion, morphine sulfate is used.

A bolus is used if the patient is in pain, and 0.5–1.5 mg morphine sulfate is titrated q5–10min to pain relief. The incremental doses for adults range from 0.5 to 2.5 mg, the lockout interval is 5 to 15 minutes, and the 4-hour drug limit is 8–30 mg. For example, morphine sulfate (1 mg/ml) is given as 1.5 mg q10min with a 4-hour limit of 15 mg. Adjunct medication is often used to potentiate pain relief. Hydroxyzine (25 mg IM) is an excellent anxiolytic drug that may be ordered as a one-time dose or for the first 48 hours.

Equianalgesic opioids are used if morphine is poorly tolerated, and meperidine, hydromorphone, fentanyl, and sufentanil have all been used successfully.

B. Sickle cell crisis

1. **Painful vaso-occlusive crises** account for nearly all the acute hospital admissions of patients with sickle cell disease, which is common in urban areas. In these patients, the episodes vary in severity and duration within the same patient as well as among individual patients. Factors known to precipitate a crisis are cold, tiredness, exertion, infection, stress, worry, dehydration, and alcohol consumption. Pain is usually undertreated in all painful conditions, but more so in sickle cell disease. These patients are children, adolescents, or young adults, for whom physicians have little information regarding analgesic usage. It affects mainly African-American and Hispanic persons who may be perceived as addiction prone. Lack of adequate pain relief in these patients tends to focus their attention on the next dose of analgesic, and encourages a hostile interaction with the health providers, who may then label these patients "manipulative." Those patients who have frequent vaso-occlusive incidents have developed some tolerance to narcotics and require larger doses of opioids to relieve pain than comparable individuals with postoperative or acute trauma pain. These patients can also develop pathologic changes in any organ as complications.

2. The authors have developed the following **protocol for pain management** of sickle cell disease with the aid of PCA. After a drug history has been taken during and between crises (i.e., preferences, amounts, route of administration, the location and intensity of pain noted, and other organic disease processes established), the opioid and the amount to be used are determined. Drugs used in PCA are morphine hydrochloride (1–5 mg/ml); meperidine (10–50 mg/ml); hydromorphone (1–2 mg/ml); and fentanyl (50 μg/ml). The 24-hour narcotic used is calculated on the basis of intramuscular drugs used in the emergency room or on admission, increased by 50%, and converted to the narcotic to be used, e.g., morphine sulfate *(X)*. One third of this calculated dose *(X)* is divided in 24 hours, and the PCA apparatus is programmed to deliver this dose as a continuous drip per hour *(Y)*.

⅔ of *X* divided by 6 = *Z*.
***Z* plus 4*Y* is the 4-hour maximum.**
***Z* divided by 8–10 is the PCA incremental dose.**
Lockout period is 8–10 minutes.

Patients are seen twice in the first 24 hours, and adjustments are made according to response.

Tapering begins usually after 48 to 72 hours. The continuous drip (over 24 hr) is discontinued first, and over the first 2 to 5 days the 4-hour maximum is decreased. Meperidine was found to be the least suitable for this protocol. Extremely high doses, more than the calculated dose, were required for adequate pain relief, probably owing to tolerance to meperidine, the opioid most frequently used in these patients.[6]

C. Cancer pain

C. Cancer pain, like other acute and chronic pain conditions, is poorly controlled; however, with proper management, 95% of patients can be made comfortable. The reasons for poor management are, among others, failure to appreciate the amount of suffering, failure to diagnose the cause of pain, use of weak analgesics, fear by both health providers and patients of addiction to opiates, and a conviction among some that cancer pain is inevitable and untreatable.

Good management of cancer pain presupposes both a positive approach that most cancer pain can be controlled at all stages and a lack of fear of the development of tolerance or addiction. Although cancer patients often become dependent on the analgesic drugs they use, they do not usually become addicted, which is an important distinction. Once severe continuous pain develops, medication must be continuous, around the clock. Co-analgesics (e.g., antidepressants, corticosteroids, and nonsteroidal anti-inflammatory drugs), have an important role in cancer pain management. If oral medication is unsuitable because of nausea, vomiting, or inability to swallow, a subcutaneous, intramuscular, or intravenous route is used. All these methods are suitable with the PCA apparatus. Usually a continuous low-dose opioid is used with further PCA doses. Narcotic requirements vary from patient to patient, and doses must be individualized. Probably the best way to establish the amount of drug needed in 24 hours is to carefully titrate the patient with intermittent (q2min) narcotic loading doses until pain relief is satisfactory and side effects (sedation, hypotension, and decreased respiratory function) are minimal. This loading dose is a good indicator of the severity and relative tolerance of pain. The portable PCA apparatus is suitable for patients in their home.

VI. Disadvantages and complications. Complications of PCA are rare. Most are related to errors in PCA setup and the potential side effects of a particular narcotic or its method of administration. The complications most frequently found are nausea, vomiting, respiratory depression, confusion, sedation, pruritus, urinary retention, constipation, and convulsions (with normeperidine). Disadvantages are the initial cost of the device and the special training required of health providers. In general, PCA has been shown to be a safe, well-tolerated form of pain control when patients are carefully selected and infusion parameters are observed.

References

1. Sechzer PH. Objective measurement of pain. *Anesthesiology* 29:209, 1968.
2. Tamsen A, Sakurada T, Wahlstom A, et al. Postoperative demand for analgesics in relation to individual levels of endorphin and substance P in cerebrospinal fluid. *Pain* 13:171, 1982.
3. Robinson JO, Rosen JM, Revill SL, et al. Self administered intravenous and intramuscular pethidine. *Anesthesia* 35:769, 1980.
4. Rosenberg PH, Heino A, Scheinin B. Comparison of intramuscular analgesia, intercostal block, epidural morphine and on-demand-IV-fentanyl in the control of pain after upper abdominal surgery. *Acta Anaesthesiol Scand* 28:603, 1984.
5. Ferrante FM, Orav EJ, Rocco AG, Gallo J. A statistical model for patient-controlled analgesia and conventional intramuscular opioid regimens. *Anesth Analg* 67:457, 1988.
6. Kepes E, Kaplan R, Claudio M, Benjamin L. Patient controlled analgesia (PCA) during sickle cell crisis. *Pain* 5 (Suppl 5):185, 1990.

Post–Cesarean Section Analgesia
David J. Wlody

I. **Background.** The principles of postoperative pain management in the patient who has undergone cesarean section are not unlike those involved in the care of any patient undergoing major abdominal surgery; however, there are other important considerations.

  A. Most cesarean section patients are healthy, do not view themselves as sick, and as such are less likely to accept significant postoperative pain.

  B. Cesarean section patients have a strong desire to interact with friends and relatives and to bond with their new baby. Therefore, they are less likely to be satisfied with methods of pain relief that produce significant sedation.

  C. For women who are breast-feeding, analgesic techniques that minimize the amount of depressant drugs in breast milk will be preferred.

  D. An increasing number of women are choosing regional anesthesia for their surgery.

II. **Conventional intramuscular narcotics**

  A. Technique and advantages

    1. The traditional method of achieving pain relief in the postoperative period is the use of **parenteral narcotics.** Because of logistical problems with the use of intravenous narcotics, in practice this has meant intramuscular injections on an as-needed basis.

    2. The primary **advantages of intramuscular narcotics** are

      a. Their familiarity

      b. Their safety

      c. The lack of need for specialized monitoring techniques

    3. A precise dose that will provide analgesia in a given patient is difficult to pinpoint, but the following **range of doses** should be appropriate.

      a. Morphine 7.5–15 mg q3h

      b. Meperidine 50–100 mg q4h

      c. Buprenorphine 0.2–0.3 mg q4h

      d. Butorphanol 1–2 mg q3h

      e. Nalbuphine 10 mg q4–6h

  B. Disadvantages

    1. In any bolus technique, such as intermittent injections, there will be a point soon after injection when the plasma level is higher than necessary to achieve analgesia. It is at that point that **undesirable sedation** can be seen. This sedation will be even more pronounced when using agents with significant kappa-agonist activity, such as nalbuphine, butorphanol, and buprenorphine. These high peak levels can also be associated with respiratory depression.

    2. As plasma levels decline, a point will be reached when analgesia is no longer effective. At this point, if the patient desires further narcotic, there may be a considerable delay before the drug is administered, and a further delay until adequate plasma levels are achieved. It is unsurprising that Harrison and associates have shown that 94% of patients receiving intramuscular analgesia reported moderate to severe **pain during the first 24 hours** after cesarean section.[1]

    3. A significant degree of **discomfort** is also attendant **with intramuscular injections.** Since the average cesarean section patient receives approximately nine intramuscular injections,[2] this is not an insignificant concern.

III. **Patient-controlled analgesia**

  A. Technique and advantages

    1. Patient-controlled analgesia (PCA) **avoids** the pharmacokinetic **shortcomings**

of intermittent intramuscular injections. By providing small intravenous boluses of narcotic on demand, PCA allows the maintenance of a relatively constant plasma drug concentration. Thus, it avoids the "peaks" that may lead to excessive sedation, as well as the "valleys" of inadequately treated pain.

2. In addition, although PCA gives somewhat less effective analgesia than neuraxial opioids, **patient satisfaction** appears to be equal, if not greater, with PCA. This may be due to a greater sense of control when the patient is able to tailor her analgesic therapy to her own desires.

3. **Morphine** is the most commonly used opioid for PCA. Initially, the bolus dose is set at 1 mg, with an 8-minute lockout. If pain is not controlled in 1 hour, the dose is increased to 1.5 mg. If pain continues after another hour, the lockout interval is decreased to 6 minutes.

4. It is important, however, to ensure that there is **adequate analgesia** before PCA is initiated.

5. It is equally as important to provide **adequate** patient **education** preoperatively, if possible. It should be explained that the goal of PCA is not total pain relief, but rather a degree of pain relief that minimizes side effects. The use of PCA should also be encouraged before predictably painful events such as ambulation.

B. Disadvantages
1. Initiation of a PCA service requires a fairly **large capital expense,** as well as a commitment to a continuing nursing education program.

2. There is a **potential for programming errors** that might lead to narcotic overdose as well as a potential for intentional abuse. PCA is contraindicated in patients with histories of drug abuse.

3. Although morphine has little effect on neonatal neurobehavioral indices, meperidine has a significant **depressant effect on breast-fed infants** of mothers receiving the drug via PCA.[3]

IV. Epidural opioids
A. Advantages compared with conventional narcotics
1. It is well established that epidural opioids provide **better analgesia** than conventional intramuscular narcotics.[1,4] Analgesia can be provided for up to 24 hours with no sympathetic, motor, or sensory blockade.[5]

2. There are **benefits other than analgesia** in patients receiving epidural opioids.
   a. Earlier ambulation
   b. Earlier return of bowel function
   c. Decreased pulmonary complications
   d. Earlier hospital discharge

B. Drugs and dosages
1. The most commonly used narcotic is **morphine;** its optimum dose appears to be 4–5 mg. This dose can be expected to provide 16 to 24 hours of pain relief. Higher doses have led to increased side effects with no added analgesic efficacy.[5]

2. Epidural **fentanyl** 50 μg has been shown to provide effective analgesia within 7 minutes, lasting up to 5 hours.[6] Because of its higher lipid solubility, fentanyl has fewer side effects than morphine.

3. Other narcotics used to provide postoperative analgesia are listed with their approximate duration of action.
   a. Hydromorphone, 1.0–1.5 mg, 16 hours
   b. Meperidine, 50 mg, 3 hours
   c. Sufentanil, 30 μg, 3 hours
   d. Butorphanol, 4 mg, 6 hours

4. **Continuous epidural infusion** of an opioid, either by itself or in combination with a local anesthetic, is another technique. This technique is of particular advantage when using fentanyl; effective pain relief with few side effects can be provided without having to perform frequent "top-ups." Typically, a solution of 5 μg/ml is infused at 5–10 ml/hr to provide adequate dermatomal spread of anesthesia. This can be combined with 0.125% bupivacaine if adequate monitoring of sympathetic block can be provided.

C. Side effects and their treatment
1. **Pruritus** has been reported to occur in as many as 90% of patients receiving epidural morphine, although this symptom appears to be sensitive to the diligence with which it is sought; a large number of patients will only report pruritus if carefully questioned. Frequently, pruritus is limited to the face. There is a suggestion that it is less commonly seen when the more lipid-soluble

agents are used. Although there is no evidence that pruritus is mediated through histamine release, parenteral antihistamines (diphenhydramine 25 mg IV) are usually effective in relieving the symptom. Alternatively, naloxone 0.04–0.1 mg IV in carefully titrated doses can eliminate pruritus without reversing analgesia. This relief may be short-lived, requiring continuous infusions of naloxone 3–5 μg/kg/hr.

2. **Nausea and vomiting** have been reported to occur in as many as 50% of women receiving epidural morphine after cesarean section, although the true incidence appears to be closer to 25%, with approximately half requiring treatment. The etiology of nausea and vomiting in this setting is thought to be direct stimulation of the chemoreceptor trigger zone due to rostral spread of opioid. Lipophilic narcotics less commonly produce nausea and vomiting.[6] Treatment options include prochlorperazine 5 mg IM, droperidol 0.625 mg IV, and metoclopramide 5–10 mg IV. There is evidence that transdermal scopolamine is effective in reducing the incidence of nausea and vomiting when used prophylactically.[7]

3. **Urinary retention** is not uncommon after the administration of epidural narcotics. The mechanism is poorly understood, but is most likely due to failure of the detrussor muscle to contract, as well as failure of the external sphincter to relax.[8] Fortunately, in the cesarean section patient, bladder catheterization is routinely used 12 to 24 hours after surgery. It is highly unusual for urinary retention to persist beyond that time; if it does, intermittent bladder catheterization is indicated, since pharmacologic measures such as naloxone are seldom effective.

4. **Reactivation of labial herpes simplex** has been reported in cesarean section patients receiving epidural morphine.[9] It has been suggested that this may be due to reactivation of latent virus by rostral spread of morphine. If this is the case, there may be an advantage to using a lipid-soluble narcotic such as fentanyl in patients with a history of recurrent labial herpes.

5. **Delayed respiratory depression**
   a. Delayed respiratory depression after epidural narcotic administration is the most serious complication of the technique. It is widely assumed that the mechanism for respiratory insufficiency is a direct depressant effect on the medullary respiratory center owing to rostral spread of the narcotic. The incidence of respiratory depression in surgical patients has been estimated to be approximately 1%. Several **patient characteristics** increase the risk of respiratory depression:
      (1) Supplemental parenteral narcotic administration
      (2) Advanced age
      (3) Preexisting pulmonary function abnormalities
      (4) Generalized debilitation
   b. Fortunately, the **incidence** of respiratory depression in cesarean section patients is considerably lower. In a study of 1000 patients who received 5 mg of epidural morphine, only four were found to have a respiratory rate of less than 10 breaths/min. Of these four, only one had significant hypercarbia.[10] Thus, the incidence of severe respiratory depression in cesarean section patients may be as low as 0.1%.
   c. Many **monitoring techniques** have been proposed for the detection of respiratory depression. Pulse oximetry is difficult to maintain on an ambulating patient, and desaturation is a relatively late sign of respiratory depression. Commercially available apnea monitors have frequent false alarms. The most sensitive technique appears to be an hourly measurement of the patient's respiratory rate and level of sedation. Significant respiratory depression does not appear de novo; it is uniformly preceded by progressive somnolence over a period of several hours.
   d. **Naloxone** should be available at the bedside of all patients receiving epidural narcotics. In the event of severe respiratory depression or apnea, nursing staff should be permitted to administer naloxone 0.4 mg IV immediately. Lesser degrees of respiratory depression or somnolence can await evaluation by an anesthesiologist and can be treated by repeated doses of naloxone 0.04 mg. Respiratory depression requiring treatment probably justifies the initiation of a continuous infusion of 3–5 μg/kg/hr.
   e. **Epidural fentanyl** has been shown to depress the carbon dioxide response curve, but life-threatening respiratory depression appears to be quite uncommon.

f. Although it is not a complication of epidural narcotics, some patients will develop **breakthrough pain.** This can be treated with small doses of parenteral narcotics, e.g., morphine 2–4 mg. Alternatively, a mixed agonist-antagonist drug such as nalbuphine 2.5–5.0 mg can be used. The advantage of such a drug is that there is little possibility that it will contribute any significant additional respiratory depressant effect and may, in fact reverse the respiratory depression produced by the spinal narcotic.

g. Previous administration of chloroprocaine has been shown to render epidural narcotics less effective. This is not due to the low pH of chloroprocaine solutions, as alkalinization of the local anesthetic will not prevent this phenomenon. Camann et al. suggest that this is a receptor-mediated phenomenon, because it is not seen when the kappa-agonist butorphanol is used, but is significant when a mu-agonist such as morphine is used.[11] This phenomenon should be considered when choosing a local anesthetic or a particular opioid.

V. Intrathecal opioids

A. Technique and advantages

1. Intrathecal morphine provides a **similar degree of analgesia** to epidural morphine.
2. The analgesia with intrathecal morphine appears to be of **longer duration** than with epidural morphine.
3. The incidence of severe respiratory depression, contrary to initial reports, appears to be no higher with intrathecal morphine than with epidural morphine, if the dose is 0.5 mg or less.
4. As the majority of regional anesthetics for cesarean section are **spinal anesthetics,** intrathecal morphine allows one to provide the same excellent analgesia in this group of patients that can be provided to patients with epidural anesthetics.
5. The **optimum dose** for intrathecal morphine is **0.2–0.3 mg.** Higher doses do not appear to provide higher-quality analgesia, nor do they significantly prolong the duration of analgesia. They do, however, increase the risk of respiratory depression.[12]
6. The doses of morphine utilized for the intrathecal approach will have **no significant accumulation in breast milk.**

B. Side effects

1. Patients receiving intrathecal morphine are subject to the **same effects as** those receiving **epidural morphine,** including nausea, urinary retention, pruritus, and respiratory depression. It is not clear whether the incidence of these complications differs between the two techniques.
2. Unless an indwelling subarachnoid catheter is placed, **analgesia cannot be prolonged** without performing a second intrathecal injection. This is less of a concern with cesarean section patients, however, because typically their pain can be managed with oral analgesics after the first postoperative day.

VI. Miscellaneous techniques

A. Wound infiltration
is infrequently utilized for postoperative analgesia, but is simple and can be surprisingly effective: 15 to 25 ml of 0.25% bupivacaine can provide 4 to 5 hours of pain relief after cesarean section.

B. Ilioinguinal nerve block
with 10 ml of 0.5% bupivacaine bilaterally can provide pain relief comparable to that with intrathecal morphine 0.15 mg for up to 24 hours.[13] Although the pain relief may not be equivalent to that with higher-dose intrathecal morphine, this may be a reasonable supplement to conventional narcotics in patients not receiving spinal opioids.

C. Nonsteroidal anti-inflammatory drugs
have become an increasingly useful method of providing postoperative anesthesia owing to the development of a parenteral formulation, ketorolac. Ketorolac is of particular utility when used in combination with a parenteral narcotic, as it has no respiratory depressant effect. This might be a significant advantage when treating patients for breakthrough pain after the administration of spinal opioids. The usual dose is 30–60 mg IM.

D. Patient-controlled epidural analgesia
is of considerable interest for pain after cesarean section. One technique utilizes a continuous infusion of fentanyl 2 µg/ml in 0.03% bupivacaine at 10 ml/hr, with the patient being permitted to self-administer a 10-ml bolus every 2 hours.[14] This provides excellent pain relief with good patient satisfaction.

References

1. Harrison DM, Sinatra R, Morgese L, et al. Epidural narcotic and patient controlled analgesia for post-cesarean section pain relief. *Anesthesiology* 68:454–457, 1988.
2. Stenkamp SJ, Easterling TR, Chadwick MS. Effect of epidural and intrathecal morphine on the length of hospital stay after cesarean section. *Anesth Analg* 68:66–69, 1989.
3. Wittels B, Scott DT, Sinatra RS. Exogenous opioids in human breast milk and acute neonatal neurobehavioral: a preliminary study. *Anesthesiology* 73:864–869, 1990.
4. Eisenach JC, Grice SC, Dewan DM. Patient-controlled analgesia following cesarean section: a comparison with epidural and intramuscular narcotics. *Anesthesiology* 68:444–448, 1988.
5. Rosen MA, Hughes SC, Shnider SM, et al. Epidural morphine for the relief of postoperative pain after cesarean delivery. *Anesth Analg* 62:666–672, 1988.
6. Naulty JS, Datta S, Ostheimer GW, et al. Epidural fentanyl for post-cesarean delivery pain management. *Anesthesiology* 63:694–698, 1985.
7. Loper KA, Ready LB, Dorman BH. Prophylactic transdermal scopolamine patches reduce nausea in postoperative patients receiving epidural morphine. *Anesth Analg* 68:144–146, 1989.
8. Durant PAC, Yaksh TL. Drug effects on urinary bladder tone during spinal morphine-induced inhibition of the micturition reflex in unanesthetized rats. *Anesthesiology* 68:325–334, 1988.
9. Crone LL, Connolly JM, Clark KM, et al. Recurrent herpes simplex virus labialis and the use of epidural morphine in obstetric patients. *Anesth Analg* 67:318, 1988.
10. Leicht CH, Hughes SC, Dailey PA, et al. Epidural morphine sulfate for analgesia after cesarean section. A prospective report of 1,000 patients. *Anesthesiology* 65:A336, 1986.
11. Camann WR, Hartigan PM, Gilbertson LI, et al. Chloroprocaine antagonism of epidural opioid analgesia: a receptor specific phenomenon? *Anesthesiology* 73:860–863, 1990.
12. Chadwick HS, Ready LB. Intrathecal and epidural morphine sulfate for post-cesarean analgesia—a clinical comparison. *Anesthesiology* 68:925–929, 1988.
13. Witkowski TA, Leighton BL, Norris MC. Ilioinguinal nerve blocks: an alternative or supplement to intrathecal morphine. *Anesthesiology* 73:A962, 1991.
14. Cohen S, Amar D, Pantuck CB. Continuous epidural-PCA post–cesarean section: buprenorphine-bupivicaine 0.03% vs fentanyl-bupivicaine 0.03%. Presented at the Society for Obstetric Anesthesia and Perinatalogy Annual Meeting, Madison, WI, May 24–26, 1990.

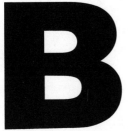

B

Pharmacologic
Management

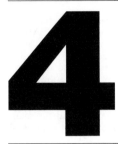

Nonsteroidal Anti-inflammatory Drugs
Vincent R. Saladini, Jr.

I. Background
  A. The nonsteroidal anti-inflammatory drugs (NSAIDs) comprise a group of medications used for mild to moderate pain. As their name implies, the NSAIDs are most effective in providing analgesia in pain syndromes that are **associated with inflammatory conditions.** Of note is that the NSAIDs are not associated with tolerance or physical dependence, and this offers an important advantage over opioid analgesics.
  B. Although the NSAIDs are often used alone in treating a variety of pain syndromes, their analgesic effects can be even further **potentiated** when they are used **in conjunction with other agents** such as the opioid analgesics or tricyclic antidepressants. When the NSAIDs are used as part of a combination drug therapy regimen, each of the medications can often be used in lower doses, thereby reducing potential side effects.
  C. Lack of effect or side effects from one NSAID does not preclude success using a different NSAID. Longer-acting NSAIDs have an obvious **advantage in chronic pain syndromes.** In some pain syndromes, such as pain of bone metastases, NSAIDs can be more effective than opioid drugs.

II. Mechanism of action. The NSAIDs provide for analgesia by **inhibition of prostaglandin synthesis.** With inflammatory conditions or tissue injury, prostaglandins are among the cellular products that are produced and released. The prostaglandins that are released subsequently stimulate peripheral nociceptors and thereby elicit the pain response. In effect, by inhibiting prostaglandin synthesis, the NSAIDs inhibit peripheral nociceptor stimulation and thus decrease pain perception.

III. Absorption is primarily in the **small intestine.** Absorption in the stomach also occurs, but to a lesser degree. High gastric pH or the presence of food in the stomach will decrease gastric absorption.

IV. Hepatic metabolism occurs **with renal excretion** of the resulting metabolites.

V. Side effects
  A. Gastric irritation can occur with the potential for ulcer formation. When NSAIDs are the only agents that can provide pain relief in a patient with a history of an ulcer or GI irritation, the addition of misoprostol (Cytotec) allows continued use of an NSAID.
  B. Prolongation of bleeding time also occurs owing to platelet dysfunction. It can last for the duration of the platelet's life span (approximately 10 days).
  C. CNS stimulation occurs with salicylate overdose. Tinnitus is one of the earliest clinical manifestations of salicylate overdose. Hyperventilation, mental confusion, seizures, and metabolic acidosis can also develop.
  D. Renal dysfunction, particularly necrosis, has been associated with long-term NSAID administration.
  E. Allergic hypersensitivity reactions, not necessarily dose-related, are rare but can occur. Clinical manifestations can appear within minutes of NSAID ingestion. The most common manifestations are rhinitis, bronchospasm, urticaria, laryngeal edema, hypotension, and circulatory collapse.
  F. Hepatic dysfunction may be induced by NSAIDs in a small percentage of the general patient population. It is usually reversed with the discontinuance of the NSAID. Mild elevation of results on one or more liver function tests (LFTs) may occur. Particular caution must be exercised in administering NSAIDs to patients in whom there is a history of hepatic dysfunction or LFT abnormalities. LFT results should be monitored periodically against baseline values (e.g., serum glutamate pyruvate transaminase) obtained before initiating NSAID therapy,

particularly if long-term treatment is the goal. If signs and symptoms of hepatic dysfunction occur, or if LFT results progressively worsen, then NSAID therapy should be discontinued.

G. **Fluid retention and edema** can occur because of the effect of prostaglandin inhibition on renal function. Prostaglandins are integrally involved in maintaining renal perfusion by their effect on the renal vascular bed. By inhibiting renal prostaglandins, renal perfusion may subsequently decrease to the point at which renal function is effectively inhibited, and this can create a negative secondary effect on the volume and electrolyte status of a patient. Renal function, urine volume, and electrolyte status should be carefully monitored in individuals with the following conditions, who are at greatest risk.

1. Baseline renal dysfunction or prerenal azotemia
2. Congestive heart failure
3. Hepatic dysfunction with a compromised intravascular volume
4. The elderly

H. **Blood dyscrasias** that have occurred from NSAIDs include agranulocytosis, aplastic anemia, and thrombocytopenia.

I. **Possible prolongation of gestation or spontaneous labor** precludes the use of NSAIDs late in pregnancy.

VI. **Drug interactions**

A. **Anticoagulants**
1. Salicylates will not affect activity.
2. Phenylbutazone will prolong prothrombin time.

B. **Digitalis.** Indomethacin can induce digitalis toxicity.

C. **Hypoglycemics** will be enhanced by NSAIDs.

D. **Antacids** will increase excretion of salicylates.

VII. **Commonly used NSAIDs**

A. **Salicylates**
1. **Aspirin**
2. **Diflunisal (Dolobid)**

B. **Propionic acid derivatives**
1. **Ibuprofen (Advil, Motrin)**
2. **Naproxen (Naprosyn, Anaprox)**
3. **Fenoprofen (Nalfon)**
4. **Ketoprofen (Orudis)**

C. **Indomethacin (Indocin)**

D. **Sulindac (Clinoril)**

E. **Tolmetin (Tolectin)**

F. **Phenylbutazone**

G. **Piroxicam (Feldene)**

H. **Diclofenac sodium (Voltaren)**

I. **Ketorolac (Toradol)**

J. **Nabumetone (Relafen)**

K. **Para-aminophenol derivatives**
1. **Acetaminophen (Tylenol)**
2. **Phenacetin**

VIII. **Specific NSAIDs**

A. **Salicylates** are among the most commonly used analgesics. They are particularly useful for the treatment of pain syndromes associated with inflammatory conditions such as rheumatoid arthritis. Because of their effectiveness and relatively low cost, they are often used as first-line agents in treating such conditions.

1. **Dosage and administration.** Although dosage and response are highly individualized, the usual dose is 650 mg q4h. Dosages up to 5–6 g/day can be given; however, dosages greater than 6 g/day may precipitate early signs of salicylate toxicity such as tinnitus.

2. **Diflunisal.** The standard dose is 500–1000 mg/day divided in twice-daily doses.

B. **Propionic acid derivatives**

1. Ibuprofen was the first agent in this class to come into existence. The most notable differences between the propionic acid derivatives involve potency and half-life. Naproxen has a particularly long half-life compared with the other agents in this class, and thus it can be administered twice a day.

2. Naproxen sodium 275 and 550 mg (Anaprox and Anaprox DS), the sodium salt derivatives of naproxen, have a more rapid absorption than their parent

compound. Indications for their usage include osteoarthritis, rheumatoid arthritis, bursitis, gout, and primary dysmenorrhea.

3. **Side effects** are similar to those experienced with the salicylates. There does, however, seem to be a somewhat lower incidence of GI irritability than with the salicylates, especially if they are taken with small amounts of food and if less than maximal total daily doses are administered.

4. **Dosage and administration** (usual daily dose and maximum daily dose)
   a. Ibuprofen 1200–1600 mg/day, divided q6–8h, maximum 3200 mg/day
   b. Naproxen
      (1) For more severe pain, such as that of osteoarthritis and rheumatoid arthritis, 500–1000 mg/day, divided q12h, or 2–4 tsp twice daily if 25 mg/ml suspension is used, maximum 1500 mg/day
      (2) For milder pain, such as with dysmenorrhea or acute gout, initial dose 750 mg, then 250 mg q8h until symptoms resolve.
   c. Naproxen sodium and naproxen sodium, double strength
      (1) For osteoarthritis and rheumatoid arthritis, 550–1100 mg/day, divided q12h, maximum 1375 mg/day (1650 mg/day for a limited time)
      (2) For acute gout or dysmenorrhea, initial dose 825 mg, then 275 mg q8h until symptoms resolve.
   d. Fenoprofen 900–2400 mg/day, divided q6–8h, maximum 3200 mg/day
   e. Ketoprofen 150–200 mg/day, divided q6–8h, maximum 300 mg/day

C. **Indomethacin**
   1. **Dosage and administration.** The usual dosage is 25 mg bid-tid up to a maximum dose of 200 mg/day for moderate to severe rheumatoid arthritis. For acute gouty arthritis, dosage is 50 mg PO tid for 3 to 5 days, while for exacerbations of bursitis or tendinitis, the dosage is 25 mg–50 mg PO tid for 7 to 10 days. There are four preparations of indomethacin (e.g., Indocin):
      a. Capsules, 25 mg and 50 mg
      b. Sustained-release capsules (Indocin D), 75 mg
      c. Suppositories, 50 mg
      d. Oral suspension, 25 mg/ml

D. **Sulindac**
   1. **Side effects** are similar to those with the other NSAIDs. As the major route of elimination of sulindac and its metabolites is via the kidneys, patients with renal dysfunction should be monitored particularly closely for signs and symptoms of potential toxicity and adverse effects due to excessive drug accumulation. A reduction in the total daily dosage of sulindac may be necessary.
   2. **Dosage and administration.** The usual dosage is 150 mg PO bid with a maximum dosage of 400 mg/day.

E. **Tolmetin** is more potent than the salicylates, but less potent than indomethacin or phenylbutazone. The usual dosage is 400 mg PO tid with a maximum dosage of 1800 mg/day.

F. **Phenylbutazone** is a very potent anti-inflammatory agent and is not recommended for use as a routine analgesic or long-term inflammatory agent because of its toxicity.
   1. **Absorption is rapid,** and complete absorption occurs after oral administration.
   2. **Hepatic metabolism** occurs **with renal excretion.** One of its metabolites, oxyphenbutazone, is also a potent anti-inflammatory agent.
   3. **Side effects.** Phenylbutazone is a notably **toxic agent** with the potential for causing anemia and agranulocytosis. Pulmonary edema may also occur secondary to its tendency to cause sodium and chloride retention, along with a decreased urine output owing to a direct effect on the renal tubules. Thus, this agent is particularly **contraindicated in patients with cardiac or renal disease.** Like the other NSAIDs, phenylbutazone may also cause GI irritation and potential CNS toxicity.
   4. **Dosage and administration.** The usual dose is 300–600 mg/day for no more than several days at a time.

G. **Piroxicam.** The major advantage of this agent is that its long half-life permits a once-a-day dosage regimen. The standard dosage is 20 mg PO once a day.

H. **Diclofenac sodium** is an NSAID with analgesic, antipyretic, and anti-inflammatory properties. It is used in the treatment of osteoarthritis and rheumatoid arthritis, for which the usual dose is 100–200 mg/day, divided q6h, q8h, or q12h. The maximal daily dose is 200 mg/day.

I. **Ketorolac** is an NSAID that is available for either intramuscular or oral use with equianalgesic potential. Its indication in either form is for **short-term use** (less than 5 days) because of the potential for increased incidence of side effects, particularly GI, beyond this time period. Ketorolac has been used extensively in postoperative pain management, and when the dosage is appropriate, it provides a level of analgesia that is comparable to that of narcotics such as meperidine and morphine without affecting opiate receptors. Its principal advantage over opiates is that it provides analgesia without having any sedative or hypnotic properties or addiction potential. As such, ketorolac has been particularly useful in managing patients in outpatient ambulatory surgery units and in providing analgesia for patients with acute or chronic pulmonary dysfunction, in whom the sedative or respiratory depressive effects of opiates might prove particularly problematic. Because it has no addiction potential, ketorolac is also an excellent agent for treating patients in whom the issue of narcotic addiction is of concern. Ketorolac administered intramusculary can be effective in the acute treatment of migraine when nausea precludes the use of oral agents. One must remember, however, that ketorolac is an NSAID with antiplatelet aggregation properties; therefore, it **should not be used as a preoperative medication.**

1. **Dosage and administration.** As noted previously, ketorolac is not indicated for chronic pain relief, and its use should not exceed 5 days in injectable form and several weeks in oral form. The usual daily dose and maximum daily dose are as follows:

   a. **Oral preparation:** 40 mg/day, divided q4–6h, maximum 40 mg/day
   b. **Intramuscular preparation:** initial dose 30–60 mg IM, then half the initial dose q6h, maximum 150 mg for first day of use, then 120 mg/day
   c. If one desires to convert from an intramuscular regimen to an **oral** regimen, then the **maximum combined dose** should not be greater than 120 mg for the day on which the conversion takes place (including a maximum oral dose of 40 mg). Thereafter, the oral regimen should be followed.

J. **Nabumetone** is an NSAID used in the management of patients with osteoarthritis and rheumatoid arthritis.

1. **Absorption is excellent** after oral administration. As opposed to many other NSAIDs, the rate of absorption of nabumetone from the GI tract is actually increased when it is taken with food.
2. **Metabolism and excretion.** After oral administration, nabumetone is **absorbed in the GI tract.** It then undergoes metabolic transformation in the liver, at which point the pharmacologically inactive parent compound is converted into its active metabolite along with several inactive metabolites. The active metabolite also eventually undergoes hepatic biotransformation to yield inactive metabolites, and ultimately, all of the **inactive metabolites undergo renal excretion.**
3. **Dosage and administration.** Dosage adjustment is not necessary in patients with renal disease because of the extent to which nabumetone and its active metabolite undergo hepatic biotransformation to yield inactive metabolites. The usual daily dose is 1000–1500 mg administered in a single dose or divided into a twice-a-day regimen. The maximum daily dose is 2000 mg.

K. **Para-aminophenol derivatives** are not NSAIDs, but because they are also used for mild to moderate pain, they are often discussed with NSAIDs. They are particularly useful analgesics for patients who are unable to tolerate salicylates. Both acetaminophen and phenacetin are mild to moderate analgesics. Their main advantage over the salicylates and other NSAIDs is that they do not cause either gastric irritation or platelet dysfunction. However, because the para-aminophenols cause only minimal inhibition of peripheral prostaglandin synthesis, they are weak anti-inflammatory agents and, therefore, are not as efficacious in the treatment of inflammatory conditions such as rheumatoid arthritis.

1. **Absorption is excellent** after oral administration.
2. Both acetaminophen and phenacetin undergo **hepatic metabolism with renal excretion.** Approximately 80% of phenacetin is dealkylated to acetaminophen. Persons with a glucose-6-phosphate dehydrogenase deficiency have a limited ability to metabolize phenacetin to acetaminophen. As a result, a greater percentage of the phenacetin is converted to toxic metabolites, which in turn can cause methemoglobinemia and hemolysis. As noted previously, acetaminophen is metabolized in the liver. If excessive doses of acetaminophen are

ingested, the metabolite N-acetyl-p-benzoquinone is formed, which can lead to hepatotoxicity.

3. **Side effects are few** as long as these agents are taken within the recommended dosages. Except for methemoglobinemia in individuals with glucose-6-phosphate dehydrogenase deficiency, the other major side effects such as hepatic necrosis and renal tubular necrosis tend to occur when excessive doses are ingested. Hepatotoxicity with acetaminophen can occur after doses of 200 mg/kg of body weight are ingested. Clinical manifestations and laboratory abnormalities consistent with hepatocellular injury occur 2 to 6 days after the toxic dose is taken.

4. **Dosage and administration**
   a. **Acetaminophen.** The standard dose is 325–650 mg PO q4h.
   b. **Phenacetin.** It is not commonly used as an individual agent because of its significant nephrotoxicity and adverse hematologic side effects.

Selected Readings

Ameer B, Greenblatt DJ. Acetaminophen. *Ann Intern Med* 87:202–209, 1977.

Flower RJ, Moncada S, Vane JR. Analgesic-Antipyretics and Anti-inflammatory Agents: Drugs Employed in the Treatment of Gout. In: Gilman A, Goodman LS (eds.), *The Pharmacological Basis of Therapeutics.* New York: Macmillan, 1985. Pp. 682–728.

Goldfinger SE. Treatment of gout. *N Engl J Med* 285:1303–1306, 1971.

Metz SA. Anti-inflammatory agents as inhibitors of prostaglandin synthesis in man. *Med Clin North Am* 65:713–757, 1981.

Smyth CJ. Therapy of rheumatoid arthritis. *Postgrad Med* 51 (Suppl):23–31, 1972.

Stoelting RK. *Pharmacology and Physiology in Anesthetic Practice.* Philadelphia: J.B. Lippincott, 1987. Pp. 240–250.

Local Anesthetics

Ellen S. Steinberg
Eric B. Fishman
Alan C. Santos

I. Background. Local anesthetics are among the most commonly used agents for providing surgical anesthesia. They are also frequently used in obstetrics or for the diagnosis and management of chronic pain syndromes. As with many pharmacologically active molecules, their structure is integrally related to their activity.

A. Structure–activity relationship of local anesthetics

1. The local anesthetic agents used in clinical practice are of two types, either **amino-esters or amino-amides.** Two typical local anesthetic molecules, procaine and lidocaine, are depicted in Figure 5-1. Alterations in any of the molecular components may alter the potency, toxicity, duration of action, protein binding, lipid solubility, or metabolism of the local anesthetic.

2. The aromatic portion, typically a benzene ring, renders the molecule **lipophilic.** An intermediate alkyl chain, which separates the benzene ring from the terminal amine, contains either an ester or an amide linkage. The terminal amine is a proton acceptor and thus is the hydrophilic polar end. Aliphatic substitutions to the aromatic ring or the tertiary amine increase lipid solubility, anesthetic potency, and duration of action. For instance, the addition of a butyl group to the tertiary amine portion of mepivacaine results in the formation of bupivacaine, a more lipophilic and potent agent. Lengthening the intermediate alkyl chain increases anesthetic potency, but also enhances systemic toxicity.

3. Local anesthetics are usually prepared as the hydrochloride salt and therefore ionize in solution to form a quaternary amine (positive charge) and a chloride ion (negative charge). Local anesthetics are weak bases existing in both ionized and unionized forms. The **degree of ionization** is dependent on the pH of the environment in relation to the pK_a of the particular drug. The pK_a is that concentration of hydrogen ion at which the concentration of charged local anesthetic (BH^+) is equal to that of the uncharged base (B). This relationship is defined by the Henderson-Hasselbach equation, which states that

$$pK_a = pH - \log (B)/(BH^+)$$

Thus, more of the drug will exist in an ionized form as the surrounding environment becomes more acidic. Those local anesthetics with a pK_a closer to physiologic pH are less ionized than those with a high pK_a. This relationship is important because it is the unionized moiety that is lipid soluble and crosses neural membranes. The charged molecule, however, is thought to be the pharmacologically active form.

4. The most common method of classifying local anesthetics is based on the presence of an amide or ester linkage between the hydrophobic and hydrophilic portions of the molecule (Table 5-1). This is also important in determining the **route of metabolism;** esters are metabolized by enzymatic hydrolysis and amides undergo hepatic metabolism.

II. Mechanism of action

A. Anatomy of the nerve and axonal membrane

1. A peripheral neuron generally consists of an **axon and cell body.** A fascicle is composed of several axons. In addition, each nerve fiber is surrounded by a Schwann cell sheath. In larger nerves, Schwann cell sheaths are often classified by whether they are myelinated or unmyelinated. Saltatory conduction is facilitated by small unmyelinated junctions between the Schwann cell sheaths (nodes of Ranvier). As each peripheral nerve generally has several connective tissue layers, a local anesthetic molecule must traverse at least four or five membranes before arriving at its site of action.

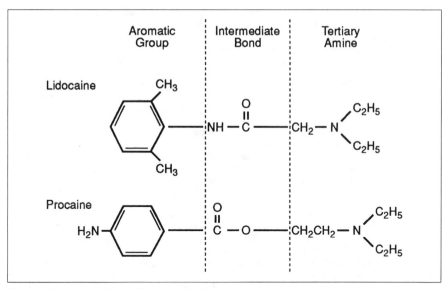

Fig. 5-1. Typical local anesthetic molecules.

Table 5-1. Physicochemical characteristics of local anesthetics

Agent	Class	pK_a	Protein binding (%)	Lipid solubility
Procaine	Ester	8.9	5.8	Low
2-Chloroprocaine	Ester	8.7	—	Low
Tetracaine	Ester	8.6	76.0	High
Prilocaine	Amide	7.7	55.0	Moderate
Lidocaine	Amide	7.7	64.3	Moderate
Mepivacaine	Amide	7.6	77.5	Moderate
Bupivacaine	Amide	8.1	95.0	High
Etidocaine	Amide	7.7	94.0	High

    2. Lipid membrane structure is best described by the "fluid mosaic model" of Singer and Nicolson,[1] in which the membrane is thought to consist of a bimolecular lipid matrix. The lipid, or nonpolar, portion is oriented toward the center of the membrane. The hydrophilic "heads" or polar sections are in contact with the surrounding intracellular and extracellular environment. Embedded within the bilayer are several proteins located interiorly or exteriorly, or completely traversing the cell membrane. The latter are thought to function as ionic channels or pores, allowing for the passage of sodium, potassium, and calcium ions, thereby causing changes in membrane surface charge that are necessary for the propagation of an action potential.

B. Physiology of nerve conduction

    1. A **voltage difference** of approximately 90 mV exists between the inner and outer surfaces of the nerve cell, the interior being negative with relation to the exterior. This voltage difference is maintained by the following mechanisms.

        a. The membrane is relatively impermeable to sodium ions compared with potassium.

        b. A sodium-potassium ATPase pump actively extrudes Na^+ ions from the cell and transports K^+ into the cell.

    2. In order for the action potential to be generated, **depolarization of the nerve** to at least a threshold potential of -55 mV must occur. Once the threshold potential is reached, the permeability of the membrane to sodium increases dramatically as the Na⁺ channels open, allowing sodium ions to move down their concentration gradient into the cell. The membrane potential briefly becomes positive, the Na⁺ channels close, and the K⁺ pores open, allowing for the restoration of the resting potential. At the completion of the action potential, the Na⁺–K⁺ pump reestablishes the proper intracellular ionic concentrations. The generation of an action potential is an "all-or-none" phenomenon in that either the critical threshold potential is achieved during a local depolarization and the action potential is generated, or the threshold is not reached and conduction of the impulse will not occur.[2]

C. Mechanism of action of local anesthetics

1. The mechanism by which a local anesthetic induces neural blockade is the **inhibition of membrane sodium conductance.**[3] There is probably more than one site at which sodium conduction can be inhibited because a wide variety of chemical compounds exhibit local anesthetic properties. Several theories explaining the mechanism of action of local anesthetics have been proposed. Of these, the most convincing is the **receptor theory,** which postulates the existence of various receptors for local anesthetics, either within the Na⁺ channel itself or on the neuronal membrane. Local anesthetic binding to these receptors inhibits sodium flux, presumably by controlling the "gating mechanisms" responsible for changes in Na⁺ conductance.[4,5] The exact location of these receptors in the membrane is unclear, but as many as three different receptor sites may exist:

   a. The external opening of the Na⁺ channel (to which tetrodotoxin and saxitoxin bind)

   b. The interior of the Na⁺ pore (to which the ionized local anesthetic moiety binds)

   c. The outer interface between the channel itself and the lipid membrane (where an uncharged base such as benzocaine would attach)[6]

2. Other investigators have suggested that only one receptor exists and that various local anesthetic molecules arrive at that site by **different pathways.**[5] This theory is attractive because it applies to all forms of the local anesthetic molecule that may be active and accounts for the property of frequency-dependent blockade (neuronal blockade by a charged local anesthetic molecule may be increased with frequent, repetitive depolarization).[7]

III. Pharmacology. Unlike many drugs that depend on systemic absorption for delivery to their respective pharmacologically active sites, local anesthetics are deposited at or near the nerves or nerve terminals to produce the desired conduction blockade. Nonetheless, these agents can be absorbed from the injection site, and systemic toxicity could result from high blood levels. Thus, factors that can modify the absorption pharmacokinetics of local anesthetic agents and, therefore, the resultant peak blood or plasma drug concentration are important.

A. The dose of drug administered is a major determinant of blood level; the larger the dose, the higher the blood level. Therefore, only the lowest possible concentration and volume of local anesthetic necessary to produce a desired nerve conduction blockade should be used. In all cases this amount should be less than the recommended maximum dose listed in Table 5-2.

B. Site of injection. The **vascularity** of the injected tissues may also affect the peak plasma concentration, as well as the rate at which it is attained. Obviously, an intravenous injection of drugs (such as lidocaine for control of ventricular arrhythmias) will result in the highest blood concentration, usually within 1 minute of administration. Application of local anesthetic agents to such highly vascular areas as the intercostal neurovascular bundle or paracervical tissues during pregnancy will result in higher blood levels than injection into relatively less vascular areas such as the peridural space. The lowest blood levels of drug are usually observed after intrathecal injection, in part because of the small doses of local anesthetic needed to produce a subarachnoid block.

C. Use of adjuvants

1. The inclusion of **vasoconstrictors,** such as epinephrine or phenylephrine, in the local anesthetic solution may prolong the latency and duration of action and reduce absorption of the drug from the injection site.

2. The **effects of vasoconstrictors are less pronounced with the longer-acting amides,** such as bupivacaine and etidocaine, than with an intermediate agent, such as lidocaine. Mepivacaine is not as potent a vasodilator as lidocaine; thus

Table 5-2. Recommended maximum dosage of local anesthetics

Drug	Dose (mg) by type of block		
	Infiltration	Major nerve block*	Epidural*
2-Chloroprocaine	800–1000	—	1000
Prilocaine	500–600	600	600
Lidocaine	300–500	500	500
Mepivacaine	300–500	500	500
Bupivacaine	175	225	225
Etidocaine	300	400	300

*Doses listed for major nerve block and epidural are for drugs with epinephrine 1:200,000. Maximum doses are slightly lower when epinephrine is not added to the solutions.

its effects are less enhanced by epinephrine. Ropivacaine is a new long-acting amide agent, similar to bupivacaine, but unlike the latter, it appears to constrict cutaneous vessels.[8]

3. The **use of vasoconstrictors may be limited by the presence of disease states** such as hypertension, coronary artery disease, or valvular heart disease. The use of epinephrine-containing solutions during **pregnancy** has been controversial because it may result in uteroplacental hypoperfusion or may inhibit uterine contractility during labor. Some physicians have advocated the inclusion of epinephrine (15 μg) in the "test dose" alone in order to detect accidental intravascular epidural needle or catheter placement. It is important to realize that even this small dose, if given intravenously to pregnant ewes, will result in decreased uterine artery blood flow lasting for approximately 2 to 4 minutes.[9] This may precipitate fetal distress in situations associated with uteroplacental insufficiency, such as diabetes mellitus. The effect of epinephrine on the fetal-maternal ratio of local anesthetic blood concentrations is inconsistent; thus its use for diminishing fetal drug exposure is discouraged.

4. **Carbonation of amide local anesthetic agents** has been used to shorten the latency and obtain more profound conduction blockade. The effect of carbonation on drug absorption has been contradictory.

D. **Physicochemical factors.**
   Lipid solubility and protein binding are also important modifiers of absorption. Those agents that are highly lipid soluble or protein bound (bupivacaine, etidocaine, and ropivacaine) penetrate tissues and bind proteins readily. Less soluble and protein-bound agents, such as lidocaine or mepivacaine, are more available for uptake into the circulation.

E. **Metabolism and excretion**
   1. Drug accumulation may also depend on how quickly a local anesthetic is cleared from the blood. This is usually the result of metabolism and excretion. In this regard, some ester-type agents, such as 2-chloroprocaine, are rapidly hydrolyzed in the plasma by pseudocholinesterase, the in vivo half-life being approximately 20 seconds.[10] Although 2-chloroprocaine has a high margin of safety, caution must be taken in patients with pseudocholinesterase deficiency or those taking exogenous inhibitors of the enzyme (i.e., echothiophate).

   2. Amide local anesthetic agents are metabolized in the liver, and the conjugated product is excreted in the urine. Renal clearance of unchanged local anesthetic is small, generally less than 2% of the administered dose.[11] For the most part, metabolism of these agents is sensitive to changes in hepatic blood flow. This is particularly true for lidocaine and prilocaine, both of which have a higher hepatic extraction ratio than that of bupivacaine. Prilocaine has the highest hepatic clearance of the amide local anesthetics; however, it is used only as a component of EMLA (eutectic mixture of local anesthetics) cream because of an association between its degradation product, o-toluidine, and the potential for methemoglobinemia.

   3. Disease states and concomitant drug administration can affect the metabolism of amide local anesthetics. Conditions that decrease hepatic blood flow, such

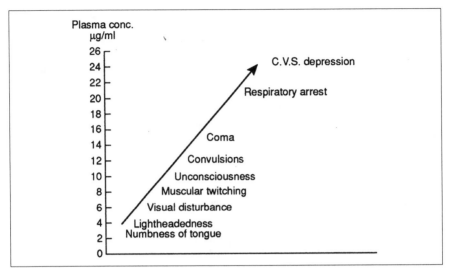

Fig. 5-2. Systemic toxicity of lidocaine with rising plasma concentrations. CVS = cardiovascular system.

as congestive heart failure, halothane anesthesia, or chronic cimetidine or propranolol administration, prolong the elimination half-life of lidocaine.

F. Systemic toxicity

1. The appearance of **signs or symptoms** consistent with local anesthetic toxicity is generally proportionate to the plasma concentration of the drug. Figure 5-2 illustrates the systemic effects of lidocaine based on different plasma concentrations.

    a. At plasma concentrations of approximately 5 µg/ml, premonitory symptoms **(tinnitus, circumoral numbness)** may become manifest.

    b. With increasing drug concentrations, **cortical disinhibition** occurs, leading to muscular twitching or even generalized convulsions.

    c. **Coma, respiratory arrest, and cardiovascular collapse** may ensue at the highest plasma concentrations of lidocaine.

2. The local anesthetic **margin of safety**, as measured by the ratio of the dose or plasma concentration resulting in cardiovascular collapse to that resulting in convulsions, is greater for intermediate-acting agents, such as lidocaine and mepivacaine, than for longer-acting amides, such as bupivacaine, etidocaine, and ropivacaine. Cardiac arrest after accidental intravenous injection of large doses of 0.75% bupivacaine intended for epidural block has been reported. Most of these patients have been refractory to cardiopulmonary resuscitation, with malignant ventricular arrhythmias a prominent feature.[12] Pregnancy appears to predispose to bupivacaine cardiotoxicity because the dose and plasma concentrations of the drug required to result in circulatory collapse are lower in pregnant than nonpregnant ewes.[13] This is not the case with lidocaine, mepivacaine, or the newer long-acting agent ropivacaine.[14] The toxicity of these agents does not appear to be enhanced by pregnancy.[15,16]

3. **Anaphylactoid reactions** to local anesthetic agents are rare and generally related to the inclusion of additives or by-products of metabolism rather than to the parent compound itself. Sensitivity to the ester agents is generally more common and caused by para-aminobenzoic acid. In most instances, hypersensitivity to amide agents is attributed to the additive methylparaben.

G. Tissue toxicity

1. Case reports of long-term **motor and sensory deficits** resulting from accidental subarachnoid injection of large doses of 2-chloroprocaine aroused concern about the possible neural toxicity of local anesthetics.[17,18] In vitro studies of the agent revealed that the combination of low pH and the use of sodium bisulfite as a preservative was responsible for the neurotoxicity, not the local anesthetic itself.[19] No further case reports of neural toxicity have been reported since the

Table 5-3. Supplies that should be readily available during local anesthetic use

Suction

Airway apparatus
Mask
Ambubag or other means of delivering positive-pressure ventilation
Oxygen supply
Laryngoscope
Cuffed endotracheal tube with stylet
Oral and nasal airways

Drugs
Pentothal or diazepam
Succinylcholine
Atropine
Vasopressor (ephedrine)

---

drug was reformulated using EDTA (ethylenediaminetetraacetic acid) as the preservative.

2. In 1991, cases of **cauda equina syndrome** after continuous spinal anesthesia (CSA) using 5% lidocaine were reported.[20,21] Common to all cases were the use of an indwelling intrathecal catheter, use of the hyperbaric preparation of 5% lidocaine in 7.5% dextrose, and relatively high doses of lidocaine injected. Subsequently, the CSA catheter was recalled by the Food and Drug Administration (FDA) and the technique of CSA was largely abandoned while investigations into the etiology of this neurologic syndrome were pursued.

Several animal studies have shown a direct, concentration-dependent, neurotoxic effect of lidocaine. At low concentrations of lidocaine (1%), only minimal effects on neuronal tissues are noted. However, at higher concentrations (5%), significant damage to nerve bundles is seen.[22-25]

It has been proposed that the combination of high lidocaine concentration, maldistribution of the drug to sacral levels preferentially, and the high dose and long duration of exposure to the drug is responsible for the development of the cauda equina syndrome in these patients.

IV. **Prevention and treatment of systemic reactions**
   A. **Prevention**
      1. Adverse systemic reactions can best be prevented by strict observance of **maximum recommended dose** guidelines. Tissue vascularity, disease states, or drug therapy may require modification of the allowable dose.
      2. When performing epidural anesthesia, aspiration of the needle or catheter, followed by administration of an **appropriate test dose** to detect unintended intravascular or subarachnoid injection, is necessary.
      3. **Fractionation of the full dose** to observe the patient for premonitory signs of toxicity is the best way of preventing severe systemic toxicity. A subarachnoid injection of an appropriate test dose will lead to profound sensory and motor blockade, alerting the clinician to improper placement and thus averting total spinal anesthesia should larger doses be administered.
   B. **Treatment.** In all instances, the **equipment and medications** necessary **to treat unexpected reactions** should be at hand. These are listed in Table 5-3.
      1. If generalized convulsions occur, effective ventilation with 100% oxygen should be immediately established to prevent hypoxemia and acidosis. In most instances this can be easily accomplished with **positive-pressure mask ventilation;** however, a **laryngoscope and endotracheal tube** should be readily available to intubate the patient should mask ventilation prove difficult or if there is a risk of inhalation of gastric contents.
      2. Early airway protection in this latter setting also includes the application of **cricoid pressure** until intubation is accomplished.
      3. If seizures continue (they are usually limited), they should be terminated with a small intravenous dose of a **rapid-acting anticonvulsant,** pentothal (50–100 mg) or diazepam (5–10 mg).
      4. Total or high spinal blockade may also require **airway protection and artificial ventilation.** Adequacy of circulation must be ensured with the use of **appropriate vasopressors** (ephedrine, phenylephrine, epinephrine) and volume expansion.

The reverse Trendelenburg position should not be used to limit subarachnoid spread of local anesthetic because it may result in cardiovascular collapse as a result of venous pooling due to total sympathectomy.

V. **Individual agents.** Local anesthetic drugs are conveniently classified according to their potency and duration of action. The agents commonly used in clinical practice in the United States are listed in Table 5-1.

A. **Cocaine** was the first local anesthetic to be isolated and used. Its toxicity and addictive potential are high, and its clinical use is now limited to topical anesthesia of the upper respiratory passages. The best-known side effect of cocaine is CNS stimulation, which results from even small doses of the drug. Cocaine blocks the reuptake of norepinephrine at adrenergic nerve endings, and thus potentiates the responses of end organs to catecholamines, resulting in vasoconstriction. This peripheral effect, combined with a central stimulating effect on the cardiovascular system, results in significant tachycardia and hypertension, which can be severe. Cocaine is also pyrogenic and can produce extremely high fevers.

B. **Procaine (Novocaine).** The many side effects and significant toxicity associated with the use of cocaine led investigators to search for a safer substitute. Procaine, considered to be the prototype ester local anesthetic, demonstrates relatively low potency and toxicity and a short duration of action (about 30 min). With the development of other safe local anesthetics possessing greater potency and longer duration of action, procaine is now most commonly used for infiltration anesthesia (0.5% or 1.0%), with or without epinephrine. It can also be used in concentrations up to 2% for peripheral nerve block, in a 10% solution alone, or in combination with 1% tetracaine for spinal anesthesia. Like all other ester local anesthetics, procaine is rapidly metabolized in the plasma by esterases.

C. **2-Chloroprocaine (Nesacaine)** is a derivative of procaine and possesses most of its desirable properties. It has the advantage of higher potency and more rapid metabolism than procaine. Its main use is for epidural anesthesia in 2% or 3% concentrations, for which its short latency and rapid metabolism prove beneficial in certain circumstances (particularly obstetrics).

D. **Tetracaine,** the longest-acting ester local anesthetic, is metabolized by plasma cholinesterases at a much slower rate than either procaine or 2-chloroprocaine. It is about eight times more potent than procaine, and is more highly protein bound. It is available in various concentrations as an ointment, cream, or solution for topical anesthesia of the eye, skin, rectum, and mucous membranes, but is most commonly used for spinal anesthesia.

E. **Benzocaine** is an ester derivative of para-aminobenzoic acid that is very poorly soluble in water and is very slowly absorbed. It is available in oily solutions, creams, ointments, and aerosols for topical application to the skin and mucous membranes only.

F. **Lidocaine** is by far the most commonly used and perhaps the best-studied local anesthetic agent. Solutions of 1% to 2% are generally suitable for peripheral nerve and peridural blockade. A 5% solution for subarachnoid administration is also available, although, as discussed earlier, its potential neurotoxicity may limit its use in the future. For intravenous regional anesthesia (Bier block) or local infiltration, a 0.5% solution may be used. Topical anesthesia can be provided with 2% to 10% solutions.

G. **Mepivacaine** (1% to 2%) is also used for nerve and peridural blockade in a manner similar to lidocaine. The drug is not available for subarachnoid block.

H. **Prilocaine** alone is no longer available for use in the United States. Although the drug is rapidly cleared from the body, concern has been expressed about a metabolic product, o-toluidine, which can cause methemoglobinemia. This may become clinically significant at doses of prilocaine in the range of 9 to 10 mg/kg of body weight in the healthy patient. However, even small amounts of methemoglobin may adversely affect a patient with already impaired oxygen uptake and delivery.

Prilocaine has found renewed use with the FDA approval of EMLA cream. EMLA is a combination of 2.5% prilocaine and 2.5% lidocaine in a 1:1 ratio by weight. The mixture results in a lowering of the melting point of the two anesthetics so that the mixture exists as an oil rather than a solid at room temperature. This results in enhanced penetration and the development of topical anesthesia in intact skin. Blood levels are well below toxic levels, even in diseased skin in which absorption is faster.[26] It should be used with caution, however, in patients susceptible to the development of methemoglobinemia (i.e., patients with glucose-

6-phosphate deficiency and patients taking oxidizing drugs such as antimalarial agents and sulfonamides). EMLA cream is being used most often in pediatric patients to ameliorate the pain associated with venipuncture.[27–29] It has also found use as an anesthetic during debridement of leg ulcers,[30] laser treatment of port-wine stains,[31] cutting split-thickness skin grafts,[32] various genital procedures,[33] and in postherpetic pain refractory to other treatments.[34]

I. Bupivacaine is approximately 4 times as potent as its parent compound, mepivacaine, with a slower onset and longer duration of action. It is available in solutions of 0.25% to 0.5% for peripheral nerve or epidural blockade and as a 0.75% hyperbaric solution for spinal anesthesia. At lower concentrations, the drug exhibits a "motor-sparing" sensory block, which makes it an ideal agent for epidural administration during labor. Concentrations even lower than 0.25% are being used in combination with narcotics to maximize pain relief with minimal motor block. When motor relaxation is required for surgery, the 0.5% or 0.75% solutions must be used. The 0.75% solution is no longer available for use in obstetrics after reports of cardiac arrest after the inadvertent intravascular injection of the drug in pregnant patients. However, even dilute solutions of bupivacaine can cause toxicity because both the total dosage of the drug and the plasma receptor concentration determine toxicity.

J. Etidocaine was synthesized from lidocaine. Like bupivacaine, the drug is highly protein bound, but it is even more lipid soluble than bupivacaine. Thus, in contrast to bupivacaine, concentrations of etidocaine below 1% result in a higher degree of muscle paralysis compared with sensory anesthesia. This phenomenon is due to rapid penetration of etidocaine into the highly lipid-soluble myelin sheath of motor neurons. With the exception of prilocaine, etidocaine has the fastest hepatic clearance of amides used in the United States. Like bupivacaine, it appears to have less of a margin of safety than the intermediate-acting drugs.

K. Ropivacaine is a new amino-amide local anesthetic agent that is structurally similar to bupivacaine. Although its potency and duration of action are like those of bupivacaine, it may be less cardiotoxic.[35,36] Of particular interest is that, unlike bupivacaine, the cardiotoxicity of ropivacaine is not enhanced by pregnancy.[16] Epidural injection of 0.5% ropivacaine provides good sensory analgesia with little motor blockade. Increasing concentrations of the drug (up to 1.07%) result in increasing motor blockade as well as duration of action (356 ± 75 min.).[37]

References

1. Singer SJ, Nicolson GL. The fluid mosaic model of the structure of cell membranes. *Science* 175:720, 1972.
2. Fozzard HA. Conduction of the action potential. In Berne RM, Sperelakis N, Gieger SR (eds.), *Handbook of Physiology.* Baltimore: Williams & Wilkins, 1979. P. 335.
3. Ritchie JM. Mechanisms of action of local anesthetic agents and biotoxins. *Br J Anaesth* 47:191, 1975.
4. Strichartz G. Molecular mechanisms of nerve block by local anesthetics. *Anesthesiology* 45:421, 1976.
5. Hille B. Local anesthetics: hydrophilic and hydrophobic pathways for the drug-receptor reaction. *J Gen Physiol* 69:497, 1977.
6. Strichartz GR, Ritchie JM. The action of local anesthetics in ion channels of excitable tissues. In Strichartz GR (ed.), *Handbook of Experimental Pharmacology.* Berlin: Springer-Verlag, 1987. P. 21.
7. Courtney KR. Mechanism of frequency-dependent inhibition of sodium currents in frog myelinated nerve by the lidocaine derivative GEA 968. *J Pharmacol Exp Ther* 195:225, 1975.
8. Kopaca DJ, Carpenter RL, Mackey DC. Ropivacaine vasoconstricts cutaneous blood vessels. *Anesthesiology* 69:A343, 1988.
9. Hood DD, Dewan DM, Rose JC, James FM III. Maternal and fetal effects of intravenous epinephrine containing solutions in gravid ewes. *Anesthesiology* 59:A393, 1983.
10. OBrien JE, Abbey V, Hinsvark O, et al. Metabolism and measurement of 2-chloroprocaine, an ester-type local anesthetic. *J Pharm Sci* 66:75, 1979.
11. Santos AC, Pedersen H, Morishima HO, et al. Pharmacokinetics of lidocaine in nonpregnant and pregnant ewes. *Anesth Analg* 67:1154, 1988.
12. Albright GA. Cardiac arrest following regional anesthesia with etidocaine and bupivacaine. *Anesthesiology* 51:285, 1979.

13. Morishima HO, Pedersen H, Finster M, et al. Bupivacaine toxicity in pregnant and nonpregnant ewes. *Anesthesiology* 63:134, 1985.

14. Santos AC, Pedersen H, Harmon TW, et al. Does pregnancy alter local anesthetics toxicity? *Anesthesiology* 70:991, 1989.

15. Morishima HO, Finster M, Arthur GR, Covino BG. Lidocaine toxicity in pregnant sheep. *Anesthesiology* 69:A672, 1988.

16. Pedersen H, Santos AC, Morishima HO, et al. Toxicity of ropivacaine in pregnant and nonpregnant ewes. *Anesthesiology* 69:A342, 1988.

17. Ravindran RS, Bond VK, Tasch MD, et al. Prolonged neural blockade following regional analgesia with 2-chloroprocaine. *Anesth Analg* 59:447–451, 1980.

18. Reisner LS, Hochman BN, Plumer MH. Persistent neurologic deficit and adhesive arachnoiditis following intrathecal 2-chloroprocaine injection. *Anesth Analg* 59(6):452–454, 1980.

19. Barsa J, Batra M, Fink BR, Sumi SM. A comparative in vivo study of local neurotoxicity of lidocaine, bupivacaine, 2-chloroprocaine, and a mixture of 2-chloroprocaine and bupivacaine. *Anesth Analg* 61:961–967, 1982.

20. Rigler ML, Drasner K, Krejcie TC, et al. Cauda equina syndrome after continuous spinal anesthesia. *Anesth Analg* 72:275–281, 1991.

21. Schell RM, Brauer FS, Cole DJ, Applegate RL. Persistent sacral nerve root deficits after continuous spinal anesthesia. *Can J Anaesth* 38:908–911, 1991.

22. Lambert DH, Hurley RJ. Cauda equina syndrome and continuous spinal anesthesia. *Anesth Analg* 72:817–819, 1991.

23. Kroin JS, Penn RD, Levy FE, Kerns JM. Effect of repetitive lidocaine infusion on peripheral nerve. *Exp Neurol* 94:166–173, 1986.

24. Kalichman MW, Moorhouse MB, Powell HC, Myers RR. Relative neural toxicity of local anesthetics. *J Neuropathol Exp Neurol* 52:234–240, 1993.

25. Bainton CR, Strichartz GR. Concentration dependence of lidocaine-induced irreversible conduction loss in frog nerve. *Anesthesiology* 81:657–667, 1994.

26. de Waard–van der Spek FB, van den Berg GM, Oranje AP. EMLA cream: an improved local anesthetic. Review of current literature. *Pediatr Dermatol* 9:126–131, 1992.

27. Hopkins CS. Pain-free injection in infants: use of a lignocaine-prilocaine cream to prevent pain at intravenous induction of general anesthesia in 1–5 year-old children. *Anesthesia* 43:198–201, 1988.

28. Cooper CM, Gerrish SP, Hardwick M, Kay R. EMLA cream reduces the pain of venipuncture in children. *Eur J Anaesthesiol* 4:441–448, 1987.

29. Soliman IE, Broadman LM, Hannallah RS, McGill WA. Comparison of the analgesic effects of EMLA (eutectic mixture of local anesthetics) to intradermal lidocaine infiltration prior to venous cannulation in unpremedicated children. *Anesthesiology* 68:804–806, 1988.

30. Holm J, Andren B, Grafford K. Pain control in the surgical debridement of leg ulcers by the use of topical lidocaine-prilocaine cream, EMLA. *Acta Derm Venereol (Stockh)* 70:132–136, 1990.

31. Ashinoff R, Geronemus RG. Effect of the topical anesthetic EMLA on the efficacy of pulsed dye laser treatment of port-wine stains. *J Dermatol Surg Oncol* 16:1008–1011, 1990.

32. Ohlsen L, Englesson S, Evers H. An anesthetic lidocaine/prilocaine cream (EMLA) for epicutaneous application tested for cutting split skin grafts. *Scand J Plast Reconstr Surg* 19:201–209, 1985.

33. van den Berg GM, Lillieborg S, Stolz E. Lidocaine/prilocaine (EMLA®) cream versus infiltration anesthesia: a comparison of the analgesic efficacy for punch biopsy and electrocoagulation of genital warts in men. *Genitourin Med* 68:162–165, 1992.

34. Stow PJ, Glynn CJ, Minor B. EMLA cream in the treatment of post-herpetic neuralgia: efficacy and pharmacokinetic profile. *Pain* 39:301–305, 1989.

35. Skerman B, Hellberg IB, Trossvik C. Primary evaluation of the local anesthetic properties of the amino-amide agent ropivacaine (LEA 103). *Acta Anaesthesiol Scand* 32:571, 1988.

36. Pedigo NW, Walmsley PN, Kasten GW, Lock RL. Relative cardiotoxicity of the long-acting local anesthetic bupivacaine and ropivacaine in dogs. *Anesth Analg* 67:S266, 1988.

37. Concepcion M, Arthur GR, Steele SM, et al. A new local anesthetic ropivacaine, its epidural effects in humans. *Anesth Analg* 70:80, 1990.

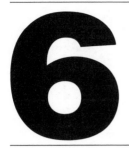

6

Psychotropic Adjuvant Analgesics for Chronic Pain

Nancy Chiyo Maruyama
William Breitbart

I. Background.

A. **Psychotropic medications** have been reported to be effective in the treatment of a variety of chronic pain syndromes. It has long been noted that pain syndromes have significant emotional and behavioral components. However, these drugs not only treat concomitant depression or anxiety but also have innate analgesic properties themselves. In addition to treating pain and psychological symptoms, their side effects can be manipulated to target symptoms such as insomnia or anxiety. The following agents are currently used as adjuvant analgesics:

1. **Antidepressants**
2. **Neuroleptics**
3. **Psychostimulants**
4. **Benzodiazepines**
5. **Antihistamines**
6. **Mood-stabilizing anticonvulsants**

B. In this chapter we review the use of psychotropic adjuvant analgesics in the **management of chronic pain syndromes,** the different classes of drugs, their indications, and how to select an agent. Specific information on the assessment of the patient before treatment, dosage and duration of treatment with psychotropic adjuvant analgesics for chronic pain, and the adverse effects of these agents are addressed.

II. Antidepressants

A. **Tricyclic antidepressants** (TCAs) have been used effectively in the management of a variety of chronic pain syndromes for 20 years. There is substantial evidence to suggest that TCAs, in particular, are analgesic and useful in the treatment of such chronic pain syndromes as diabetic neuropathy, postherpetic neuralgia, headache, facial pain, low back pain, and, in combination with opioids, cancer pain. Amitriptyline is the TCA most studied and has proved effective as an analgesic in a large number of clinical trials addressing a wide variety of pain syndromes.[1-5] Other TCAs shown to be effective as analgesics are imipramine,[6-8] desipramine,[9,10] nortriptyline,[11] clomipramine,[12,13] doxepin,[14] and maprotiline.[15]

TCAs serve as primary analgesics in chronic neuropathic pains such as postherpetic neuralgia or painful polyneuropathy when pain is characterized as lancinating, shooting, or burning. More recent controlled studies suggest TCAs have a role not only in the treatment of the lancinating component of neuropathic pain, but also in the continuous dysesthetic component.[1,16] (See Table 6-1 for a summary of studies of antidepressants in chronic pain.) Their role in arthritis and in pain of mixed etiologies is less clear.

B. **Other antidepressants,** including the monoamine oxidase inhibitors (MAOIs) such as phenelzine, the atypical antidepressants such as trazodone, and the newer serotonin-specific reuptake inhibitors (SSRIs), fluoxetine, paroxetine, and sertraline, may also have a role in the management of chronic pain, although the results of clinical trials of their efficacy as analgesics have been equivocal.[9,36,37,42] Trazodone has been found to be analgesic in a cancer pain population; however, a trial for dysesthetic pains from traumatic myelopathy failed to show efficacy. Fluoxetine has not been demonstrated to have clinically significant analgesic properties in patients with diabetic neuropathy when compared with desipramine and amitriptyline.[9] Paroxetine, recently released on the U.S. market, is the first SSRI to be shown effective in neuropathic pain.[43] Sertraline's analgesic properties have not yet been studied.

The use of MAOIs in patients with chronic pain is complicated by their potential

Table 6-1. Antidepressants in chronic pain

Pain syndrome	Antidepressant	Dose (mg)	Benefit[a]	Studies (ref. no.)
Headache				
Chronic tension	Amitriptyline	30–110	+	Diamond and Frietag (17); Lance and Curran (18)
Migraine	Amitriptyline	10–175	+	Gomersall and Stuart (19); Couch and Hassanein (20)[b]; Anthony and Lance (21)
	Phenelzine	45	+	
Mixed vascular tension	Doxepin	100	+	Morland et al. (22)
Headache in Parkinson's disease	Amitriptyline	50	+	
"Psychogenic"	Doxepin	30–50	+	Okasha et al. (23)
	Amitriptyline	30–50	+	
Facial pain				
Various etiologies, "psychogenic"	Phenelzine	45	+	Lascelles (24); Feinmann et al. (25)
	Doxepin		+	
Trigeminal neuralgia	Clomipramine	20–75	+	Watson et al. (5,15); Watson and Evans (26)
	Amitriptyline	30–110	+	
Postherpetic neuralgia	Amitriptyline	25–150	+	Watson et al. (5, 15); Watson and Evans (26)
	Desipramine	173 (mean)	+	
	Maprotiline	200	+	
Diabetic neuropathy	Amitriptyline	25–150	+	Turkington (27); Kvinesdal et al. (6); Max et al. (1); Sindrup et al. (8)
	Imipramine	100	+	
	Paroxetine	40	+	
Arthritis, rheumatic pain	Imipramine	50–75	+	McDonald-Scott (28); Gringas (29); Glick and Fowler (30)
	Clomipramine	25	–	
Low back pain	Imipramine	75	–	Jenkins et al. (31); Alcoff et al. (32); Hameroff et al. (14)
	Imipramine	150	+	
	Doxepin	2.5 mg/kg	+	

Condition	Drug	Dose	Benefit	Reference
Fibromyalgia	Amitriptyline	50	−	Walsh (33–35); Ventafridda et al. (36); Magni et al. (37)[b]
	Doxepin	75	+	
Cancer pain	Imipramine	50–150	+	
	Trazodone	20–60	+	
	Amitriptyline	50–150	+	
	Clomipramine	50–150	+	
	Doxepin			
Mixed pain and depression	Amitriptyline	150–300	+	
	Imipramine	150–300	+	
	Desipramine	150–300	+	
	Doxepin	150–300	+	
Mixed organic and "psychogenic" pain	Zimelidine	200	+	Johansson and von Knorring (38)
Pain without organic etiology	Amitriptyline	150	−	Pilowsky et al. (3)
Pain in depression	Doxepin	150	−	Evans et al. (39); Ward et al. (40); Raft et al. (41)
	Doxepin	150	+	
	Desipramine		+	
	Phenelzine	1.5 mg/kg		
Painful poly- and mononeuropathies	Clomipramine	150	+	Langohr et al. (12)
Dysesthetic pain, posttraumatic myelopathy	Trazodone	150	−	Davidoff et al. (42)

[a]Benefit (+) is defined as more than 50% of patients reporting pain relief, or significantly more than with placebo.
[b]Uncontrolled study.

adverse interactions with opioids and other psychotropic medications and their dietary restrictions. Despite these limitations they may have a role in the treatment of chronic pain. Lascelles, in a placebo-controlled trial, found phenelzine to be efficacious in atypical facial pain.[24] There have been several favorable uncontrolled trials of phenelzine and tranylcypromine. Anthony and Lance demonstrated analgesic efficacy of phenelzine in cases of severe migraine.[21]

C. **Mechanisms of action. No single mechanism** explains the analgesic effects of antidepressants. Initially the effects of TCAs on chronic pain were attributed only to their antidepressant activity. Though relief of mood symptoms does contribute to the analgesic properties of these medications, this is neither the only mechanism nor the most important. Antidepressants are effective as adjuvants in chronic pain through several proposed mechanisms that include antidepressant activity,[44] potentiation or enhancement of opioid analgesia,[45-47] and direct analgesic effects.[48]

  1. **Antidepressant activity.** Relief of depression in patients with chronic pain results in reported pain relief.[49] The antidepressant effects of the TCAs and other antidepressants probably do make an important contribution to the analgesic properties of this class of drugs, although studies have shown that pain relief can occur in the absence of relief of depression.[38]

  2. **Potentiation of opioid analgesia.** Antidepressants also potentiate the analgesic effects of the opioid drugs by acting directly on the CNS. This is mediated through serotonergic, catecholaminergic, and possibly even anticholinergic effects.[45] Manipulation of CNS serotonin can dramatically influence the degree of analgesia produced by opioid analgesics such as morphine. Increasing levels of CNS serotonin results in greater degrees of analgesia produced by opioid drugs, while depletion of CNS serotonin results in decreased opioid analgesia.[45] Modulation of the noradrenergic and cholinergic systems in the brain also has profound effects on opioid analgesia.[45,50,51] Antidepressants can also potentiate the analgesic effects of opioids through pharmacokinetic mechanisms. Imipramine, orally administered, can increase the bioavailability of morphine by reducing its rate of elimination.[52] Desipramine can elevate methadone levels in serum.[53]

  3. **Direct analgesic effects.** Antidepressants have direct analgesic properties of their own.[51,54] A leading hypothesis for the mechanism of innate or direct antidepressant analgesia is that descending serotonergic and noradrenergic pathways originate in the brain stem and synapse on the dorsal horn of the spinal cord at every level.[15,50,54]

  4. **Summary.** The various classes of antidepressants, TCAs, atypical, SSRIs, and MAOIs, have both short- and long-term effects on a number of neurotransmitters and their receptors.[55] Amitriptyline, for example, elevates levels of serotonin and noradrenaline in the nervous system by blocking synaptic reuptake of serotonin and norepinephrine. As such, amitriptyline is a mixed noradrenergic and serotonergic agent. Other antidepressants have been demonstrated to have more specific serotonergic or noradrenergic properties. Many antidepressants with mixed or predominantly serotonergic activity such as amitriptyline, imipramine, nortriptyline, clomipramine, doxepin, and trazodone have been shown to have direct analgesic effects. This led some researchers to hypothesize a serotonergically mediated mechanism of analgesia, although newer SSRIs such as zimelidine (never released in the United States) and fluoxetine, as well as the serotonin partial agonist, buspirone (marketed as an anxiolytic), have proved disappointing in clinical studies of neuropathic pain.[9,26,56] Maprotiline and desipramine, both rather selective noradrenergic agents, have now also been demonstrated to have direct analgesic properties.[10,15] At present, the mechanism of analgesia shared universally by all antidepressants is not agreed upon, and variations among individuals in pain response seem to be important variables. Other possible mechanisms include adenosinergic effects,[57,58] antihistaminic or anticholinergic effects,[31] and direct neuronal effects that inhibit paroxysmal neuronal discharge or decrease the sensitivity of adrenergic receptors on damaged nerves.[7]

D. **Selecting an agent** often depends not only on the type of pain present but also on the drug's side effect profile (Table 6-2), the patient's existing medical problems, the nature of depressive symptoms, if present, and the patient's past response to specific antidepressants. For example, sedating drugs such as amitriptyline, imipramine, or trazodone can be utilized at bedtime for the patient who has insomnia complicating the presence of pain and depression. The more activating agents such as fluoxetine, nortriptyline, or desipramine can be used for the patient troubled by fatigue. Highly anticholinergic agents such as amitriptyline or imipramine can be helpful in drying respiratory secretions in some patients, but should be avoided in the patient troubled by constipation or prostatic hypertrophy. For these patients the clinician should select a less anticholinergic agent such as nortriptyline or desipramine. Alternatively, the clinician might select an antidepressant that does not have anticholinergic properties, for example, trazodone or one of the serotonin reuptake inhibitors.

Agents that have a high incidence of orthostatic hypotension such as amitriptyline, imipramine, or the MAOIs should be used with caution in elderly patients at higher risk of injury should they fall. Agents less likely to cause orthostasis such as nortriptyline, desipramine, trazodone, or an SSRI should be chosen. For patients with significant cardiac conduction abnormalities, an agent that does not affect cardiac conduction, such as an SSRI or trazodone, should be selected rather than the TCAs, which prolong cardiac conduction. If a particular agent has been helpful in the past, it should be considered again.

III. Tricyclic antidepressants
A. Assessment of the patient
1. Before prescribing a TCA, a **medical history and physical examination** should be performed, paying particular attention to cardiac conduction system disease. Those patients over 40 years or with a history of cardiac disease should have an ECG. Tricyclic antidepressants (amitriptyline, imipramine, nortriptyline, desipramine, doxepin, and clomipramine) should not be used for patients with bifascicular block, left bundle branch block (LBBB), or prolonged QT interval, though they may be used in patients with first-degree heart block. If there is a question of safety, a cardiologist should evaluate the patient before beginning the trial.
2. **Educate the patient** before initiating the medication trial about the possible need for sequential drug trials and the delay of sometimes 4 to 6 weeks before the full analgesic effects may be appreciated. Patients should be warned of common side effects and the need for determining serum drug levels. This can improve patient compliance.
3. The clinician should be aware of the patient's **concurrent medications.** TCAs have a quinidinelike effect, prolonging cardiac conduction, and can result in dangerous additive cardiotoxicity if used with quinidine or other type II antiarrhythmics. When administered in conjunction with antihistamines or over-the-counter cold medications, TCAs can cause anticholinergic toxicity. Concurrent use with beta-adrenergic blockers such as alpha-methyldopa or clonidine can potentiate the hypotensive effects of TCAs. The effects of warfarin (Coumadin) may be increased by use with cyclic antidepressants.[59,60]

B. **Dose ranges** vary from 20 to 300 mg of amitriptyline or imipramine, but the most frequently used doses are between 50 and 100 mg. Some physicians report low doses (10–30 mg) of TCAs such as amitriptyline to be as effective as high doses (75–150 mg).[4] Zitman et al.,[61] however, demonstrated only modest analgesic results from low-dose amitriptyline. Watson et al.[62] believed there was a "therapeutic window" (20–100 mg amitriptyline) for analgesia. More recently, there has been compelling evidence that the therapeutic analgesic effects of amitriptyline correlate with serum levels just as antidepressant effects do, and that analgesic treatment failure is due to low serum levels.[1,2] A regimen of up to 150 mg of amitriptyline or higher is suggested.[6,26]

In healthy adults, initial doses of 50 mg of amitriptyline or imipramine may be used. The medication can be taken at bedtime, and the dose is increased in increments of 25–50 mg every 3 to 4 days, as side effects allow, up to 150 mg of amitriptyline or imipramine or their equivalent. Nortriptyline, which is twice as potent, is begun at 25 mg and increased up to 75 mg as tolerated. For debilitated or elderly patients, treatment should be initiated at a low dose and gradually increased until therapeutic blood levels are achieved. For example, begin amitriptyline at 10–25 mg at bedtime in an elderly patient and increase it by 10–25 mg every 2 to 4 days as side effects allow, until 100–150 mg. Other TCA dosage recommendations can be found in Table 6-3.

C. **Serum levels,** at the very least, confirm patient compliance and ensure that adequate trials are given. Before drawing plasma to determine drug levels the clinician should wait until the drug reaches steady state levels (approximately

Table 6-2. Antidepressant effects

Drug	Initial amines affected		Anticholinergic	Antihistamine	Orthostasis	Sedation	Heart block
TCAs							
Amitriptyline	5HT	++	+++	++ (H₁,H₂)	+++	+++	+++
	NE	+/−					
	DA	0					
Nortriptyline	5HT	+/−	++	+	+	++	+++
	NE	++					
	DA	0					
Imipramine	5HT	+	++	+	+++	++	+++
	NE	+					
	DA	0					
Desipramine	5HT	0	+	+	+	+	+++
	NE	+++					
	DA	0					
Doxepin	5HT	+	+++	+++	+++	+++	++
	NE						
	DA	0					
Clomipramine	5HT	+++	+++		+++	+++	+++
	NE						
	DA						
Maprotiline	5HT	0	++	++	+	++	++
	NE	++					
	DA	0					

Atypical						
Bupropion	5HT	+/−	0	0	None	Stimulant low
	NE	+/−				
	DA	++				
Trazodone	5HT	+	Very low	+	++	+++	Insig.
	NE	0				
	DA	0				
SSRI						
Fluoxetine	5HT	+++	0	0	None	Stimulant activating	Insig.
	NE	0				
	DA	0				
Sertraline	5HT	+++	0	0	None	+/−	Insig.
	NE	0				
	DA	0				
Paroxetine	5HT	+++	0	0	None	+/−	Insig.
	NE	0				
	DA	0				
MAOIs						
Phenelzine	5HT	++	0	0	+++	+
	NE	++				
	DA	++				

5HT, serotonin; NE, norepinephrine; DA, dopamine. The number of symbols represents a relative estimate of the intensity of the effect.
Source: Adapted from the AMA *Drug Evaluations Manual*, 1992.[60]

Table 6-3. Psychotropic adjuvant analgesics

Generic name (trade name)	Approximate daily dosage range (mg)	Route*
Tricyclic antidepressants		
Amitriptyline (Elavil)	50–150	PO, IM
Nortriptyline (Pamelor)	25–60	PO
Imipramine (Tofranil)	50–150	PO, IM
Desipramine (Norpramin)	50–150	PO
Doxepin (Adapin, Sinequan)	50–150	PO
Clomipramine (Anafranil)	50–150	PO
Atypical antidepressants		
Trazodone (Desyrel)	50–300	PO
Fluoxetine (Prozac)	20–60	PO
Paroxetine (Paxil)	10–40	PO
Sertraline (Zoloft)	50–200	PO
MAOI		
Phenelzine (Nardil)	45–75	PO
Psychostimulants		
Methylphenidate (Ritalin)	2.5–20 bid	PO
Dextroamphetamine (Dexedrine)	2.5–20 bid	PO
Phenothiazines		
Fluphenazine (Prolixin)	1–3	PO, IM
Methotrimeprazine (Levoprome)	10–20 q6h	IM, IV
Butyrophenones		
Haloperidol (Haldol)	1–3	PO, IM, IV
Pimozide (Orap)	2–6 bid	PO
Antihistamines		
Hydroxyzine	50 q4–6h	PO, IM, IV
Benzodiazepines		
Lorazepam (Ativan)	0.5–2.0 tid	PO, IM, IV
Alprazolam (Xanax)	0.25–2.0 tid	PO
Clonazepam (Klonopin)	0.5–4.0 bid	PO
Anticonvulsants		
Carbamazepine (Tegretol)	400–1600	PO
Valproate (Depakote, Depakene)	950	PO

*The routes of administration are those approved for use in the United States. Intravenous infusions of tricyclic and noncyclic agents are used outside of the United States.

five half-lives, which should be 5 days in healthy adults and longer in elderly or debilitated patients). Plasma to determine drug levels should be drawn 10 to 14 hours after the last dose. Titration should be resumed and continued until therapeutic levels are achieved.

There is compelling evidence that the analgesic effects of amitriptyline are correlated with serum levels as they are in the treatment of depression. Treatment failure may be due to low serum levels.[1,2] Only imipramine, desipramine, nortriptyline, and amitriptyline have been studied adequately to draw conclusions about the relation between serum levels and response of depression.

1. In the treatment of depression, studies suggest a linear relation between blood levels of **imipramine** and its metabolite **desipramine.** A combined imipramine and desipramine level of more than 225 ng/ml correlates with a better clinical response than lower levels.

2. For **desipramine,** too, these appears to be a linear relation between the patient's response and serum levels above 125 ng/ml.
3. **Nortriptyline** seems to have a "therapeutic window" with a curvilinear relation between patient response and levels between 50 and 150 ng/ml; the best response appears to occur at a level around 110 ng/ml.
4. For **amitriptyline,** the relation has been less clear; some describe a linear relation, others a curvilinear, and still others describe no relation at all. Serum levels of amitriptyline measure the sum of the levels of amitriptyline and its metabolite nortriptyline.

D. **Duration of treatment.** One can see early analgesic effects of antidepressants within hours or days. These analgesic effects are most likely mediated by inhibition of neuronal reuptake of such neurotransmitters as serotonin and norepinephrine.[13,45,48] However, further analgesic effects may occur as late as 4 to 6 weeks after therapeutic blood levels are achieved. These may correlate with changes in neurotransmitter receptors. In animal studies long-term administration of antidepressants decreases beta- and $alpha_2$-adrenergic receptor sensitivity and the number of 5-hydroxtryptamine$_2$ receptors, while $alpha_1$-adrenergic receptor sensitivity and the number of muscarinic receptors appear to stay the same.[1,3] Because these receptor changes take 3 to 6 weeks to take place, an adequate trial of an antidepressant for analgesia may require 4 to 6 weeks.

E. **Side effects**
1. The most common side effects of TCAs are due to their **anticholinergic and alpha-adrenergic blocking properties** (see Table 6-2). These side effects include diaphoresis, dry mouth, blurred vision, constipation, tachycardia, and hypotension. Antidepressants have varying degrees of anticholinergic activity. Sedation is another common CNS effect of the more anticholinergic agents. For patients troubled by insomnia, a more sedating agent should be chosen and given at bedtime. More serious anticholinergic effects include urinary retention, adynamic ileus, and even a toxic delirium in which patients may become "mad as a hatter, red as a beet, dry as a bone." For patients with baseline cognitive deficits, less anticholinergic agents such as desipramine or nortriptyline, or agents that are not anticholinergic such as the SSRIs or trazodone should be selected.
2. The most common cardiovascular side effect of TCAs is **orthostatic hypotension,** an effect that is mediated by the $alpha_1$-antagonist property of the medications. TCAs should be used with caution in elderly patients who are at greater risk of injury from potential falls. Nortriptyline and desipramine are the least likely of the TCAs to cause orthostatic hypotension. The clinician should monitor orthostatic BP before initiating a TCA and regularly during titration of the medication.
3. **Cardiotoxicity** is the most serious potential adverse effect of TCAs, which have a quinidinelike activity and delay intraventricular cardiac conduction. The clinician should elicit a careful history, looking for preexisting cardiac disease and concurrent antiarrhythmic medication use from patients. Those patients who have significant cardiac conduction abnormalities such as LBBB, bifascicular block, or prolonged QT intervals should be excluded, and a less cardiotoxic agent such as an SSRI should be selected. The clinician should monitor ECGs before and during treatment for patients who are over 40 years or have preexisting heart disease.
4. TCAs can precipitate **narrow-angle glaucoma.** Ophthalmology evaluation and follow-up for patients with glaucoma are recommended.
5. All cyclic antidepressants, particularly maprotiline, can **lower seizure threshold** and should be avoided in patients with a history of seizure disorder. Desipramine reportedly lowers seizure threshold the least.[60]
6. One problem with dosing TCAs in chronic pain patients with depression in whom suicide risk is an issue is the **potential lethality** of TCAs **in overdose.** Ingestion of more than 1 g of imipramine or amitriptyline or their equivalent may cause fatal cardiac arrhythmias. Overdose is a medical emergency, and patients will require cardiac monitoring. The risk can be reduced by administering the medication on a weekly basis and closely monitoring plasma levels and compliance. When suicide is a serious consideration, the clinician should

select a medication with less potential for lethality in overdose, such as the SSRIs.

7. TCAs, SSRIs, and MAOIs all appear to be associated with a high incidence of **sexual dysfunction,** including impairment of arousal and orgasm. Males may have problems with both erection and ejaculation; delayed, inhibited, and retrograde ejaculation have been described.

IV. **Atypical antidepressants: Trazodone.** Trazodone has alpha-adrenergic blocking activity and, at therapeutic doses, inhibits serotonin reuptake. It has no MAO inhibitory activity and little anticholinergic activity. Trazodone can be initiated at 50–75 mg/day and gradually increased to 200–300 mg/day, with some doses as high as 400–500 mg/day. It is given at bedtime to take advantage of its sedating properties. It does not appear to have effects on cardiac conduction, though further studies must be undertaken. Men should be forewarned that priapism can occur, usually early in the treatment course. If a patient experiences priapism, the medication should be discontinued immediately, and the physician consulted.

V. **Serotonin-specific reuptake inhibitors (SSRIs).** Unlike the TCAs, fluoxetine, sertraline, and paroxetine are highly specific inhibitors of serotonin reuptake.

A. **Fluoxetine**

1. **Indications.** Fluoxetine (Prozac) has become extremely popular for the treatment of **depression** because of its lack of anticholinergic or cardiac side effects and its safety in overdose. Its role and that of the other SSRIs in the treatment of pain is less clear.

2. **Dosage.** Fluoxetine is given in a single 10- or 20-mg dose with breakfast. It is activating and, if given later in the day, can cause insomnia. Some patients respond on alternate-day dosing (20 mg every other day).

3. **Side effects.** Fluoxetine has a long elimination half-life—1 to 4 days for fluoxetine and 7 to 10 days for its active metabolite desmethylfluoxetine—and this may pose problems for some patients. It may require weeks for some of the side effects to subside following cessation of the medication. A 5-week washout period must elapse after stopping fluoxetine and before starting an MAOI because of potentially dangerous drug interactions. Its more common side effects are

   a. **Anxiety**
   b. **Agitation**
   c. **Insomnia**
   d. **Restlessness**
   e. **GI distress**

4. **Mechanism of action.** Fluoxetine and other SSRIs are **highly protein bound** and may interact with other protein-bound medications such as digoxin and warfarin by displacing them and increasing plasma levels of active drug, thereby causing adverse effects. Levels of digoxin or bleeding parameters (prothrombin time and partial thromboplastin time) should be monitored when such medications are used concurrently with fluoxetine or other SSRIs, and doses of medications should be adjusted.

B. **Sertraline**

1. **Dosage.** Sertraline has a shorter half-life than fluoxetine, and its metabolite has much less activity than the parent compound. Doses begin at 50 mg/day in the morning or evening, and are increased if necessary to 200 mg. The precise dosage in treating depression is not established, and sertraline's use in the treatment of chronic pain has not been studied.

2. **Side effects.** As with fluoxetine, a washout period before initiation of an MAOI is required because adverse interactions can occur with other medications. The most common side effects of sertraline are

   a. **GI distress**
   b. **Nausea**
   c. **Diarrhea or dyspepsia**
   d. **Tremor**
   e. **Dizziness**
   f. **Insomnia**
   g. **Primary ejaculatory delay**

C. **Paroxetine**

1. **Dosage.** Paroxetine, the only SSRI with demonstrated analgesic efficacy,[43] is begun at 20 mg/day in either the morning or evening for healthy adults and

10 mg/day in the elderly and debilitated. As with sertraline, paroxetine has a shorter half-life than fluoxetine.

2. **Side effects.** Paroxetine's side-effect profile is similar to that of **sertraline**, but reportedly it is less anxiogenic. As with fluoxetine and sertraline it requires a washout period before initiation of an MAOI.

VI. Monoamine oxidase inhibitors. Phenelzine is the most commonly used MAOI for patients with chronic pain. Other MAOIs available in the United States are tranylcypromine (Parnate) and isocarboxazid (Marplan).

A. **Assessment of the patient**

1. The clinician must evaluate the patient for concurrent use of sympathomimetic agents or opioids as well as previously used long-acting agents such as fluoxetine that might interact dangerously with an MAOI.
2. Patients must be educated about maintaining a tyramine-free diet and avoiding medications such as over-the-counter cold and flu preparations that might contain sympathomimetic amines such as pseudoephedrine, which can precipitate a hyperadrenergic crisis.

B. **Dosage.** Phenelzine is started at 15 mg PO bid, and increased by 15 mg every 3 to 4 days to a dose of 45 mg/day. Should there be no response, the dose can be increased to 60 to 75 mg, in increments of 15 mg/wk. Titration may be limited by side effects such as postural hypotension and sedation, although tolerance can develop for some of these. Phenelzine irreversibly binds monoamine oxidase; amine levels do not return immediately to normal after cessation of the drug. Patients should therefore continue the tyramine-free diet for 2 weeks after stopping the medication.

C. **Side effects**

1. The most **common side effects** of MAOIs are
   a. **Sedation**
   b. **Weight gain**
   c. **Dizziness**
   d. **GI symptoms**
   e. **Sexual dysfunction** such as delay of orgasm and ejaculation
   f. **Orthostatic hypotension**
2. MAOIs have **adverse interactions with tyramine and other amines.** Medications that alter amine levels, antidepressants, and opioids have all been reported to interact with MAOIs in a dangerous and potentially lethal fashion. MAOIs inactivate intestinal and hepatic monoamine oxidase type A, which preferentially metabolizes norepinephrine and serotonin and elevates levels of catecholamines. Use with some opioids such as meperidine (Demerol) or the antidepressant fluoxetine and most likely other SSRI antidepressants is contraindicated because of potentially lethal "serotonergic crisis" characterized by nausea, confusion, hyperthermia, autonomic hyperactivity, and rigidity.[63,64] Because of the long half-life of fluoxetine, the clinician must wait 3 to 4 weeks before introducing an MAOI.
3. **Hyperadrenergic crisis** following ingestion of tyramine-containing foods or medications containing sympathomimetic amines is the most serious side effect and should be treated as a medical emergency. Symptoms include hypertension, hyperpyrexia, autonomic hyperactivity, and cardiac arrhythmias. Phentolamine 5 mg IV is used to block adrenergic receptors.

VII. Psychostimulants

A. **Indications**

1. Controlled single-dose studies have established the analgesic efficacy of the stimulant drugs methylphenidate and dextroamphetamine. They are particularly useful as adjuvant analgesics used in conjunction with opioids, for **postoperative pain, cancer pain, and pain associated with Parkinson's disease.**[65–68] In patients with cancer, psychostimulants have been demonstrated to diminish sedation secondary to opioids as well as potentiate their analgesic effects.[66,67,69]
2. Pemoline is an alternative psychostimulant, chemically unrelated to amphetamine. No studies of pemoline's potential as an adjuvant analgesic have yet been conducted.
3. Methylphenidate has been reported to improve functioning on a number of neuropsychological tests, including tests of memory, mental speed, and concentration, in patients who are being administered continuous infusion of opioids for cancer pain.[69] Methylphenidate and dextroamphetamine can also stimulate

appetite, improve weakness and fatigue, as well as boost mood in depressed, medically ill patients. When effective, these medications work rapidly, unlike the cyclic and noncyclic antidepressants, which may require more than 7 to 10 days to take effect. There is no established use for psychostimulants in patients with chronic noncancer pain, but they can probably be used in a similar fashion. However, the problems of dependence and tolerance, which are often not problematic for patient with cancer pain, may be important issues for patients with chronic noncancer pain.

B. Mechanism of action. The psychostimulants cause **release of norepinephrine, dopamine, and serotonin from presynaptic nerve terminals and act as agonists at postsynaptic receptors.** They also inhibit reuptake of norepinephrine and dopamine and inhibit monoamine oxidase. Some postulate that their analgesic effects are mediated through norepinephrine- or serotonin-containing descending pain pathways.[68]

C. Assessment of patients. Before starting treatment, patients should have a physical examination with evaluation of BP, heart rate, and heart rhythm. Stimulants can elevate BP and pulse and should be monitored carefully in patients with hypertension or tachycardia. However, in general, the psychostimulants' cardiovascular side-effect profile is safer than that of TCAs.

D. Dosage

1. Methylphenidate or dextroamphetamine can be initiated at a dose ranging from 2.5 to 5.0 mg given early in the day (i.e., 8 AM and 1 PM) to avoid insomnia. The dose may be increased by 5 to 10 mg every 2 to 4 days to a maximum dose ranging from 30 mg/day to 60 mg/day, or until unwanted side effects intervene.
2. Pemoline is started at 18.75 mg at 8 AM and noon, and gradually increased to 75 mg/day or less.
3. Patients are well maintained on methylphenidate for 1 to 3 months, with some patients being maintained for longer periods. Tolerance can develop, and dose adjustment may be necessary.

E. Abuse and withdrawal. The use of methylphenidate and dextroamphetamine is limited by their abuse potential. Although there are no observable physical signs of withdrawal, there may be psychological symptoms of increased fatigue and depression. Abrupt discontinuation of these agents may be complicated by the development of some depressive symptoms.

F. Side effects. In general, psychostimulants have a safer cardiovascular profile than TCAs. There have been reports of transient, reversible liver function abnormalities developing in patients on pemoline, and so it should be used with caution in patients with liver disease.

1. **The most common side effects** of psychostimulants are
   a. **Anxiety**
   b. **Insomnia**
   c. **Restlessness**
   d. **Overstimulation**
   e. **Tics**
2. **The less common side effects** include
   a. **Involuntary movements**
   b. **Myoclonus or tremors**
   c. **Confusion**
   d. **Paranoia**
   e. **Tachycardia**
   f. **Mild elevations of BP** in patients with underlying hypertension

VIII. Benzodiazepines

A. Indications

1. There is **no clear evidence of specific analgesic properties** for benzodiazepines, and various studies have shown antidepressants to be superior to benzodiazepines in the treatment of chronic tension headaches, painful diabetic neuropathy, and idiopathic psychogenic pain.[18,23,27,70] Furthermore, long-term use, such as might be required to treat chronic pain, is complicated by problems of tolerance, dependency, and withdrawal. Nevertheless, benzodiazepines have a role in the treatment of patients with chronic pain.
2. Benzodiazepines are used to **reduce anxiety and relieve insomnia associated with pain** and can decrease a patient's emotional reactivity to pain.[71,72] Diazepam and other benzodiazepines are commonly used as muscle relaxants for

Table 6-4. Commonly prescribed benzodiazepines

Drug	Elimination Half-life (hr)	Active metabolite	Dosage equivalency (mg)
Short to intermediate half-life			
Alprazolam (Xanax)	6–20	Yes	0.50
Chlonazepam (Klonopin)	18–50	No	0.25
Lorazepam (Ativan)	10–20	No	1.00
Midazolam (Versed)	2–3		
Oxazepam (Serax)	5–15	No	15.00
Temazepam (Restoril)	8–20	No	30.00
Triazolam (Halcion)	1–5	Yes	0.25
Long half-life			
Clorazepate (Tranxene)	30–200	Yes	7.50
Chlordiazepoxide (Librium)	30–100	Yes	10.00
Diazepam (Valium)	20–100	Yes	5.00

Source: Adapted from Arana GW, Hyman SE. *Handbook of Psychiatric Drug Therapy.* Boston: Little, Brown, 1991.

acute and chronic musculoskeletal pain and for the muscle spasms that accompany local trauma and nerve damage. Some physicians believe the anticonvulsant effects of benzodiazepines give them a role in the treatment of neuropathic pain. Clonazepam, in particular, may be useful for the cancer patient in the management of lancinating neuropathic pains as well as for the patient with trigeminal neuralgia, posttraumatic neuralgia, and headache.[73,74]

B. **Mechanism of action.** Benzodiazepines bind to a site on the **gamma-aminobutyric acid (GABA) receptor** and allosterically modify its structure so that it has increased affinity to GABA, the major inhibitory neurotransmitter of the brain. GABA opens a chloride channel, allowing chloride ions to flow in, hyperpolarizing and thereby inhibiting the neuron. Some pharmacologists attribute the different effects of benzodiazepines to its action on GABA neurons at different brain sites (limbic system, brain stem, cortex). These, in turn, act to inhibit presynaptic release of other neurotransmitters, such as norepinephrine and serotonin. Some have shown that GABA agonists and various inhibitors of GABA uptake decrease the analgesia of morphine while activation of GABA reduces morphine analgesia.[75]

C. **Selecting an agent.** A benzodiazepine is best selected on the basis of potency and pharmacokinetic principles. Only diazepam, lorazepam, and midazolam are available in parenteral preparations. The various benzodiazepines have different rates of onset and elimination (Table 6-4). Many of the agents have active metabolites, and with repeated dosing, the medication and its active metabolites can accumulate in the body, making the duration of their effect significantly longer than simple half-life might indicate. The drugs are metabolized in the liver, and doses should be adjusted for patients with liver disease. Only lorazepam, oxazepam, and temazepam are metabolized in a single step—glucuronidation—which, unlike the other processes in the metabolism of benzodiazepines, is relatively spared in the elderly and in those with liver disease. Thus, lorazepam, oxazepam, and temazepam should be used preferentially in those populations. Such patients may develop confusion several weeks after a dose increase of a longer-acting agent owing to accumulation of the drug and its active metabolites. High-potency drugs are more likely to cause tolerance; and when this is combined with a short half-life, an interdose rebound of symptoms can occur. Longer-acting agents are less likely to be associated with withdrawal but can cause oversedation and, as described previously, accumulate in the elderly and those with liver disease.

Table 6-5. Neuroleptics in chronic pain

Syndrome	Drug	Dose (mg)
Headaches	Trifluoperazine	1
	Fluphenazine	1
Thalamic pain	Chlorpromazine	50–400
Trigeminal neuralgia	Pimozide	2–12
Facial pain	Haloperidol (with behavior modification)	2–6
Neuropathic pains	Fluphenazine (with tricyclic antidepressants)	
Postherpetic neuralgia	Chlorprothixene	100–200
	Perphenazine (with antidepressant)	6
	Fluphenazine (with antidepressant)	3
Delusional disorder with pain	Chlorpromazine	400

   D. **Dosage.** Benzodiazepines should be started in low doses. Lorazepam is started at 0.5 mg tid and increased to a maximum of 6–8 mg/day. Clonazepam, which may have a role in neuropathic pain, is begun at 0.25 mg tid and may be titrated up to 6 mg and higher per day. One should, however, first take into account a tolerance to benzodiazepines when estimating starting doses of such agents for analgesic and other purposes. The timing of doses may be adjusted according to symptoms and side effects.
   E. **Withdrawal.** These medications must be tapered on discontinuation to avoid withdrawal, a syndrome characterized by extreme anxiety, palpitations, autonomic hyperactivity, and possibly seizures. Following abrupt termination of an agent with a short half-life, withdrawal can appear within 1 to 2 days. For longer-acting agents, withdrawal may occur after 2 to 5 days, or later.
   F. **Side effects.** The most common side effects of benzodiazepines are **sedation and fatigue.** They also can impair motor and cognitive performance. Before starting benzodiazepine treatment, patients should be warned not to drive or operate machinery. Disinhibition is another adverse effect that occurs in some patients.
IX. **Neuroleptics**
   A. **Indications.** With the exception of methotrimeprazine and pimozide, there are limited data to support the analgesic potential of neuroleptics. Table 6-5 lists various neuroleptic agents and their use in chronic pain. Although inconclusive, many case reports have described **low doses** of neuroleptic alone, **or in conjunction with antidepressants, as useful in a variety of chronic pain states.**
      1. Several controlled studies have shown that the phenothiazine **methotrimeprazine** (15 mg) **is equianalgesic to morphine** (10 mg) for patients with acute postoperative pain or myocardial infarction. Others have found it beneficial in controlling cancer pain, pleurisy, and postherpetic pain.[76–78] It has none of the opioid effects on gut motility and thus can be used when ileus limits use of opioids. It is a dopamine blocker and so has antiemetic as well as anxiolytic effects and can prove helpful when nausea and vomiting are problematic.
      2. **Other phenothiazines,** such as chlorpromazine, **are useful as antiemetics** but probably have little use as analgesics. Besides methotrimeprazine, only pimozide and fluphenazine have been demonstrated in controlled studies to have analgesic potential.[79] One double-blind controlled study of 50 patients showed significant reduction of chronic tension headaches by fluphenazine 1 mg/day.[80] A double-blind crossover trial comparing pimozide (4–12 mg/day) with carbamazepine in the treatment of trigeminal neuralgia suggested greater efficacy with pimozide, but with significant side effects, including parkinsonian symptoms and mental slowing.[81]
      3. **Haloperidol is the drug of choice in managing delirium or psychosis** and has clinical usefulness as a co-analgesic for patients with cancer pain.[82]
   B. **The mechanism of action of methotrimeprazine is unknown,** although some hypothesize that alpha-adrenergic blockade is important.[78,83] Animal studies

suggest that D_1 and D_2 antagonists can potentiate opioid analgesia, leading some to hypothesize that dopaminergic pathways modulate endogenous pain pathways.[84]

C. Assessment of the patient. The clinician should evaluate each patient for liver disease, parkinsonism, or other movement disorders before initiating a neuroleptic trial. Because the elderly, women, and patients with preexisting brain damage are at particular risk of developing tardive dyskinesia, this needs to be considered when selecting a neuroleptic. In cases of refractory neuropathic pain treatment, options may be so limited that the risks of these agents can be justified.[79] Baseline CBC, liver function tests (LFTs), and, for patients over 40 years, ECG should be documented. Because methotrimeprazine is available only in a parenteral preparation, is highly sedating, and can cause orthostatic hypotension, it should be considered for the patient with pain from advanced cancer who is largely bedridden and has intravenous access.[79]

D. Dosage

1. Doses for methotrimeprazine range from 12.5 to 50 mg q4–8h up to 300 mg/day. Because methotrimeprazine can cause sedation, anticholinergic symptoms, and orthostatic hypotension, it should be administered cautiously by slow intravenous or subcutaneous infusion. Larger doses can be given at bedtime to take advantage of its sedating properties and to minimize the risk of injury from falls because of orthostatic hypotension.

2. Fluphenazine and haloperidol are commonly used in low doses (2–8 mg/day).

3. Pimozide has been used for neuropathic pain in doses ranging from 4 to 12 mg/day.

E. Side effects

1. Different agents have varying degrees of anticholinergic activity. Haloperidol (Haldol), fluphenazine (Prolixin), and pimozide (Orap) are the least anticholinergic, while thioridazine (Mellaril) and chlorpromazine (Thorazine) are more anticholinergic. **Anticholinergic effects** include
   a. Dry mouth
   b. Blurred vision
   c. Constipation
   d. Urinary retention

2. **Extrapyramidal side effects,** listed below, can be managed by lowering the dose or by adding an anticholinergic agent such as benztropine (Cogentin) 2–6 mg/day, or trihexyphenidyl (Artane) 2–6 mg/day, or diphenhydramine (Benadryl) 50 mg.
   a. **Parkinsonian syndrome** of bradykinesia, cogwheel rigidity, tremor, festinating gait, and drooling, which are more common with the higher-potency drugs
   b. **Acute dystonias and akathisia,** which are also more common with the higher-potency drugs

3. All neuroleptics, particularly with long-term use, can cause abnormal **involuntary movement disorders** such as tardive dyskinesia and tardive dystonia. While under neuroleptic treatment, patients should be monitored for signs of dyskinesia. The Abnormal Involuntary Movement Scale (AIMS) can be administered periodically. Discontinuation of neuroleptics may be followed initially by worsening of the dyskinesia, but this usually improves over 2 to 3 months.[60,85] Tardive dsyskinesia has the following characteristics:
   a. **Orofacial, buccolingual dyskinetic movements**
   b. **Choreiform movements of the extremities**
   c. **Nonrhythmic truncal movements**

4. Neuroleptics cause varying degrees of **sedation.** When sedation is desirable, in patients with insomnia, for example, a more sedating agent should be chosen and given at bedtime.

5. Neuroleptics more likely to produce **postural hypotension** should not be chosen for use in patients at risk of injury from falls.

6. Neuroleptics result in a **lowered seizure threshold** and should be used with caution in patients with seizure disorder. Molindone (Moban) may be less likely to lower the seizure threshold.

7. **Weight gain**

8. **Dermatoses**

9. **Sexual dysfunction** with the following characteristics, which are usually reversible with cessation of drug:
   a. **Loss of libido**

  b. Inability to achieve orgasm
  c. Erectile and ejaculatory difficulties
 10. **Neuroleptic malignant syndrome** is a rare but life-threatening side effect.
  a. Characteristics
   (1) Severe muscle rigidity
   (2) Hyperthermia
   (3) Autonomic instability and rhabdomyolysis
   (4) Elevated serum creatinine phosphokinase
   (5) Myoglobinuria
  b. The neuroleptic should be stopped, and some of the following **supportive measures** instituted:
   (1) Hydration
   (2) Antipyretics
   (3) Cooling blankets, if necessary
   (4) Respiratory support
   (5) Possibly dialysis
   (6) Dantrolene 0.8–2.5 mg/kg IV q6h
   (7) Bromocriptine 7.5–50 mg PO every day.[60]

X. Antihistamines

 A. Indications. Animal studies have demonstrated analgesic properties for several antihistamines, and some studies have shown that antihistamines in conjunction with acetaminophen, morphine, or meperidine are more effective than those agents alone. However, clinical experience with these agents as adjuvant analgesics has been disappointing, and only hydroxyzine is utilized as an adjuvant analgesic.[63] Hydroxyzine's mild anxiolytic properties make it useful in the anxious cancer patient with pain,[86] and it has antiemetic activities as well. Most of the clinical use of antihistamines is **in combination with other analgesics for the short-term treatment of headache and other musculoskeletal pains.**

 B. Mechanism of action. Some propose that histamine acts centrally in pathways mediating endogenous pain modulation. Others hypothesize it has peripheral effects on inflammatory pain. For example, histamine influences substance P actions on vasculature and leads to the release of bradykinins and prostaglandins.

 C. Dosing. The analgesic activity of 100 mg of parenteral hydroxyzine approaches that of 8 mg of morphine and has additive analgesic effects when combined with morphine. The clinician can add hydroxyzine (25–50 mg PO, IV, or SQ q4–6h) to a patient's opioid regimen to relieve anxiety, provide sedation, and act as an antiemetic.

 D. Side effects. Antihistamines can be used to dry secretions in some patients and target insomnia in others. They can be additive with other centrally acting agents. Their most common side effects are
  1. Dry mouth
  2. Sedation

XI. Anticonvulsants

 A. Indications. The anticonvulsant drugs carbamazepine and valproate and the benzodiazepine clonazepam are now widely prescribed not only by neurologists but also by psychiatrists, who use them as **mood-stabilizing agents** for acute mania, rapid-cycling bipolar disorder, and bipolar disorder prophylaxis. The anticonvulsants are first-line agents in the **treatment of the lancinating, lightninglike, jabbing component of neuropathic pain,** as contrasted to the continuous dysesthetic component. Together data from the studies described below present a compelling argument for the role of anticonvulsants in neuropathic pain.[79,87,88]

  1. Controlled trials have demonstrated the benefit of carbamazepine in the treatment of trigeminal neuralgia, postherpetic neuralgia, and painful diabetic neuropathy.[89-93] Case reports and uncontrolled studies suggest benefit in glossopharyngeal neuralgia, tabetic lightning pains, paroxysmal pains in multiple sclerosis, postsympathetectomy pain, "flashing" dysesthesias in patients with spinal cord injury, postlaminectomy stabbing pains, as well as lancinating pains associated with cancer and posttraumatic mononeuropathy.[74,79,94-101]

  2. Uncontrolled studies indicate a role for valproate in the management of lancinating neuropathic pains of trigeminal neuralgia and postherpetic neuralgia.

 B. Mechanism of action. The actual mechanism by which the anticonvulsants produce analgesia is **unknown.** Some propose that when incoming sensory neurons are disrupted, such as in "deafferentation pain syndromes," the postsynaptic pain-transmitting neurons become hyperexcitable. This hyperexcitability is akin to seizurelike activity and is the target of anticonvulsant agents. Carbamazepine has membrane-stabilizing effects only at high doses. At therapeutic doses it decreases the repetitive firing of neurons. Some propose that its mechanism of action in pain is related to its molecular similarity to imipramine, the TCA. Like imipramine, it blocks norepinephrine reuptake and potentially can affect descending pain pathways. Because it has affinity for temporal and limbic areas of the brain that may regulate affect, some feel that its analgesia may result from its psychotropic as well as its anticonvulsant properties.[79,102]

C. Selecting an agent. Most clinicians begin with a trial of carbamazepine for lancinating neuropathic pains. Because patient response is variable, a trial of other medications such as phenytoin, valproate, and clonazepam is useful for patients who fail to respond to carbamazepine or have intolerable side effects.

D. Assessment of the patient. Patients facing a trial of either carbamazepine or valproate should have a medical examination screening for hematologic or hepatic abnormalities. Baseline CBC and screening profile should be documented with particular attention to WBCs, sodium levels, and LFTs. Both medications are associated with rare severe blood dyscrasias and hepatic abnormalities. Carbamazepine is contraindicated for patients with WBC less than 4000. An ECG should be obtained for patients who are over 40 years or have a history of cardiac abnormalities; carbamazepine can cause intraventricular cardiac conduction delay and is contraindicated in patients with a high degree of heart block.

E. Dosage

1. Carbamazepine should be started at low doses (100–200 mg bid) and gradually titrated upward (200 mg every 2 to 3 days) as side effects allow. The clinician should wait 5 days, leaving the medication at a stable dose until it achieves steady state levels. Then plasma should be drawn to determine a drug level just before the morning dose. CBC and LFTs should be documented at baseline before treatment and monitored every week for the first 2 months of treatment and quarterly thereafter. A WBC less than 4000 is a contraindication to use. Should the WBC drop below 3000 or the absolute neutrophil count below 1500, carbamazepine should be discontinued.

2. Before initiating a trial of valproate, baseline LFTs should be documented. A test dose of 250 mg of valproate can be given with a meal. Over several days, the dose is increased gradually in 250-mg increments to 250 mg tid. Serum levels are drawn at trough, the time before the patient's morning dose.

F. Side effects

1. **Carbamazepine**

   a. **Common side effects.** These side effects do not necessitate discontinuation of treatment, but the dose should be reduced. During initiation of treatment, they can be minimized by slow titration.

      (1) **Sedation**

      (2) **Ataxia**

      (3) **Blurred vision**

      (4) **Nausea**

      (5) **Vomiting**

      (6) **Mild elevations of LFTs**

      (7) **Slowing of intracardiac conduction.** Carbamazepine should be avoided in patients with a high degree of heart block.

   b. **Less common side effects** are listed below. Carbamazepine is relatively contraindicated in patients with hematologic abnormalities, with a WBC less than 4000, or in the cancer patient with pain who faces bone marrow suppression from chemotherapy.

      (1) **Rashes**

      (2) **Hyponatremia secondary to syndrome of inappropriate antidiuretic hormone (SIADH) or hepatitis**

      (3) **Aplastic anemia**

      (4) **Other severe blood dyscrasias**

2. **Valproate** can cause

   a. **Transient elevations of SGOT and SGPT** that do not require discontinuation of treatment

   b. **Sedation**

   c. **Nausea**

   d. **Vomiting**

   e. **Hand tremor,** with long-term use

   f. Thrombocytopenia or platelet dysfunction, at high doses
   g. Fatal hepatotoxicity in rare cases—prior to treatment it is wise to screen
   patients for liver disease and draw baseline LFTs
   h. A Hyperammonemia syndrome that is very rare
XII. Summary. Several principles should guide the use of psychotropic adjuvant analgesics:
   A. The clinician should be familiar with the pharmacokinetic and pharmacodynamic
   principles that influence the distribution, metabolism, and clearance of these
   agents and concomitant side effects.
   B. Most of the drugs should be started in low doses and titrated slowly to minimize
   side effects and maximize benefits.
   C. Clinicians should provide medication trials of adequate duration and dosage.
   Sometimes maximal analgesic effects are not seen until 4 to 6 weeks after therapeutic levels of drug are achieved.
   D. Before starting a medication, clinicians should educate patients about the potential delay in action of these drugs. Patients should be informed that serial drug
   trials may be required before the most effective drug or combination of drugs is
   found to provide a satisfactory analgesic response.

References

1. Max MB, Culnane M, Schafer SC, et al. Amitriptyline relieves diabetic-neuropathy pain in patients with normal and depressed mood. *Neurology* 37:589–596, 1987.
2. Max MB, Schafer SC, Culnane M, et al. Amitriptyline, but not lorazepam, relieves postherpetic neuralgia. *Neurology* 38:427–1432, 1988.
3. Pilowsky I, Hallett EC, Bassett DL, et al. A controlled study of amitriptyline in the treatment of chronic pain. *Pain* 14:169–179, 1982.
4. Sharav Y, Singer E, Schmidt E, et al. The analgesic effect of amitriptyline on chronic facial pain. *Pain* 31:199–209, 1987.
5. Watson CP, Evans RJ, Reed K, et al. Amitriptyline versus placebo in post herpetic neuralgia. *Neurology* 32:671–673, 1982.
6. Kvindesal B, Molin J, Froland A, Gram LF. Imipramine treatment of painful diabetic neuropathy. *JAMA* 251:1727–1730, 1984.
7. Young RJ, Clarke BF. Pain relief in diabetic neuropathy: the effectiveness of imipramine and related drugs. *Diabet Med* 2:363–366, 1985.
8. Sindrup SH, Ejlertsen B, Froland A, et al. Imipramine treatment in diabetic neuropathy: relief of subjective symptoms without changes in peripheral and autonomic nerve function. *Eur J Clin Pharmacol* 37:151–153, 1989.
9. Max MB, Kishore-Kumar R, Schafer SC, et al. Efficacy of desipramine in painful diabetic neuropathy: a placebo-controlled trial. *Pain* 45:3–10, 1991.
10. Kishore-Kumar R, Max MB, Schafer SC, et al. Desipramine relieves postherpetic neuralgia. *Clin Pharmacol Ther* 47:305–312, 1990.
11. Gomez-Perez FJ, Rull JA, Dies H, et al. Nortriptyline and fluphenazine in the symptomatic treatment of diabetic neuropathy. A double-blind cross-over study. *Pain* 23:395–400, 1985.
12. Langohr HD, Stohr M, Petruch F. An open and double-blind crossover study on the efficacy of clomipramine (Anafranil) inpatients with painful mono- and polyneuropathies. *Eur Neurol* 21:309–315, 1982.
13. Tiegno M, Pagnoni B, Calmi A, et al. Chlorpromazine compared to pentazocine as a unique treatment in postoperative pain. *Int J Clin Pharmacol Res* 7:141–143, 1987.
14. Hammeroff SR, Cork RC, Scherer K, et al. Doxepin effects on chronic pain, depression and plasma opioids. *J Clin Psychiatry* 2:22–26, 1982.
15. Watson WPN, Chipman M, Reed K, et al. Amitriptyline versus maprotiline in post herpetic neuralgia: a randomized, double-blind, cross over trial. *Pain* 48:29–36, 1992.
16. Max MB, Portenoy R, Laska E. The design of analgesic clinical studies. In Max MB, Portenoy R, Laska E (eds.), *Advances in Pain Research and Therapy*, Vol. 18. New York: Raven, 1991.
17. Diamond S, Frietag FG. The use of fluoxetine in the treatment of headache. *Clin J Pain* 5:200–201, 1989.
18. Lance JW, Curran DA. Treatment of chronic tension headache. *Lancet* 1:1236–1239, 1964.

19. Gomersall JD, Stuart A. Amitriptyline in migraine prophylaxis. *J Neurol Neurosurg Psychiatry* 36:684–690, 1973.
20. Couch JR, Hassanein RS. Amitriptyline in the prophylaxis of migraine. *Neurology* 36:695–699, 1979.
21. Anthony M, Lance JW. MAO inhibition in the treatment of migraine. *Arch Neurol* 21:263, 1969.
22. Morland TJ, Storli OV, Mogstad TE. Doxepin in the treatment of mixed vascular and tension headaches. *Headache* 19:382–383, 1979.
23. Okasha A, Ghaleb HA, Sadek A. A double-blind trial for the clinical management of psychogenic headache. *Br J Psychiatry* 122:181–182, 1973.
24. Lascelles RG. Atypical facial pain and depression. *Br J Psychol* 122:651–659, 1966.
25. Feinmann C, Harris M, Cawley R. Psychogenic facial pain: presentation and treatment: *Br Med J* 288:436–438, 1984.
26. Watson CP, Evans RJ. A comparative trial of amitriptyline and zimelidine in postherpetic neuralgia. *Pain* 23:387–394, 1985.
27. Turkington RW. Depression masquerading as diabetic neuropathy. *JAMA* 243: 1147–1150, 1980.
28. McDonald-Scott WA. The relief of pain with an antidepressant in arthritis. *The Practitioner* 202:802–807, 1969.
29. Gringas M. A clinical trial of Tofranil in rheumatic pain in general practice. *J Int Med Res* 4:41–49, 1976.
30. Glick EN, Fowler PD. Imipramine in chronic arthritis. *Pharmacol Med* 1:94–96, 1979.
31. Jenkins DB, Ebbutt AF, Evans CD. Tofranil in the treatment of low back pain. *J Int Med Res* 4:28–40, 1976.
32. Alcoff J, Jones E, Rust P, et al. A trial of imipramine for chronic low back pain. *J Fam Pract* 14:841–846, 1982.
33. Walsh TD. Controlled study of imipramine and morphine in chronic pain due to advanced cancer [abstract]. American Society of Clinical Oncology, May 4–6, Los Angeles, 1986.
34. Walsh TD. Antidepressants and chronic pain. *Clin Neuropharmacol* 6:271–295, 1983.
35. Walsh TD. Adjuvant analgesic therapy in cancer pain. In Foley KM, Bonica JJ, Ventafridda V, Callaway MV (eds.), *Advances in Pain Research and Therapy*, Vol. 16. New York: Raven, 1990. Pp. 155–165.
36. Ventafridda V, Bonezzi C, Caraceni A, et al. Antidepressants for cancer pain and other painful syndromes with deafferentation component: comparison of amitriptyline and trazodone. *Ital J Neurol Sci* 8:579–587, 1987.
37. Magni G, Arsie D, DeLeo D. Antidepressants in the treatment of cancer pain. A survey in Italy. *Pain* 29:347–353, 1987.
38. Johansson F, von Knorring L. A double-blind controlled study of a serotonin uptake inhibitor (zimelidine) versus placebo in chronic pain patients. *Pain* 7:68–78, 1979.
39. Evans W, Gensler F, Blackwell B, et al. The effects of antidepressant drugs on pain relief and mood in the chronically ill. *Psychosomatics* 14:214–219, 1973.
40. Ward GN, Bloom VL, Friedel RO. The effectiveness of tricyclic antidepressants in the treatment of coexisting pain and depression. *Pain* 7:331–341, 1979.
41. Raft D, Davidson J, Wasik J, et al. Relationship between response to phenelzine and MAO inhibition in a clinical trial of phenelzine, amitriptyline and placebo. *Neuropsychobiology* 7:122–126, 1981.
42. Davidoff G, Guarracini M, Roth E, et al. Trazodone hydrochloride in the treatment of dysesthetic pain in traumatic myelopathy: a randomized, double-blind, placebo-controlled study. *Pain* 29:151–161, 1987.
43. Sindrup SH, Gram LF, Brosen K, et al. The selective serotonin reuptake inhibitor paroxetine is effective in the treatment of diabetic neuropathy symptoms. *Pain* 42:135–144, 1990.
44. France RD. The future for antidepressants: treatment of pain. *Psychopathology* 20:99–113, 1987.
45. Botney M, Fields HC. Amitriptyline potentiates morphine analgesia by direct action on the central nervous system. *Ann Neurol* 13:160–164, 1983.
46. Malseed RT, Goldstein FJ. Enhancement of morphine analgesics by tricyclic antidepressants. *Neuropharmacology* 18:827–829, 1979.
47. Ventafridda V, Bianchi M, Ripamonti C, et al. Studies on the effects of antidepressant drugs on the antinociceptive action of morphine and on plasma morphine in rat and man. *Pain* 43:155–162, 1990.

48. Spiegel K, Kalb R, Pasternak GW. Analgesic activity of tricyclic antidepressants. *Ann Neurol* 13:462–465, 1983.
49. Bradley JJ. Severe localized pain associated with depressive syndrome. *Br J Psychiatry* 109:741–745, 1963.
50. Basbaum AI, Fields HL. Endogenous pain control mechanisms: review and hypothesis. *Ann Neurol* 4:451–462, 1978.
51. Gram LF. Antidepressants: receptors, pharmacokinetics and clinical effects. In Burrows GD, Norman TR, Davies B (eds.), *Antidepressants*. Elsevier Science, Amsterdam: 1983. Pp. 81–95.
52. Feinmann C. Pain relief by antidepressants: possible modes of action. *Pain* 23:1–8, 1985.
53. Liu SF, Wang RIH. Increased analgesia and alterations in distribution and metabolism of methadone by desipramine in the rat. *J Pharmacol Exp Ther* 195:94–104, 1975.
54. Fields HL, Basbaum AI. Endogenous pain control mechanisms. In Wall PD, Melzak R (eds.), *Textbook of Pain*. London: Churchill Livingston, 1984.
55. Charney DS, Meukes DS, Heniuger PR. Receptor sensitivity and the mechanism of action of antidepressant treatment. *Arch Gen Psychiatry* 38:1160–1180, 1981.
56. Kishore-Kumar R, Schafer SC, Lawlow BA, et al. Single doses of the serotonin agonists buspirone and m-chlorophonyl piperazine do not relieve neuropathic pain. *Pain* 37:223–227, 1989.
57. Salter MW, Henry JL. Evidence that adenosine moderates the depression of spinal dorsal horn neurones induced by peripheral vibration in the rat. *Neuroscience* 22:631–650, 1987.
58. Merskey H, Hamilton JT. An open trial of possible analgesic effects of dipyridamole. *J Pain Symptom Manage* 4:34–37, 1989.
59. Arana GW, Hyman SE. *Handbook of Psychiatric Drug Therapy* Boston: Little, Brown, 1991.
60. American Medical Association, Division of Drugs and Toxicology, Department of Drugs. *Drug Evaluations Manual*. Chicago: American Medical Association, 1992. Pp. 207–347.
61. Zitman FG, Linssen ACG, Edelbroek PM, Stijnen T. Low dose amitriptyline in chronic pain: the gain is modest. *Pain* 42:35–42, 1990.
62. Watson CP, Evans RJ, Reed K, et al. "Therapeutic window" for amitriptyline analgesia. *Can Med Assoc J* 130:105, 1984.
63. Stack CG, Rogers P, Linter SPK. Monoamine oxidase inhibitors and anaesthesia. *Br J Pharmacol* 60:222–227, 1988.
64. Wells DG, Bjorksten AR. Monoamine oxidase inhibitors revisited. *Can J Anaesth* 36:64–74, 1989.
65. Forrest WH, Brown BW, Brown CR, et al. Dextroamphetamine with morphine for the treatment of postoperative pain. *N Engl J Med* 296:712–715, 1977.
66. Bruera E, Chadwick S, Brennels C, et al. Methylphenidate associated with narcotics for the treatment of cancer pain. *Cancer Treat Rep* 71:67–70, 1987.
67. Bruera E, Brenneis C, Paterson AH, MacDonald RN. Use of methylphenidate as an adjuvant to narcotic analgesics in patients with advanced cancer. *J Pain Symptom Manage* 4:3–6, 1989.
68. Cantello R, Aguggia M, Gilli M, et al. Analgesic action of methylphenidate on parkinsonian sensory symptoms. Mechanisms and pathophysiological implications. *Arch Neurol* 45:973–976, 1988.
69. Bruera E, Miller MJ, MacMillan K, Kuehn N. Neuropsychological effects of methylphenidate in patients receiving a continuous infusion of narcotics for cancer pain. *Pain* 48:163–166, 1992.
70. Singh PN, Sharma P, Gupta PK, et al. Clinical evaluation of diazepam for relief of postoperative pain. *Br J Anaesth* 53:831, 1981.
71. Chapman CR, Reather BW. Effects of diazepam on human pain tolerance and pain sensitivity. *Psychosom Med* 35:330–340, 1973.
72. Gracely RH, McGrath P, Dubner R. Validity and sensitivity of ratio scales of sensory and affective verbal pain descriptors: manipulation of affect by diazepam. *Pain* 5:19–29, 1978.
73. Caccia MR. Clonazepam in facial neuralgia and cluster headache: clinical and electrophysiological study. *Eur Neurol* 13:560–563, 1975.
74. Swerdlow M, Cundill JG. Anticonvulsant drugs used in the treatment of lancinating pains: a comparison. *Anesthesia* 36:1129–1134, 1981.

75. Mantegazza P, Tammiso R, Vicentine L, et al. The effects of GABAergic agents on opiate analgesia. *Pharmacol Res Commun* 12:239–247, 1980.
76. Lasagna L, DeKornfeld JJ. Methotrimeprazine: a new phenothiazine derivative with analgesic properties. *JAMA* 178:887–890, 1961.
77. Montilla EE, Frederick W, Cass L. Analgesic effects of methotrimeprazine and morphine. *Arch Intern Med* 111:725–728, 1963.
78. Beaver WT, Wallenstein SL, Houde RW, et al. A comparison of the analgesic effect of methotrimeprazine and morphine in patients with cancer. *Clin Pharmacol Ther* 7:436–446, 1966.
79. Portenoy RK. Adjuvant analgesics in pain management. In Doyle K, Hanks GW, MacDonald N (eds.), *Oxford Textbook of Palliative Medicine.* Oxford, UK: Oxford University Press, in press.
80. Hakkarainen H. Fluphenazine for tension headache: double-blind study. *Headache* 17:216, 1977.
81. Lechin F, van der Dijs B, Lechin ME, et al. Pimozide therapy for trigeminal neuralgia. *Arch Neurol* 9:960–964, 1989.
82. Maltbie AA, Cavenar JO, Sullivan JL, et al. Analgesia and haloperidol: a hypothesis. *J Clin Psychiatry* 40:323–326, 1979.
83. Moore JA, Dundee JW. Alterations to somatic pain associated with anesthesia: VII. The effects of nine phenothiazine derivatives. *Br J Anaesth* 33:422–431, 1961.
84. Kiritsy-Roy JA, Standish SM, Terry LC. Dopamine D-1 and D-2 receptor antagonists potentiate analgesic and motor effects of morphine. *Pharmacol Biochem Behav* 32:717, 1989.
85. Monks R, Mersky H. Psychotropic drugs. In Wall PD, Melzack R (eds.), *Textbook of Pain,* 2nd ed. New York: Churchill Livingstone, 1989. Pp. 702–721.
86. Beaver WT, Feise G. Comparison of the analgesic effects of morphine, hydroxyzine and their combination in patients with post-operative pain. In Bonica JJ, Albe-Fesard DG, Fink BR, Jones LE (eds.), *Advances in Pain Research and Therapy,* vol. 1. New York: Raven, 1976.
87. Peiris JB, Perera GL, Devendra SV, et al. Sodium valproate in trigeminal neuralgia. *Med J Aust* 2:278, 1980.
88. Raftery H. The management of postherpetic pain using sodium valproate and amitriptyline. *J Irish Med Assoc* 72:399, 1979.
89. Campbell FG, Graham JG, Zilkha KJ. Clinical trial of carbamazepine (Tegretol) in trigeminal neuralgia. *J Neurol Neurosurg Psychiatry* 29:265, 1966.
90. Rockliff BW, Davis EH. Controlled sequential trials of carbamazepine in trigeminal neuralgia. *Arch Neurol* 15:129, 1966.
91. Killian JM, Fromm GH. Carbamazepine in the treatment of neuralgia: use and side effects. *Arch Neurol* 19:129, 1968.
92. Nicol CF. A four year double-blind study of carbamazepine interfacial pain. *Headache* 9:54, 1969.
93. Rull JA, Quibrera R, Gonzalez-Millan H, et al. Symptomatic treatment of peripheral diabetic neuropathy with carbamazepine (Tegretol): double-blind cross-over trial. *Diabetologia* 5:215, 1969.
94. Taylor PH, et al. Glossopharyngeal neuralgia with syncope. *J Laryngol Otol* 91:859, 1977.
95. Raskin NH, Levinson S, Hoffman PM, et al. Postsympathectomy neuralgia: amelioration with diphenylhydantoin and carbamazepine. *Am J Surg* 128:75, 1974.
96. Ekbom K. Carbamazepine in the treatment of tabetic lightning pains. *Arch Neurol* 26:374, 1972.
97. Elliot F, Little A, Milbrandt W. Carbamazepine for phantom limb phenomena. *N Engl J Med* 295:678, 1976.
98. Espir MLE, Millac P. Treatment of paroxysmal disorders in multiple sclerosis with carbamazepine (Tegretol). *J Neurol Neurosurg Psychiatry* 33:528, 1970.
99. Mullan S. Surgical management of pain in cancer of the head and neck. *Surg Clin North Am* 53:203, 1973.
100. Dunsker SB, Mayfield FH. Carbamazepine in the treatment of flashing pain syndrome. *J Neurosurg* 45:49, 1976.
101. Martin G. Recurrent pain of a pseudodiabetic variety after laminectomy for a lumbar disc lesion. *J Neurol Neurosurg Psychiatry* 43:283, 1980.
102. Weinberger J, Nicklas WJ, Berl S. Mechanism of action of anticonvulsants. *Neurology* 26:162, 1976.

C

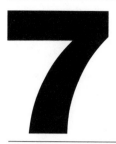

Regional Anesthetic Techniques for Chronic Pain Management
May L. Chin

I. Background. Nerve blocks are useful in the management and diagnosis of patients with certain chronic pain conditions. It is important to understand that nerve blocks alone are seldom adequate in treating these patients. In many instances, the inclusion of other treatment modalities, such as physical therapy and psychological counseling, is essential to effectively manage patients with chronic pain.

Certain risks are associated with the performance of regional techniques and with the use of local anesthetics. Neurotoxicity and CNS, cardiovascular, or respiratory complications can occur, for example, as a result of gross overdose of local anesthetics or as a result of injecting the local anesthetic into the "wrong" place (i.e., intravascular or intrathecal space). Careful dosing of local anesthetics; patient vigilance; and verification of needle placement by peripheral nerve stimulators, fluoroscopy, or CT scan help minimize these risks. Depending on the type of nerve block, patients may need an intravenous line for sedation and for emergency drugs. Routine monitors such as those for ECG, BP, and oxygen saturation are recommended whenever the patient receives intravenous sedation. In addition, equipment for managing the airway, oxygen, and suction should be readily available.·

II. Sympathetic blockade

A. Stellate ganglion block. The cervical sympathetic chain lies on either side of the vertebral column and is composed of three ganglia: the superior cervical ganglion (at C1–3), the middle cervical ganglion (at C6), and the stellate or cervicothoracic ganglion (at C7). The stellate ganglion, which consists of the inferior cervical and first thoracic ganglia, lies just anterior to the transverse process of the seventh cervical vertebra. A stellate ganglion block produces a sympathetic block of the head, neck, upper extremity, and chest.

1. Indications
a. Diagnosis and treatment of **sympathetic dystrophy** of the upper extremity
b. Treatment of **vascular insufficiency** (upper extremity)
c. Treatment of **herpes zoster** (head, neck, upper thorax)

2. Technique
a. Position the patient supine and extend the neck with the help of a small roll placed under the shoulders. Ensure a functioning intravenous line. Stand on the side to be blocked.
b. At the level of the cricoid cartilage, move the index and the third finger of the nondominant hand in unison off the midline laterally and locate the anterior tubercle of the C6 vertebra (Chassaignac's tubercle). This is the entry site for the needle. The common carotid artery is lateral to this site and may have to be retracted. The block can also be carried out at the level of C7 instead of at C6, using the same technique (Fig. 7-1).
c. Prepare the skin for aseptic technique. Find the entry site as described, and infiltrate the skin with local anesthetic. Use a short 22- or 23-gauge needle with a clear hub. Insert the needle perpendicular to the skin and direct it posteriorly until bone is contacted (Fig. 7-2). Withdraw the needle 1 to 2 mm and stabilize the needle with the nondominant hand. Inject 10 ml of local anesthetic in small increments, aspirating each time, to prevent intravascular or intrathecal injection. The patient is asked not to verbalize during the block, so a form of hand signal should be established ahead of time (e.g., "raise your right hand if you feel OK"). This allows continuous assessment of the mental status during the injection. If the injection is carried out at C6 rather than C7, remove the roll and raise the head of the bed 15 to 30 degrees after the block to facilitate diffusion of the local anesthetic

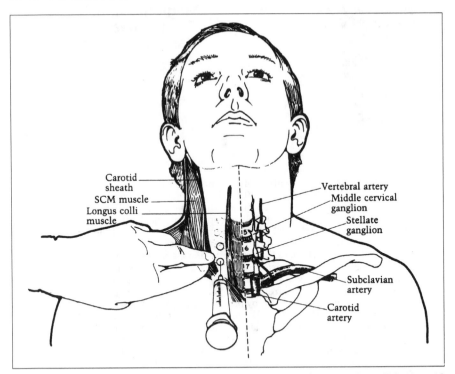

Fig. 7-1. Stellate ganglion block. The sternocleidomastoid (SCM) muscle and the carotid sheath are retracted laterally with one hand while the needle is introduced directly onto the lateral border of the seventh vertebral body, just medial to the transverse process. After contacting bone, the needle is withdrawn slightly and careful aspiration is performed before incremental injection. (From Mulroy MF. *Regional Anesthesia: An Illustrated Procedural Guide.* Published by Little, Brown and Company. Copyright © 1989. P. 142.)

caudally. Local anesthetics: 0.5% or 1% lidocaine (for initial or diagnostic block), or 0.25% bupivacaine (for repeat blocks).

3. **Side effects and complications**
   a. **Horner's syndrome,** which indicates a successful sympathetic block of the head and neck but not necessarily of the upper extremity
   b. **Seizures**
   c. **Loss of consciousness** due to injection of local anesthetic (as little as 0.5 ml) into the vertebral artery
   d. Total spinal resulting in **severe hypotension** and respiratory compromise
   e. **Hoarseness** from blocked recurrent laryngeal nerve
   f. **Brachial plexus block**
   g. **Unilateral phrenic nerve block**
   h. **Pneumothorax** (increased risk at C7)
4. **Assessing sympathetic blockade**
   a. **Skin blood flow changes**
      (1) **Plethysmography** can be traced with a digital clip on the affected extremity. Record tracings of pulsatile flow before and after the block.
      (2) **Change in temperature** of the affected limb or site measured with a thermocouple skin probe.
   b. **Pain evaluation**
      (1) Pain score
      (2) Analgesic requirements
      (3) Physical activity
B. **Celiac plexus block.** The celiac plexus is a conglomeration of autonomic nerves that lie in the retroperitoneal space at the level of the L1 vertebra. The aorta is

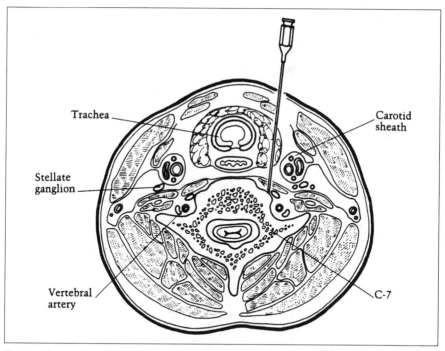

Trachea

Carotid sheath

Stellate ganglion

Vertebral artery

C-7

Fig. 7-2. Stellate ganglion block, cross section. The needle is shown resting on the anterior border of the seventh cervical vertebra. The vascular structures of the carotid sheath as well as the vertebral artery are in close proximity. The vertebral artery is passing posteriorly at this level to enter its canal in the transverse processes, but here lies near the level of intended injection. The brachial plexus roots are also just posterior and lateral to the intended site of injection. (From Mulroy MF. *Regional Anesthesia: An Illustrated Procedural Guide.* Published by Little, Brown and Company. Copyright © 1989. P. 143.)

situated posterior to the plexus and the inferior vena cava anterolateral on the right. The celiac plexus contains the sympathetic innervation of the abdominal viscera. Preganglionic nerves that arise from T5 to T12 synapse in the celiac plexus before continuing on to the abdominal organs. The postganglionic sympathetic nerves travel with the visceral afferent fibers from the abdominal organs.

1. Indications

    a. Primarily indicated in the treatment of **painful abdominal malignancy,** in particular, gastric and pancreatic cancer.

    b. It can be applied in selected cases of **chronic abdominal pain.**

2. Technique. The celiac plexus can be blocked by placing the local anesthetic solution posterior and cephalad to the diaphragmatic crura (retrocrural). This is the classic and most frequently utilized technique. Another approach deposits the local anesthetic solution in front of the aorta at the level of the celiac plexus, anterior to the diaphragmatic crura (anterocrural). In this case, the needle can be placed either posteriorly through one crus of the diaphragm or anteriorly through the abdominal wall to reach the celiac plexus.

a. Classic (retrocrural) approach

    (1) Position the patient prone and place a roll under the hip to flatten out the lumbar curvature. Ensure a functioning intravenous line. Most patients will require intravenous sedation for this block.

    (2) Mark the spinous processes of T12 and L1. Confirm this with fluoroscopy. Mark the inferior border of the twelfth ribs. Draw parallel lines 7 to 8 cm from the midline on either side. Mark the points A where the parallel lines cross the lower border of the twelfth ribs. Join the two A's with a horizontal line.

    (3) Mark B, which is in the midline between the T12 and L1 spinous

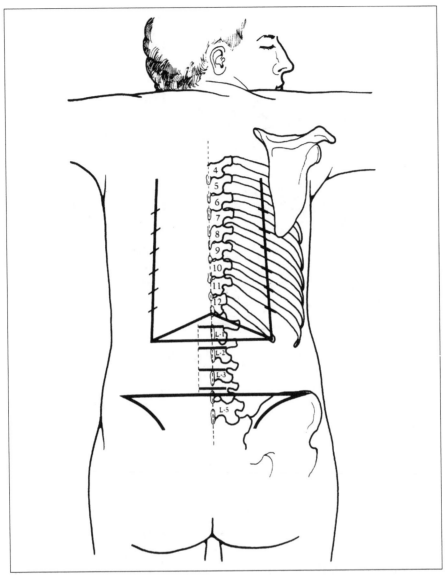

Fig. 7-3. Celiac plexus block, surface landmarks. (From Mulroy MF. *Regional Anesthesia: An Illustrated Procedural Guide.* Published by Little, Brown and Company. Copyright © 1989. P. 124.)

processes. Complete an isosceles triangle by joining the two A's and B (Fig. 7-3).

(4) Prepare the skin for aseptic technique. Anesthetize the skin at the two points marked A immediately below the twelfth rib. Insert a 15-cm 20-gauge needle at A and advance along the direction of the side of the isosceles triangle toward point B. Start with an angle of about 45 degrees from the skin and direct the needle to contact the L1 vertebral body. Once bone is contacted, withdraw the needle to subcutaneous tissue, steepen the angle, and advance the needle to contact the vertebral body again. Repeat this maneuver until the needle slips off the L1 vertebral body anteriorly. Once the needle has slipped off the vertebral body, the

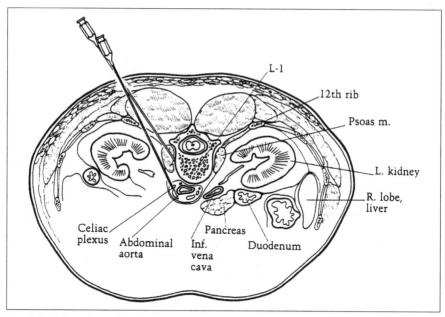

Fig. 7-4. Celiac plexus block, cross section. (From Mulroy MF. *Regional Anesthesia: An Illustrated Procedural Guide.* Published by Little, Brown and Company. Copyright © 1989. P. 144.)

tip of the needle is advanced 2 cm on the right. On the left, the needle is advanced about 1 cm or until aortic pulsations are felt (Fig. 7-4). If bony contact is made at a superficial level, this is likely to be the transverse process and not the vertebral body.

(5) Verify the position of the needles by fluoroscopy using both anteroposterior and lateral views. Aspirate and inject a 2-ml test dose of local anesthetic on each side. If negative for intravascular or intrathecal injection, proceed with a slow injection of 10 to 15 ml of local anesthetic through each needle.

(6) Local anesthetics are 1% lidocaine for diagnostic block or 0.25% bupivacaine for a block of longer duration. If a neurolytic block is planned, a diagnostic or prognostic block with local anesthetics is recommended before using neurolytic agents (50% to 100% alcohol or 6% phenol). Alcohol can produce severe pain on injection and can be mixed with a local anesthetic such as 0.25% bupivacaine before injection. Phenol can be combined with iodinated contrast medium, which enables the distribution of the solution to be observed during injection. Neurolytic agents do not spread as easily as local anesthetic solution; hence a higher volume of injectate in the range of a total of 50 ml is recommended when performing neurolysis.

b. Anterocrural approach. Follow steps described in section **II. B.2.a.(1).** In step **(2),** rather than 7 to 8 cm from the midline, shorten the distance to 5 or 6 cm. The needle is inserted on the right side at an angle of more than 45 degrees to contact the vertebral body of L1. After contact, the needle is withdrawn and redirected until it "walks off" the anterolateral edge of the vertebral body. Fluoroscopy is used to guide the needle tip anterior to the crus of the diaphragm. Inject 30 ml of local anesthetic solution through this needle. This technique places most of the injected solution anterior to the aorta where the celiac plexus is located.

c. Transaortic approach. This technique, described by Ischia et al. (1983), places the needle immediately anterior to the aorta. Use the same landmarks and techniques for the posterior placement of a left-sided needle. Once the L1 vertebral body is "walked off," the needle is carefully advanced until the tip is in the preaortic connective tissue. Attach a syringe filled with normal saline to the advancing needle. Resistance is felt as the posterior aortic wall is penetrated; within the aortic lumen blood is aspirated easily. Resistance is felt again during passage through the anterior wall; beyond that, a new loss of resistance indicates that the tip of the needle is in the preaortic area where the celiac plexus resides. Confirm needle placement with contrast medium.

    d. Anterior approach. This is often performed by a radiologist or with the assistance of one. Using CT scan guidance, the point of needle insertion to reach the L1 body is determined. The patient is supine, which is more comfortable than the prone position, and may require less sedation. The advantages of this technique are decreased chances of epidural or intrathecal injection or neurologic injury to somatic nerve roots due to retrocrural spread of the injected solution. Risks associated with this approach are infection, hemorrhage, fistula, or abscess formation.

  3. Side effects and complications

    a. Hypotension, from vasodilation of the splanchnic bed. This may be avoided with careful volume loading. Orthostatic hypotension may persist for a few days after a neurolytic block.

    b. Back pain, as a result of needles traversing muscle layers. A heating pad or muscle relaxant may help.

    c. Subarachnoid injection through a dural cuff

    d. Local anesthetic toxicity with intravascular injection

    e. Retroperitoneal hematoma from puncturing large vessels. Aorta puncture is not uncommon and rarely serious.

    f. Somatic nerve root (L1) injury or block producing numbness or paresthesia

    g. Renal puncture leading to hemorrhage of fistula formation

    h. Pneumothorax

    i. Aortic tear, occult retroperitoneal hemorrhage with transaortic technique

C. Lumbar sympathetic block. The lumbar sympathetic chains lie in a fascial plane at the anterolateral border of the vertebral bodies. They are separated from the somatic nerves by the psoas muscles. The sympathetic ganglia to the lower extremities lie along the second, third, and fourth lumbar vertebrae and contain preganglionic axons arising from T10 to L3.

  1. Indications

    a. Diagnosis and treatment of **reflex sympathetic dystrophy or causalgia of the lower extremity**

    b. Peripheral vascular insufficiency

    c. Acute herpes zoster

  2. Technique. The lumbar sympathetic chain can be blocked using either the lateral or the paravertebral approach. The technique used in the lateral approach is similar in concept to that of the celiac plexus block. In this approach the injection of local anesthetic solution through a single needle allows the solution to spread in the fascial plane surrounding the lumbar sympathetic chain.

    Position the patient prone and place a roll under the hip to flatten out the lumbar curvature. Ensure a functioning intravenous line. Most patients require intravenous sedation for this block.

    a. Lateral approach. Mark the spinous processes of the lumbar vertebrae. Measure 9 to 10 cm lateral to the L2 spinous process. This is the entry point for the needle. Prepare the skin for aseptic technique and infiltrate with local anesthetic. Insert a 15-cm 20-or 22-gauge needle toward the body of the L2 vertebral body. If bone is contacted at a superficial level (about 3 cm), this is likely to be the transverse process and not the body of the vertebra. Redirect the needle slightly cephalad or caudad to the transverse process and attempt again to contact the vertebral body. Walk the needle off the anterolateral surface of the vertebral body by changing to a steeper angle each time the vertebral body is contacted. Once the needle tip slides off the vertebral body, advance 1 cm. Alternatively, a loss-of-resistance technique using a glass syringe can be used to identify the fascial plane (Fig. 7-5). Inject 20 ml in increments after negative aspiration for blood or cerebrospinal fluid.

    b. Paravertebral approach. The spinous processes of L2, L3, and L4 are marked, and each is bisected with a perpendicular line. Along this line measure

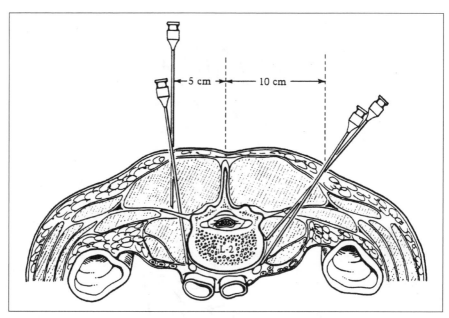

Fig. 7-5. Lumbar sympathetic block, cross section. (From Mulroy MF. *Regional Anesthesia: An Illustrated Procedural Guide.* Published by Little, Brown and Company. Copyright © 1989. P. 146.)

5 cm from the midline. Insert the needle at this point. Angle the needle at 45 degrees cephalad and advance to contact the transverse process. Measure 5 cm up the needle shaft. Withdraw the needle to subcutaneous tissue and advance the needle to the measured depth. This time the needle is perpendicular to skin and angled slightly medially to approximate the anterolateral border of the vertebral body (see Fig. 7-5). If the vertebral body is contacted, the needle is redirected as described in section **II.C.2.a** to slide off the vertebral body. Inject 10 ml of local anesthetic solution through each of the three needles after negative aspiration for blood or cerebrospinal fluid.

   c. Local anesthetics are 0.5% or 1% lidocaine for diagnostic block; 0.125% or 0.25% bupivacaine for repeat blocks.

   d. A diagnostic block with local anesthetic agents should be performed prior to using a neurolytic agent (6% phenol). Some authors recommend injecting small volumes at several needle placements. The needle placement for a neurolytic block should be confirmed with fluoroscopy and contrast injection of 1 to 3 ml. The anteroposterior view should show the contrast close to the paramedian plane and should not show any tracking along the psoas muscle. A volume of 5 ml of aqueous 6% phenol is injected after verifying needle placement.

  3. Side effects and complications
   a. Local anesthetic toxicity with intravascular injection
   b. Hypotension
   c. Subarachnoid injection
   d. Somatic nerve block
 D. Hypogastric plexus block. The hypogastric plexus lies in the retroperitoneal space, just below the aortic bifurcation, anterior to the fifth lumbar vertebra and the first sacral vertebral body. It consists of the superior hypogastric plexus, which divides left and right and continues into the pelvis as the inferior hypogastric plexus. The hypogastric plexus is in continuation with the celiac plexus and the lumbar sympathetic chains above. The hypogastric nerves supply the pelvic viscera and contain afferent pain fibers and postganglionic sympathetic fibers as well as preganglionic parasympathetic fibers.
  1. Indications

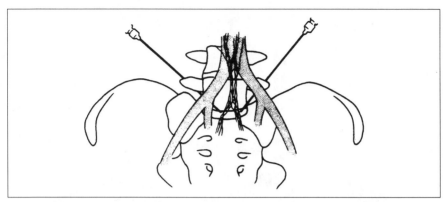

Fig. 7-6. Pelvis, anterior view illustrating location of hypogastric plexus and correct bilateral needle placement. (From Patt RB. *Cancer Pain.* Philadelphia: J.B. Lippincott, 1993. Pp. 1–15.)

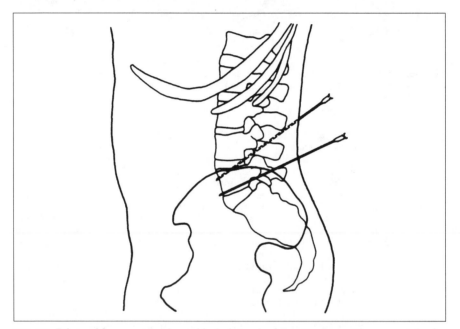

Fig. 7-7. Bilateral hypogastric plexus block, lateral schematic view with paravertebral needles positioned with their tips just anterior to the sacral promontory. (From Patt RB. *Cancer Pain.* Philadelphia: J.B. Lippincott, 1993. Pp. 1–15.)

  a. Pain control in patients with cancer-related pelvic pain
  b. Diagnostic block in patients with chronic pelvic pain
2. **Technique**
  a. Position the patient prone. Ensure a functioning intravenous line. Most patients require intravenous sedation for this block.
  b. Identify the L4–5 interspace. Draw a horizontal line through this interspace. Mark two lateral points on the horizontal line, each 5 to 7 cm from the midline. At each of the two lateral sites, insert a 15-cm 20- or 22-gauge needle using aseptic technique and direct it approximately 45 degrees medial and caudal toward the midline, aiming for the anterolateral surface of the L5 vertebral body. Once the needle has walked off the vertebral body, advance 1 cm (Fig. 7-6 and Fig. 7-7). Use fluoroscopy to confirm needle placement.

    c. For a diagnostic block, inject 8 ml of local anesthetic solution through each needle. Use 1% lidocaine or 0.25% bupivacaine.

    d. For a neurolytic block, confirm needle placement with contrast injection before injecting 8 ml of 6% phenol through each needle.

  3. Side effects and complications

    a. Bowel, bladder, and sexual dysfunction

    b. Paralysis

    c. Local anesthetic toxicity with intravascular injection

E. Intravenous regional sympathetic block. Guanethidine, reserpine, and bretylium can block the sympathetic nervous system by preventing release and/or reuptake of norepinephrine. With bretylium, the initial release of norepinephrine can cause pain.

  1. Indications: reflex sympathetic dystrophy or causalgia of the upper or lower extremity

  2. Technique

    a. The Bier block technique is used. Ensure a functioning intravenous line in the nonblock arm. Most patients require intravenous sedation in order to tolerate manipulation of the painful extremity. Insert a small intravenous catheter (20 or 22 gauge) in the extremity to be blocked. Place a tourniquet on this extremity. Exsanguinate the extremity and keep the tourniquet inflated for 30 minutes after injection of the drug. Inject the drug mixed in a volume of 50 ml for the upper extremity and a volume of 80 ml for the lower extremity. This volume of solution is a mixture of 0.5% lidocaine and normal saline in equal parts.

    b. Drugs used for the sympathetic block

      (1) Reserpine, 1 mg for the upper extremity and 1.5 mg for the lower extremity

      (2) Bretylium, 1.5 mg/kg

      (3) Guanethidine, 20 mg for the upper extremity and 40 mg for the lower extremity

  3. Side effects and complications

    a. Hypotension

    b. Local anesthetic toxicity

    c. Headache (with reserpine)

III. Epidural blockade

A. General description. In the adult, the spinal cord ends at L1–2. The dural sac surrounds the spinal cord and extends from the foramen magnum to the S2 vertebra. The epidural space surrounds the dural sac and contains fat and blood vessels. The vertebral column consists of 7 cervical, 12 thoracic, 5 lumbar, 5 fused sacral vertebrae, and the coccyx. Anterior and posterior ligaments support the vertebrae. The posterior ligaments from without to within consist of the supraspinous, interspinous, and the ligamentum flavum. These ligaments are thickest in the lumbar region. The epidural space can be approached from the cervical, thoracic, lumbar, or the caudal route.

  1. Indications

    a. Epidural steroid injection

    b. Sympathetic blockade

    c. Diagnostic block (see differential block)

  2. General technique. An intravenous line should be placed if local anesthetics are used. The epidural space can be reached via the midline or paramedian approach. A 20-gauge Tuohy needle can be used for a single-bolus technique, and a 17-gauge Tuohy needle for a continuous technique.

    a. The midline approach. Prepare a sterile field and infiltrate the skin over the chosen interspace. Engage the epidural needle in the interspinous ligament. The needle is advanced slowly to identify the epidural space using one of several techniques of "loss of resistance":

      (1) A well-lubricated syringe filled with air can be advanced with gentle ballottement on the plunger.

      (2) A syringe can be filled with saline and constant pressure applied to the plunger as the needle is advanced.

      (3) In the hanging-drop technique, the lumen of the needle is filled with a solution which is visible at the hub of the epidural needle. When the needle tip is advanced into the epidural space, the drop of solution at the hub is perceived to be "sucked in."

b. In postlaminectomy patients, it is not uncommon to encounter cerebrospinal fluid when performing an epidural. In such patients, **use of saline** instead of air in the loss-of-resistance technique may reduce the incidence of "wet tap." In the event of a wet tap, air is not introduced into the intrathecal space if saline is used.

B. Cervical epidural technique. The patient can either be sitting or lying on one side, with the neck flexed forward. To mark the level of the interspace, identify the prominent spinous process of the C7 vertebra. The interspaces can be well delineated with good neck flexion. The spinous processes are not steeply angulated, and the **midline** approach is commonly used.

C. Thoracic epidural technique

1. General technique. The patient can either sit slouched with the head flexed or lie in a lateral position with the upper back curved out. Identify and confirm the thoracic interspace by counting down from the cervical spine (C7 spinous process); by marking the tips of the scapulae, which lie at the same level as the T7 spinous process; or by counting up from the lumbar spinous processes. The **midline approach** may be difficult because of the steep angulation of the thoracic spines. The angulation is much less below T9. If a catheter is threaded for the continuous technique, it should be inserted only 2 to 3 cm into the epidural space.

2. Paramedian approach. Identify the intervertebral space. Mark the spine on either side of the chosen interspace. Infiltrate the skin at about 2 cm lateral to the inferior border of the spine (opposite the chosen interspace). Insert the epidural needle perpendicular to the skin. On contacting bone, the epidural needle is withdrawn and redirected cephalad and slightly medially until bony contact is lost. Advance the needle and identify the epidural space using the loss-of-resistance technique as previously described.

D. Lumbar epidural technique

1. General technique. The patient can sit slouched with knees flexed and feet on a stool or lie in a lateral position with the knees drawn up and the back curved out. To identify the lumbar interspace, imagine a line drawn between the iliac crests. In general this line bisects the L4 vertebral body or the L4–5 interspace. The **midline or paramedian** approach can be used; the latter is indicated in patients who, because of pain or degenerative arthritis, have difficulty in attempting a favorable position for the block.

2. Paramedian approach. Identify the lumbar interspace. Mark the spinous processes on either side of the interspace. Infiltrate the skin at 3 cm lateral to the caudal aspect of the spine (opposite the chosen interspace). Insert the epidural needle at an angle of 10 degrees toward the midline and 45 degrees cephalad. Advance the epidural needle with the loss-of-resistance technique.

E. Continuous technique

1. General technique. An epidural catheter can be inserted for short-term use (days) for postoperative analgesia or for long-term use (weeks) for control of chronic or cancer pain. Long-term catheters can be tunnelled subcutaneously to maintain catheter cleanliness and to avoid being dislodged from the epidural space. Several manufacturers provide kits specifically for the insertion of epidural or intrathecal catheters for long-term use.

2. The catheters can be directly connected to an external or internal **drug-dispensing pump.** Preservative-free narcotics such as morphine sulfate are commonly prescribed for long-term pain control using this method.

F. Caudal technique. In this technique the epidural space is approached through the sacral hiatus. This is a useful block when the lumbar approach is extremely difficult or almost impossible to perform: for example, when there are fused lumbar vertebrae or multiple back operations. Larger volumes in the range of 20 to 25 ml are required for cephalad spread when injecting solutions into the caudal space.

1. Position the patient prone. Flatten out the lumbar curve by placing a small roll under the pelvis. This block can also be done with the patient in the lateral position, with the upper leg flexed. Ensure a functioning intravenous line if use of a local anesthetic is planned.

2. Identify the sacral hiatus. The patient should spread the legs slightly and rotate the toes inward. This relaxes the gluteal muscles and may help identify the sacral hiatus. The sacral cornu can be felt on either side of the sacral hiatus (Fig. 7-8).

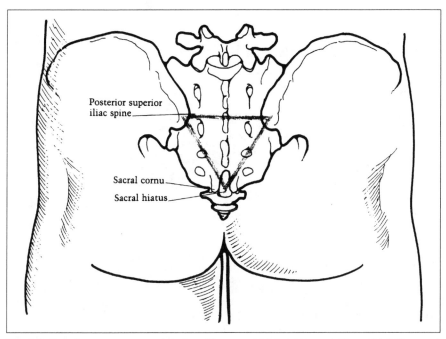

Fig. 7-8. Sacral anatomy, posterior view. The sacral hiatus is covered by a thick ligament that lies between and slightly inferior to the two prominent sacral cornua. A triangle drawn between the posterior superior iliac spines and this foramen is usually equilateral in shape. (From Mulroy MF. *Regional Anesthesia: An Illustrated Procedural Guide.* Published by Little, Brown and Company. Copyright © 1989. P. 117.)

3. **Prepare the skin for aseptic technique.** Palpate the sacral hiatus with the nondominant hand and infiltrate the skin. For a single-injection technique use a short 22-gauge needle or a 20-gauge Tuohy needle. Advance the needle in a cephalad direction through the sacral hiatus at a 45-degree angle until a decrease in resistance is felt. This may take several tries with a change in the angulation of the needle each time. If bone is contacted, the needle has advanced beyond the epidural space and is on the dorsum of the sacrum. Once there is loss of resistance, lower the angle of the needle until it is almost parallel to the sacral bone. Advance the needle into the sacral or caudal canal approximately 2 cm. Note that the dural sac ends at S2 in adults (Fig. 7-9).
4. **Malposition of the needle** can be subcutaneous, intravascular, intrathecal, or subperiosteal.
   a. To rule out **subcutaneous** placement of the needle, inject 5 ml of air or saline through the needle. At the same time, place the other hand palm down over the sacrum. If crepitus with air, or a "swelling," with saline injection is felt under the palm, the needle is positioned subcutaneously.
   b. A test dose with a local anesthetic should be carried out to rule out **intravascular or intrathecal** injection.
   c. If the needle is **subperiosteal,** there will be increased resistance and pain on injection.
G. **Epidural blood patch**
   1. **Indications.** The treatment of **postdural puncture headache** when conservative means such as bed rest, analgesics, and hydration have failed. The headache is typically aggravated by moving and/or changing positions and is often relieved by lying down.
   2. **Technique.** Place the patient in the lateral position and mark the interspace of the original puncture. Identify the epidural space at this level. Draw 10 to 15 ml of blood under sterile conditions from the patient. Inject the blood into

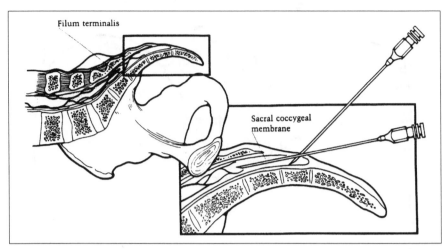

Fig. 7-9. Sacral anatomy, lateral view. A needle directed through the sacral-coccygeal membrane at a 45-degree angle will usually "pop" through the ligament and contact the anterior bone of the sacral canal. The needle should be rotated so that the bevel does not scrape the periosteum of this layer, and the angle of advancement should be changed to allow passage directly 2 to 3 cm up the canal without contacting bone again. This space is generously endowed with blood vessels, and the terminal point of the dural sac extends a variable distance into the sacral canal, but usually lies at the S2 level. (From Mulroy MF. *Regional Anesthesia: An Illustrated Procedural Guide.* Published by Little, Brown and Company. Copyright © 1989. P. 118.)

the epidural space and turn the patient supine. The procedure may be repeated in 24 hours if symptoms persist.

H. Drugs for epidural steroid injection

    1. Triamcinolone 50 mg or methylprednisolone 80 mg. Mix the steroid with preservative-free saline or a very low concentration of local anesthetic, e.g., 0.1% lidocaine (10 mg lidocaine in a total volume of 10 ml) **or** 0.1% bupivacaine (10 mg bupivacaine in a total volume of 10 ml).

    2. A higher concentration of local anesthetic may be used if the patient is in acute or severe pain or if one desires confirmation of injection into the epidural space.

    3. Total volume of injectate varies depending on the site of injection: 5 ml in the cervical region, 6 to 8 ml in the thoracic region, 10 ml in the lumbar region, and 15 to 20 ml in the caudal canal.

I. Side effects and complications

    1. Hypotension

    2. Intravascular injection with risk of local anesthetic toxicity

    3. Intrathecal injection with risk of a total or high spinal block

    4. Post–dural puncture headache

    5. Epidural hematoma

    6. Spinal cord damage (cervical and thoracic approach)

IV. Somatic nerve block

A. Paravertebral block. Thoracic and lumbar nerve roots can be blocked as they emerge from the spinal canal through the intervertebral foramina.

    1. Indications

        a. Diagnostic block for thoracic or abdominal wall pain

        b. Fractured ribs

        c. Acute herpes zoster

    2. Technique

        a. Position the patient prone. Place a roll under the abdomen to flatten out the lumbar curve. Ensure a functioning intravenous line.

        b. Mark the spinous processes. Draw a transverse line over the top of the spinous process. Draw a vertical line parallel to the midline 3 to 4 cm

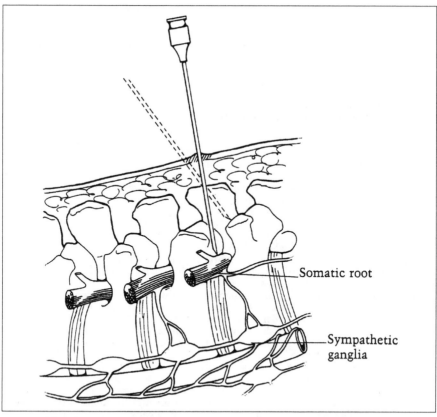

Fig. 7-10. Lumbar paravertebral block, lateral view. (From Mulroy MF. *Regional Anesthesia: An Illustrated Procedural Guide.* Published by Little, Brown and Company. Copyright © 1989. P. 134.)

laterally for lumbar and 3 cm laterally for thoracic paravertebral block. The entry point for the needle is at the intersection of these two lines.

c. Prepare the skin and infiltrate with local anesthetic. Insert a 10-cm 22-gauge needle in a slightly cephalad direction to come into contact with the transverse process. This may require several tries with a slight change in the angle of the needle each time. Note the depth of the needle with a marker once bone is contacted. Withdraw the needle to a subcutaneous level and redirect it caudal to the transverse process, and slightly medially, to a point 2 cm beyond the marker (Fig. 7-10). Inject 5–10 ml of local anesthetic solution in small increments to rule out intravascular or intrathecal injection.

d. Local anesthetics are 1% lidocaine or 0.25% or 0.5% bupivacaine. Add epinephrine depending on total dose to be used and duration of block required.

3. **Side effects and complications**
   a. **Subarachnoid or epidural injection**
   b. **Sympathetic block**
   c. **Local anesthetic toxicity** with intravascular injection
   d. **Pneumothorax** (thoracic approach)

B. **Intercostal block.** The intercostal nerves are the ventral branches of the thoracic nerves from T1 to T12. The nerves emerge from the intervertebral foramen into the paravertebral space (site of paravertebral block) and, with the exception of the twelfth nerve, continue in the costal groove of their respective ribs. The intercostal nerves run inferior to the intercostal vessels in the costal groove. Just after they exit from the intervertebral foramen, the intercostal nerves give off preganglionic sympathetic fibers through the white rami communicantes and receive postganglionic sympathetic fibers via the gray rami communicantes. At the anterior axillary line, the intercostal nerve gives off a lateral cutaneous branch. Near the sternum, the intercostal nerve gives off an anterior cutaneous branch.

1. Indications
  a. Posttraumatic: **rib fractures**
  b. Postthoracotomy, postnephrectomy **incisional pain**
  c. Acute herpes zoster
  d. Differentiation between somatic and visceral pain

2. Technique
  a. Position the patient prone with the arms hanging over the edge of the stretcher to allow the scapulae to move as lateral as possible. Place a roll under the abdomen to smooth out the lumbar curvature. If the patient is unable to lie prone, the block can be carried out in the lateral or semiprone position. If bilateral intercostal blocks are planned at multiple levels, start an intravenous line for sedation.
  b. Mark the lower edge of the ribs starting with the twelfth rib. Mark the angle of the ribs posteriorly. If there is difficulty palpating the ribs, mark 7 cm from the midline at the level of the twelfth rib and mark 5 cm from the midline at the level of the sixth or seventh rib. Join these marks to form a paramedian line that is slightly angled medially in the upper thorax. The intersection of the paramedian line with the lower border of the ribs marks the needle entry sites (see Fig. 7-3).
  c. Prepare and drape the skin. Stand on the left side of the patient if one is right-handed. Prepare the skin for aseptic technique. Infiltrate the skin over the lower border of the rib with local anesthetic. Straddle the rib on either side of the skin wheal with the index and middle fingers of the nondominant hand and retract the skin cephalad so that the skin wheal lies over the rib.
  d. Insert a short 22-gauge needle between the two fingers in a cephalad angle (about 30 degrees) to contact the rib. Release the skin slowly to allow the needle to walk off the lower edge of the rib. This may take several "releases." Once the needle is off the edge of the rib, lower the angle of the needle to 20 degrees cephalad and advance 2 mm. Steady the needle by holding the needle shaft at the skin between the thumb and index fingers. Aspirate before injecting 4 to 5 ml of local anesthetic.
  e. Another approach is to block the intercostal nerve at the mid or posterior axillary line with the patient in the supine position. The lateral cutaneous branch may be missed with this approach.
  f. Local anesthetics are 1% lidocaine or 1% mepivacaine, or 0.25% or 0.5% bupivacaine. Epinephrine 1:200,000 should be added to the local anesthetic solution to reduce systemic absorption when multiple levels or higher concentrations of local anesthetics are used.
  g. For longer duration of pain relief
    (1) Neurolytic agents, 6% to 10% phenol or 100% alcohol. Inject 2 to 3 ml. These injections may induce pain from neuritis.
    (2) Cryoanalgesia (see section **XIV**). Before proceeding with these options, it is important to perform a diagnostic or prognostic block with local anesthetics.

3. Side effects and complications
  a. Pneumothorax
  b. Local anesthetic toxicity from systemic absorption

V. Facet block. The facet or zygapophyseal joint is the articulation of a superior articular facet of one vertebra on an inferior articular facet of the adjoining vertebra. The joint lies adjacent to the neural foramen and the nerve root. The facet joint is innervated by a branch (nerve of von Luschka) of the paravertebral somatic nerve as it exits from the intervertebral foramina. It also receives a branch from the level above. Hence each facet joint has innervation from two levels.
  1. Indication: diagnosis and treatment of **lumbar facet syndrome,** which can present as low back pain with or without sciatica
  2. Technique. Multiple-level disease is not infrequent. In addition, because of the dual nerve supply of the joint, two or more levels may be blocked at a time. X-ray is used to localize the facet joint and confirm needle placement.

a. Place the patient in a prone position and place a roll under the hip to flatten out the lumbar curvature. Identify the facet joints and determine the optimum oblique view under fluoroscopy. This is generally 30 or 45 degrees. The L5–S1 facet joint may be difficult to access because of the posterior superior iliac crest.

b. Mark on the skin the points of entry for the needles. Prepare a sterile field and anesthetize the skin over the areas marked. Begin with the most cephalad facet joint. Use a 10-cm 22-gauge needle and advance it directly toward the facet joint. Use fluoroscopy to guide the needle into the joint. When the needle can no longer advance, the needle tip is in or near the facet joint.

c. After negative aspiration for blood or cerebrospinal fluid, 1 ml of contrast medium is injected to confirm the position of the needle in the joint. Then inject a total volume of 2 ml consisting of 1 ml of local anesthetic (0.5% bupivacaine) and 1 ml of cortisone (25 mg triamcinolone) into the facet joint. The patient frequently expresses immediate relief if the facet joint injected has been the cause of the pain.

3. Side effects and complications
   a. Intrathecal or intravascular injection
   b. Rupture of the joint capsule from facet joint injection: the diffusion of the solution into tissues outside the joint may be therapeutic in some cases

VI. Sacroiliac joint injection. The sacroiliac joint can be strained by certain physical activities such as heavy lifting.
   1. Indication: to diagnose or treat **sacroiliac joint syndrome**
   2. Technique. The joint is irregular and can be difficult to inject directly. The patient lies prone. With use of x-ray guidance, insert a 6-cm 22-gauge needle into the posterior portion of the joint surface. After negative aspiration, inject a mixture of 2 ml consisting of 1 ml of local anesthetic (0.5% bupivacaine) and 1 ml of cortisone (25 mg triamcinolone).

VII. Interpleural block. The space between the visceral and parietal pleura extends from the apex of the lung to about L1. Local anesthetic solution instilled in the interpleural space is thought to diffuse across the parietal pleura and intercostal muscles to reach the intercostal nerves. Blocking these nerves results in multiple levels of unilateral intercostal blocks. With positioning, the local anesthetic solution can also diffuse through the pleura into the paravertebral groove to block sympathetic nerves along the thoracic spine (splanchnic nerves), or the solution can diffuse through the apex of the lung into the paracervical area to block the cervical sympathetic chain.
   1. Indications
      a. Unilateral chest wall analgesia for **chest wall pain; fractured ribs**
      b. Abdominal pain from malignancy (pancreatic) or from acute, subacute, or chronic pancreatitis
      c. Reflex sympathetic dystrophy of the upper extremity
      d. Herpes zoster of the head, neck, and upper thorax
   2. Technique
      a. Position the patient lateral with the side to be blocked uppermost. Ensure a functioning intravenous line.
      b. Mark the seventh and eighth ribs. Prepare the skin for aseptic technique and infiltrate the skin between the marked ribs (seventh intercostal space) at a distance of 10 cm from the midline posteriorly. Advance a Tuohy needle over the superior edge of the eighth rib and identify the pleural space using the loss-of-resistance technique with either air or saline in the syringe. Alternatively, attach a well-lubricated air-filled syringe to the Tuohy needle. When the needle is in the pleural space, the negative pressure causes the plunger to fall. Once the needle is in position, a catheter can be threaded 6 to 8 cm into the pleural space.
      c. Dosages for an interpleural catheter
         (1) Bolus: 20 ml 0.5% bupivacaine with epinephrine, q6–8h prn.
         (2) Continuous infusion: bolus as above, and follow with 0.25% bupivacaine at 0.1 mg/kg/hr. There is a high incidence of incomplete analgesia with a continuous infusion.
   3. Side effects and complications
      a. Pneumothorax
      b. Local anesthetic toxicity

c. Catheter malposition
d. Pleural effusion
e. Horner's syndrome
f. Infection

VIII. Upper extremity blocks

A. **Brachial plexus block.** The brachial plexus comprises the anterior branches of the C5 to T1 nerve roots. The roots emerge from the intervertebral foramina to form three trunks sandwiched between the anterior and middle scalene muscles. As the trunks pass under the clavicle and over the first rib, they each divide into two divisions. In the axilla, the divisions join to form three cords—lateral, medial, and posterior—named according to their relation to the axillary artery. These cords give rise to the major nerves in the arm: radial from the posterior cord, median from the lateral and medial cords, ulnar from the medial cord, and musculocutaneous from the lateral cord. The brachial plexus can be approached in several ways: interscalene, supraclavicular, infraclavicular, or axillary.

1. **Indications**

a. Diagnosis and treatment of **sympathetic dystrophy of the upper extremity**
b. Treatment of **severe vasospasm**

2. **Technique.** Place the patient supine and ensure a functioning intravenous line. A peripheral nerve stimulator may be used to locate the brachial plexus.

a. **Interscalene technique**

(1) Mark the cricoid cartilage to indicate the C6 level. Turn the patient's head away from the side to be blocked. Prepare the neck for aseptic technique and stand on the side to be blocked. Have the patient lift his or her head off the table to enable identification of the lateral border of the sternocleidomastoid muscle. Roll the fingers of the nondominant hand under the muscle. Find the interscalene groove at the C6 level by slowly moving the fingers posteriorly.

(2) Insert a short 22- or 23-gauge needle in the interscalene groove in a slightly caudal and posterior direction in a plane perpendicular to the skin. Advance the needle until paresthesia is elicited. Stabilize the needle at this point. Aspirate and inject 30 to 40 ml of local anesthetic solution in increments, frequently aspirating and maintaining verbal contact with the patient.

(3) If bone is contacted, redirect the needle to search for paresthesia. Avoid the medial or cephalad direction when redirecting the needle.

b. **Supraclavicular technique**

(1) Turn the patient's head away from the side to be blocked. Place the arms alongside and stand on the side to be blocked. Mark the clavicle. Find the interscalene groove as previously described and follow it to the clavicle. The needle entry site is posterior to the midpoint of the clavicle.

(2) Prepare the skin for aseptic technique and infiltrate with local anesthetic. At the entry site described insert a 5-cm 22-gauge needle in a caudal direction. Keep the needle direction parallel to the patient's head and neck. Advance the needle to elicit paresthesia. Redirect the needle if, after advancing 3 to 4 cm, no paresthesia is elicited. If bone or first rib is contacted without eliciting paresthesia, withdraw and redirect the needle. Keep in mind the rib is in the anteroposterior plane. Walk along the rib until paresthesia is elicited. Avoid the medial direction, which is toward the cupula of the lung.

(3) When paresthesia is elicited, inject 30 ml of local anesthetic solution in increments, frequently aspirating and maintaining verbal contact with the patient.

c. **Infraclavicular technique**

(1) Identify the midpoint of the clavicle and anesthetize the skin just below the clavicle. Using a 10-cm 22- or 20-gauge needle, advance the needle under the clavicle in a lateral direction toward the humeral head until paresthesia is encountered.

(2) Inject 30 ml of local anesthetic solution in increments, frequently aspirating and maintaining verbal contact with the patient.

d. **Axillary technique**

(1) Abduct and externally rotate the arm to be blocked 90 degrees and flex the elbow. Stand on the side to be blocked. Prepare the skin for aseptic technique. Palpate the axillary artery as far up in the axilla as possible

with the index and middle fingers of the nondominant hand. Keep the fingers on the artery. After skin infiltration, insert a short 23-gauge needle just above the artery, directing the needle toward the apex of the axilla. If paresthesia is elicited, stabilize the needle and inject 40 ml of local anesthesia in increments while aspirating.

(2) If the artery is punctured, continue to advance the needle while aspirating, until the needle is just past the posterior wall of the artery. Then inject 20 ml of local anesthetic in increments, frequently aspirating. After withdrawing the needle back into the vessel, continue to aspirate until the needle is just beyond the artery anteriorly. Then inject 20 ml of local anesthetic in increments. On withdrawing the needle further, inject 3 to 5 ml of local anesthetic in the subcutaneous tissue over the artery to block the intercostobrachial nerve.

(3) Immediately adduct the arm and maintain digital pressure on the artery for a few minutes after the block. Lowering the humeral head removes obstruction to the cephalad flow of the local anesthetic solution. Digital pressure helps prevent the solution from spreading distally.

e. Continuous technique. A catheter can be inserted using the interscalene, infraclavicular, or axillary approach to provide prolonged analgesia or sympathectomy. Avoid a transarterial approach with the axillary technique if catheter insertion is planned. The catheter can be secured and left in for several days. The infraclavicular approach provides the most stability in terms of securing the catheter. The local anesthetic can be given as a bolus or a continuous infusion can be used.

3. Dose of local anesthetics for brachial plexus blocks
   a. Single dose: 30 to 40 ml of 1% lidocaine or 1% mepivacaine for diagnostic block; 30 to 40 ml of 0.125% bupivacaine for sympathetic block or 0.25% bupivacaine for a block of longer duration.
   b. Continuous infusion: bolus as described above and then infuse 0.125% or 0.25% bupivacaine at 0.1 mg/kg/hr.
4. Side effects and complications
   a. Local anesthetic toxicity from intravascular injection
   b. Spinal, subdural, and epidural injections
   c. Pneumothorax (notably with supraclavicular approach)
   d. Hemidiaphragm paresis with interscalene, supraclavicular blocks
   e. Catheter malposition
   f. Neurovascular injury
B. Peripheral nerve blocks: upper extremity. The ulnar, radial, and median nerves can each be blocked at the elbow or wrist. **Indication:** diagnosis and treatment of pain in the region of distribution. In all three blocks the patient is in the supine position with the arm to be blocked abducted at 90 degrees at the shoulder. Local anesthetics: 1% lidocaine or 0.25% or 0.5% bupivacaine can be used with volumes of 3 to 5 ml.
   1. Ulnar nerve block. The ulnar nerve originates from the medial cord of the brachial plexus. At the elbow the ulnar nerve is located in the groove between the medial epicondyle of the humerus and the olecranon process. At the wrist the ulnar nerve lies between the flexor carpi ulnaris tendon and the ulnar artery. The tendon is most medial.
      a. To block at the elbow, the arm is flexed at the elbow and the ulnar groove is palpated. Draw a line to join the medial condyle and the olecranon process. Insert the needle 1 cm proximal to this line. Use a short 25- or 27-gauge needle and inject 3 to 5 ml of local anesthetic. If paresthesia is elicited, withdraw the needle slightly before injection.
      b. To block at the wrist, flex the wrist to identify the tendon flexor carpi ulnaris. Palpate the ulnar artery lateral to the tendon. Use a short 25- or 27-gauge needle and insert this perpendicular to the wrist between the tendon and the artery. Inject 3 to 5 ml of local anesthetic solution.
   2. Median nerve block. At the elbow the median nerve lies medial to the brachial artery. The artery is felt medial to the biceps tendon. At the wrist the median nerve lies between the tendon palmaris longus and the tendon flexor carpi radialis.
      a. To block at the elbow, a line is drawn to join the medial and lateral epicondyles. The brachial artery is palpated and the needle is inserted immediately medial to the artery. Use a short 25- or 27-gauge needle. Inject 3 to 5 ml

of local anesthetic if paresthesia is elicited. If paresthesia is not elicited, inject another 2 or 3 ml of the local anesthetic medial to the artery.

b. To block at the wrist, make a fist and flex the wrist to identify the palmaris longus tendon and the tendon flexor carpi radialis. Insert a short, blunt, small-gauge needle between the tendons and inject 3 to 5 ml of local anesthetic solution.

3. Radial nerve block. At the elbow the radial nerve lies between the brachialis and brachioradialis muscle. At the wrist the radial nerve has already divided into a number of branches.

a. To block at the elbow, identify the biceps tendon and the groove between the tendon and the brachioradialis muscle. A short 25- or 27-gauge needle is inserted and directed slightly proximally at the lateral epicondyle. Inject 3 to 5 ml of local anesthetic. If no paresthesia is elicited, inject another 3 ml in a fanlike manner in the groove.

b. To block at the wrist, allow subcutaneous infiltration of local anesthetic around the anatomic snuff-box, which is identified by having the patient extend the thumb.

c. Side effects and complications. Nerve injury resulting in neuropathy from intraneural injection or compression injury. Most of the nerves described are contained in tight fascial compartments and large volumes of local anesthetic may cause high pressure and therefore nerve injury.

4. Digital nerve block

a. In the hand, raise a skin wheal between the metacarpal bones on the dorsum of the hand. Insert a short 25- or 27-gauge needle through the skin wheal between the metacarpal heads. Inject 2 ml of local anesthetic solution (1 ml at the ventral head and 1 ml at the dorsal head).

b. In the finger, infiltrate the base of the finger with 3 ml of local anesthetic solution.

c. Local anesthetics are 1% lidocaine or 0.25% or 0.5% bupivacaine. Use small volumes and **avoid epinephrine**-containing solutions.

IX. Occipital nerve block. The greater and lesser occipital nerves arise from C2 and C3. The greater occipital nerve supplies the medial posterior portion of the scalp, and the lesser, the lateral aspect of the scalp. The greater occipital nerve becomes superficial at the superior nuchal line just medial to the occipital artery.

1. Indication: diagnosis and treatment of **occipital neuralgia**

2. Technique

a. Place the patient sitting with the head flexed. Palpate the external occipital exuberance in the midline and the mastoid process laterally. The superior nuchal line joins these two landmarks.

b. About one third the distance from the midline palpate the occipital artery on the superior nuchal line. Clean the scalp with alcohol swabs. Just medial to the artery insert a short 23-gauge needle perpendicular to skin until bone is encountered. Inject 3 to 4 ml of local anesthetic in the area in a fanwise distribution. Aspirate before injection.

c. To block the lesser occipital nerve, infiltrate the skin starting from the area described above and move laterally toward the mastoid process. Inject 6 to 8 ml of local anesthetic.

d. Local anesthetic: 0.25% or 0.5% bupivacaine. A small amount of cortisone, 25 mg (1 ml) triamcinolone, can be mixed with the local anesthetic for injection.

3. Side effects and complications: intravascular injection

X. Inguinal blocks. The nerves that supply the inguinal region are the ilioinguinal, iliohypogastric, and genitofemoral nerves. The ilioinguinal and iliohypogastric nerves originate primarily from L1. These nerves follow the ilium, becoming superficial as they end in the inguinal region. The genitofemoral nerve arises from L1 and L2. It pierces the psoas muscle and divides into femoral and genital branches. The femoral branch accompanies the femoral artery under the inguinal ligament. The genital branch in the male accompanies the spermatic cord to the scrotum. In the female, this nerve runs in the inguinal canal and supplies the round ligament and the skin of the labium majora.

1. Indications: diagnosis and treatment of **pain in the inguinal region**

2. Technique

a. Ilioinguinal and iliohypogastric nerves. Position the patient supine. Mark the anterior superior iliac spine. Mark 3 cm medial and 3 cm inferior to the spine. Using aseptic technique infiltrate the skin with local anesthetic at this needle entry point. Insert a 10-cm 22-gauge needle in a cephalolateral direction to contact the ilium. Inject 10 ml of local anesthetic solution as the needle is withdrawn slowly. Reinsert the needle at a steeper angle to penetrate the abdominal muscles. Repeat the injection as the needle is withdrawn.

b. Genitofemoral nerve. The patient is supine. A short 22-gauge needle is used for the block. The inguinal ligament is identified. To block the femoral branch, infiltrate 3 to 5 ml of local anesthetic solution subcutaneously below the middle third of the inguinal ligament. To block the genital branch, insert the needle just lateral to the pubis and direct it through soft tissue down to the inguinal ligament. Inject 2 to 3 ml of local anesthetic.

c. Local anesthetics are 1% lidocaine or 1% mepivacaine or 0.25% bupivacaine.

3. Side effects and complications: local anesthetic toxicity if several other blocks are done at the same time

XI. Lower extremity nerve blocks. The nerve supply to the lower extremity arises from two major nerve plexuses, namely, the lumbar plexus and lumbosacral plexus. The former innervates the ventral aspect of the lower extremity, and the latter primarily innervates the dorsal aspect of the lower extremity. The lumbar plexus originates from the ventral divisions of the first to fourth lumbar nerves. The lumbosacral plexus originates from ventral divisions of the fourth and fifth lumbar and the first, second, and third sacral nerves. The three major nerves of the lumbar plexus are the femoral, lateral femoral cutaneous, and obturator nerves. The main nerve from the lumbosacral plexus is the sciatic nerve.

A. Sciatic nerve block. The sciatic nerve originates from the ventral divisions of the lumbosacral plexus (L4–S3). It leaves the pelvis through the greater sciatic notch and lies posteriorly between the ischial tuberosity and the greater trochanter of the femur. As it leaves the pelvis the sciatic nerve lies anterior to the pyriformis muscle. The nerve continues to descend along and posterior to the femur. At the apex of the popliteal fossa, it divides into the tibial nerve and the peroneal nerve.

1. Indication: diagnosis and treatment of **pain in the lower leg, ankle, and foot**

2. Technique. The sciatic nerve can be approached in three ways. The classic posterior approach requires the patient to lie on the side. For patients who are in significant pain and cannot be positioned laterally, the anterior approach or lithotomy approach can be attempted.

a. Posterior or classic approach

(1) The patient is placed in the lateral position with the side to be blocked uppermost. The nondependent or uppermost hip is flexed about 30 degrees and the knee is flexed at 90 degrees.

(2) Draw a line to join the posterior superior iliac spine and the midpoint of the greater trochanter. Bisect this line and mark a point 5 cm caudad on this line. This is the entry point of the needle (Fig. 7-11). A 10-cm 22-gauge needle is inserted at right angles to the skin until paresthesia is elicited. If the bone of the sciatic notch is contacted before paresthesia, the needle is redirected along a line that joins the sacral hiatus and the greater trochanter. When paresthesia is elicited, inject 20 to 25 ml of local anesthetic after negative aspiration. Local anesthetics are 1% lidocaine for diagnostic block; 0.25% or 0.5% bupivacaine for a block of longer duration.

b. Anterior approach. The patient is placed in the supine position. Draw a line to join the anterior superior iliac spine and the pubic tubercle. Divide this line into thirds. Another line is drawn parallel to the first line, extending from the greater trochanter medially. At the junction of the middle and medial thirds on the first (upper) line, drop a perpendicular line to intersect with the second (lower) line. This is the entry point for the needle. A 10-cm 22-gauge needle is inserted and directed slightly laterally to contact the femur. When bone is contacted the needle is redirected slightly medially until it just slides off the femur. Once off the femur the needle is advanced another 5 cm, seeking paresthesia. When paresthesia is elicited, inject 20 to 25 ml of local anesthetic solution after negative aspiration. Use lidocaine or bupivacaine as described in section **XI.A.2.a.(2)** above.

c. Lithotomy approach. The patient is supine. An assistant holds the hip flexed, and the leg flexed at 90 degrees. Draw a line joining the greater trochanter and the ischial tuberosity. The entry point of the needle is at the

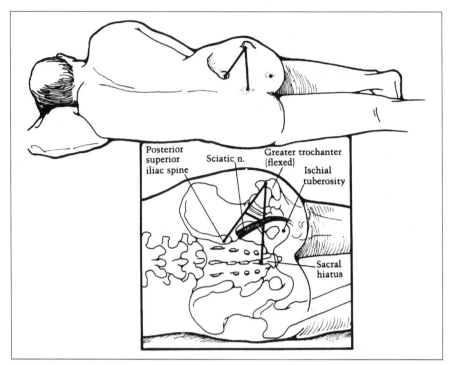

Fig. 7-11. Sciatic nerve block, classic posterior approach. With the patient in the lateral position and the hip and knee flexed, the muscles overlying the sciatic nerve are stretched to allow easier identification. The nerve lies beneath a point 5 cm caudad along the perpendicular line that bisects the line joining the posterior superior iliac spine and the greater trochanter of the femur. This point is also usually the intersection of that perpendicular line with another line joining the greater trochanter and the sacral hiatus. (From Mulroy MF. *Regional Anesthesia: An Illustrated Procedural Guide.* Published by Little, Brown and Company. Copyright © 1989. P. 191.)

midpoint of this line. Insert a 10-cm 22-gauge needle perpendicular to skin and advance it, seeking paresthesia. If paresthesia is not elicited, move the needle fanwise from medial to lateral until paresthesia is obtained. Inject 20 to 25 ml of local anesthetic after negative aspiration. Use lidocaine or bupivacaine as described in Section **XI.A.2.a.(2)** above.

3. Side effects and complications

   a. Potential nerve injury or dysesthesia as a consequence of eliciting paresthesia for the block

   b. Local anesthetic toxicity, especially if the block is done in conjunction with several other peripheral nerve blocks

   c. Patients should be warned of a **potentially prolonged block** when bupivacaine is used.

B. Femoral nerve block. The femoral nerve is the largest branch of the lumbar plexus. It passes under the inguinal ligament within the groove between the psoas and iliacus muscle. At this point it is posterior and lateral to the femoral artery. Thereafter it divides into several branches supplying the muscle and skin of the hip joint, anterior thigh, and knee.

   1. Indication: diagnosis and treatment of pain in the anterior thigh and medial aspect of the leg

   2. Technique

   a. The patient is in the supine position. Draw a line joining the anterior superior iliac spine and the pubic tubercle. Palpate the femoral artery on this line.

    b. The entry site of the needle is immediately lateral to the femoral artery. Mark the femoral artery pulsation with a finger. Advance a 5-cm 22-gauge needle perpendicular to the skin. Paresthesia is rarely elicited and not necessary for the block. The proximity of the needle to the artery should cause the needle to move with each pulsation of the femoral artery.

    c. Inject 20 ml of local anesthetic in a fanlike manner from medial (next to the artery) to lateral using a slight up-and-down motion. Use 1% lidocaine or 0.25% or 0.5% bupivacaine.

C. Obturator nerve block. The obturator nerve originates from the ventral divisions of L2, L3, and L4. It descends through the psoas muscle into the pelvis and leaves via the obturator canal to enter the thigh. It supplies the adductor muscles, the skin on the medial aspect of the thigh, and the hip and knee joints.

  1. Indications

    a. Diagnosis and treatment of pain in the area of distribution, in particular, **hip pain**

    b. Evaluation of **muscle spasm** in the lower extremity

  2. Technique

    a. The patient is supine with the legs slightly apart. Identify the pubic tubercle. Mark a point 1.5 cm lateral and 1.5 cm caudal to the tubercle. This is the entry point for the needle.

    b. Insert a 5-cm 22-gauge needle perpendicular to skin until the horizontal ramus of the pubic bone is contacted. Withdraw the needle and direct it laterally. Insert the needle 2 to 3 cm deeper than the initial contact with bone. Inject 15 ml of local anesthetic solution after negative aspiration. Move the needle back and forth slightly while injecting. Local anesthetics are 1% lidocaine for diagnostic block or 0.25% bupivacaine for a block of longer duration.

  3. Side effects and complications

    a. Local anesthetic toxicity from intravascular injection (the obturator canal is vascular) or from using large volumes of local anesthetics when other blocks are done in conjunction

    b. Nerve injury

D. Lateral femoral cutaneous nerve. This nerve originates from L2 and L3. It emerges along the lateral border of the psoas muscle and passes laterally beneath the rim of the pelvis to enter the thigh close to the anterior superior iliac spine behind the inguinal ligament.

  1. Indications

    a. Sensory analgesia of the lateral thigh

    b. Diagnosis and treatment of **meralgia paresthetica**

  2. Technique

    a. Position the patient supine. Mark the anterior superior iliac spine. Mark another point 2.5 cm medial to the spine and then 2.5 cm caudal just inferior to the inguinal ligament. This is the point of needle insertion.

    b. Prepare the skin for aseptic technique and infiltrate the skin with local anesthetic. Introduce a 5-cm 22-gauge needle through the skin and advance it until a "pop" is felt as it pierces the fascia lata. Inject 15 ml of local anesthetic in a fanlike manner from medial to lateral, above and below the fascia lata. Local anesthetics used: 1% lidocaine or 1% mepivacaine or 0.25% bupivacaine.

  3. Side effects and complications: local anesthetic toxicity, especially if done in conjunction with several other blocks

E. Lumbar plexus block (three-in-one block). The three principal nerves of the lumbar plexus are the femoral nerve, the obturator nerve, and the lateral femoral cutaneous nerve. They all emerge from the pelvis anteriorly. The intent is to block all three nerves using a single injection. Presumably, local anesthetic solution injected in a large volume near the femoral nerve will travel along fascial planes proximally to anesthetize the lumbar plexus.

  1. Indication: diagnosis and treatment of **pain in the hip, thigh or knee**

  2. Technique

    a. The patient lies supine. Palpate the femoral artery just below the inguinal ligament. Insert a 5-cm 22-gauge needle lateral to the femoral artery in a cephalad angle until femoral paresthesia is obtained.

    b. When paresthesia is elicited, fix the needle in position and digitally compress the distal femoral sheath. With frequent aspiration inject a total of 40 ml of local anesthetic solution. Local anesthetics used are 1% lidocaine for diagnostic block or 0.25% bupivacaine for a block of longer duration.

3. Side effects and complications: local anesthetic toxicity

F. Popliteal fossa block. The popliteal fossa is located behind the knee and is somewhat diamond shaped. The upper two sides (of the diamond) are made up of the semitendinous muscle medially and the biceps femoris laterally. The lower two sides consist of the two heads of the gastrocnemius muscle. The sciatic nerve divides at the cephalad end of the popliteal fossa to form the tibial and the peroneal nerves.

1. Indication: diagnosis and treatment of **pain in the foot and ankle**

2. Technique

   a. The patient is placed in the prone position. Flex the knee on the side to be blocked to help define the borders of the popliteal fossa. Outline the medial border formed by the semimembranous tendon and the lateral border formed by the biceps femoris. Draw a line through the skin crease behind the knee to mark the base of the triangle.

   b. Bisect the triangle with a perpendicular line from the base to the apex. Measure 6 cm up this line and 1 cm laterally. This is the entry site for the needle. Use a 10-cm 22-gauge needle and direct it 45 degrees cephalad to try to elicit paresthesia. When paresthesia is obtained, inject 30 to 40 ml of local anesthetic solution after negative aspiration. Local anesthetics used: 1% lidocaine or 1% mepivacaine or 0.25% bupivacaine.

3. Side effects and complications

   a. Local anesthetic toxicity

   b. Hematoma formation

G. Ankle block. The nerve supply to the foot is predominantly from the sciatic nerve. In the popliteal fossa the sciatic nerve divides into the tibial and common peroneal nerves. The tibial nerve divides into the posterior tibial nerve, which supplies the sole of the foot, and the sural nerve, which supplies the lateral aspect of the foot and ankle. The common peroneal nerve divides into deep and superficial peroneal nerves, which supply the dorsum of the foot. The femoral nerve sends a branch, the saphenous nerve, which runs superficial to the medial malleolus to supply the medial aspect of the foot and ankle.

1. Indication: diagnosis and treatment of **pain in the foot and ankle**

2. Technique. The patient is supine with a roll under the leg on the side to be blocked. Alternatively, the patient may be prone for the posterior tibial and sural nerve block and repositioned supine for the peroneal and saphenous nerves (Fig. 7-12). It is probably easier to keep the patient supine for the entire block, as this is an uncomfortable block and intravenous sedation is often necessary.

Paresthesia is not sought in blocking each of the five branches of the tibial and common peroneal nerves. Use a short 23-gauge needle for the blocks. Local anesthetics are 1% or 1.5% lidocaine or 1% or 1.5% mepivacaine for diagnostic blocks or 0.25% or 0.5% bupivacaine for blocks of longer duration. Avoid epinephrine-containing solutions.

   a. Posterior tibial nerve. The posterior tibial artery is palpated behind the medial malleolus. Direct the needle just behind the artery perpendicular to skin. If paresthesia is elicited, inject 3 ml of local anesthetic solution. If there is no paresthesia, advance to contact bone and then withdraw slightly. After negative aspiration inject 8 ml of local anesthetic solution.

   b. Sural nerve. Infiltrate 5 ml of local anesthetic solution subcutaneously between the lateral malleolus and Achilles' tendon.

   c. Deep and superficial peroneal nerves and saphenous nerve. These three nerves can be blocked using one needle entry site. At the level of an imaginary line joining the two malleoli, insert the needle in a perpendicular direction between the tendons of the anterior tibial and the extensor hallucis longus muscles. Contact bone and withdraw slightly. Inject 5 ml of local anesthetic solution after negative aspiration. Using the same needle entry site, infiltrate the skin along the imaginary line laterally to reach the lateral malleoli. This blocks the superficial peroneal nerve. The saphenous nerve is blocked by subcutaneous injection from the original needle entry site in the medial direction to reach the medial malleolus. Inject 5 ml of local anesthetic for each block.

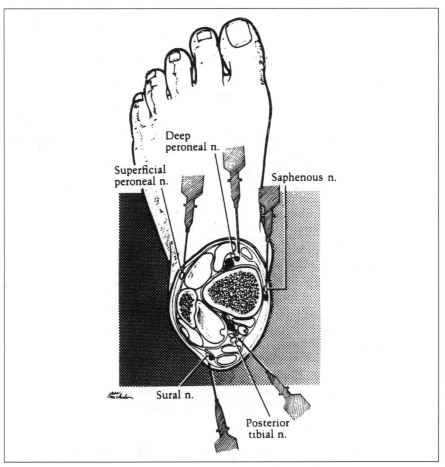

Fig. 7-12. Ankle block. Injections are made at five separate nerve locations. The superficial peroneal nerve, the sural nerve, and the saphenous are usually blocked simply by subcutaneous infiltration because they may have already generated many superficial branches as they cross the ankle joint. Paresthesias can be sought in the posterior tibial nerve or the deep peroneal, but the bony landmarks will usually provide adequate localization for the deeper injections. (From Mulroy MF. *Regional Anesthesia: An Illustrated Procedural Guide.* Published by Little, Brown and Company. Copyright © 1989. P. 203.)

      3. Side effects and complications: nerve injury or neuropathy
XII. Differential block. In the evaluation of pain, a differential nerve block can be useful in determining whether the pain is sympathetic, somatic, or centrally mediated. The differential blocks can be central blocks (e.g., spinal, epidural) or plexus blocks (e.g., brachial plexus block).

  A. Differential spinal or epidural blocks are indicated in patients with lower extremity pain, low back pain, lower abdominal pain, or pelvic pain. Patients should be experiencing pain at the time of the block. Rather than use of four different solutions (saline and 0.25%, 0.5%, and 1% procaine), a modified approach using two solutions (saline and 5% procaine) is described. The last approach does not entail waiting for the injected solution to wear off before proceeding with the next concentration and is more practical for use in outpatients.

     Place the patient in a lateral position for the block. Ensure a functioning intravenous line. Attach BP and ECG monitors. Record the temperature of the painful area.

1. For spinal block

a. Prepare two syringes, each containing 2 ml of solution. One has normal saline and the other 5% procaine. Inject the normal saline (placebo) first.

b. If pain is relieved with injection of saline, this can imply a psychiatric component to the pain manifestation, particularly if the placebo response is prolonged.

c. If pain is not relieved after 20 minutes, inject 2 ml of 5% procaine. Remove the needle and turn the patient supine. Test for sensory and motor block.

d. If pain is not relieved despite the presence of sensory and motor block, the cause is proximal to the peripheral nerves; i.e., the pain is central in origin and may be secondary to an organic lesion. There could also be an overlying psychiatric or emotional component. In either case, surgery or nerve blocks will not be helpful.

e. If pain continues to be relieved after the sensory block has worn off, the pain is likely to be sympathetically mediated.

2. For epidural block

a. Inject 20 ml of normal saline first.

b. If pain is not relieved, inject 20 ml of 3% 2-chloroprocaine or 2% lidocaine with epinephrine. Observe as described above in **section XII.A.1.**

B. Differential brachial plexus block is indicated in patients with upper extremity pain. Similarly, as with differential spinal or epidural blocks, patients should be experiencing pain at the time of the block.

1. Inject 40 ml of normal saline (placebo).

2. If there is no relief, inject 40 ml of 1.5% lidocaine. Test for sensory and motor block.

3. If pain relief outlasts the length of the sensory block, a sympathetic mechanism is confirmed.

4. If pain relief lasts only as long as the sensory block, a somatic mechanism is diagnosed.

XIII. Neurolytic spinal blockade is reserved for patients who have a life expectancy of less than 6 months, are bedridden, and have severe, intractable, localized somatic pain. Patients with a tumor causing obstruction in the spinal canal are not candidates for spinal neurolysis. Before considering spinal neurolysis, a prognostic block with local anesthetic should be performed. Patients should be advised that a repeat injection may be necessary.

1. Technique. Proper positioning is key to the success of these blocks because the agent used is either phenol, which is hyperbaric, or alcohol, which is hypobaric. These neurolytic agents cause demyelination and degeneration of the dorsal nerve roots.

a. For a hyperbaric block using phenol, the patient is positioned with the painful side down. Once spinal fluid is obtained, the patient is tilted posteriorly at an angle of 45 degrees to the horizontal surface (Fig. 7-13). For a lumbosacral block to relieve pelvic and perineal pain, the patient is positioned sitting and the lumbar puncture performed at L4–5 or L5–S1. To block the sensory roots, the patient is tilted backward at an angle of 45 degrees when the phenol is injected. Phenol 6% in glycerin is injected in very small amounts of 0.1 to 0.2 ml slowly up to a maximum of 0.6 ml (cervical), 1.0 ml (thoracic), and 0.5 ml (lumbar).

b. For a hypobaric block using alcohol, the patient is positioned with the painful side uppermost. The table is flexed to place the nerve roots to be blocked at the highest point. The patient is tilted slightly anteriorly at a horizontal angle of 45 degrees. This position allows the sensory roots to be blocked when the hypobaric alcohol is injected (Fig. 7-14). Absolute alcohol is injected slowly in 0.2 ml increments at intervals of 1 to 2 minutes up to a maximum of 2 ml at one time.

2. Side effects and complications

a. Paralysis

b. Sphincter incompetence

XIV. Cryoanalgesia. This can be applied to block most peripheral nerves and, frequently, the intercostal nerves. Cryoanalgesia uses the expansion of gas (nitrous oxide) under pressure to create an iceball ($-70°C$) at the tip of a probe. Placement of this iceball on the nerve causes a freeze injury to the nerve. The myelin and the axon are damaged, but the perineurium and the epineurium remain intact. This is a

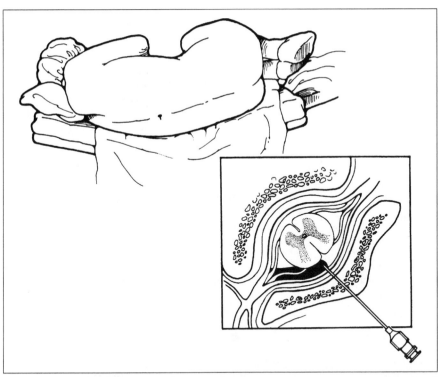

Fig. 7-13. Position for spinal phenol injection. Phenol is hyperbaric, so the patient is placed with the painful side down and rotated posteriorly so that the injection will once again be concentrated on the dorsal root nerve fibers. (From Mulroy MF. *Regional Anesthesia: An Illustrated Procedural Guide.* Published by Little, Brown and Company. Copyright © 1989. P. 270.)

reversible block with an effect reported to last anywhere from days to months. Cryoanalgesia can be performed on outpatients.

1. Technique

a. Percutaneous application of the cryoprobe requires a tract to be created first, preferably with a stiff catheter large enough to accommodate the cryoprobe (a 14-gauge intravenous catheter can be used, although this is not as stiff as one would like). Once the position of the nerve is located with the catheter, the stylet of the catheter is removed and the cryoprobe is inserted. It is important to have marked exactly how far to insert the probe so that the tip of the probe is just protruding from the end of the catheter. The probe is also connected to a peripheral nerve stimulator, which can be used to confirm the placement of the tip of the probe near the nerve.

b. Once the probe is in place, an alternating freeze-thaw cycle can take place. The cycle consists of freezing for 2 minutes and thawing for 1 minute. This can be repeated two or three times. Allow about 1 minute for the tip of the probe to thaw before removing the probe completely.

2. Side effects and complications: pneumothorax (intercostal block)

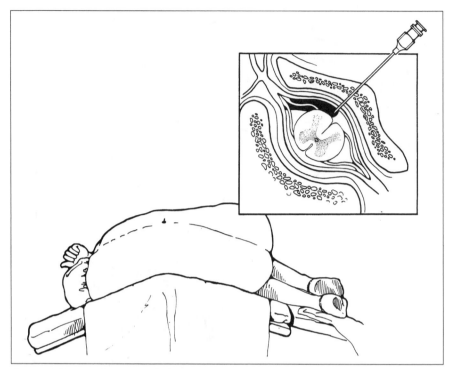

Fig. 7-14. Position for spinal alcohol injection. The patient is placed with the painful side up and rotated slightly anterior so that the involved dorsal roots are uppermost and receive the bulk of the hypobaric injection. (From Mulroy MF. *Regional Anesthesia: An Illustrated Procedural Guide.* Published by Little, Brown and Company. Copyright © 1989. P. 269.)

Selected Readings

Brown DL. *Atlas of Regional Anesthesia.* Philadelphia: W.B. Saunders, 1992.

Ischia S, Luzzani A, Ischia A. A new approach to the neurolytic block of the coeliac plexus: the transaortic technique. *Pain* 16:333–341, 1983.

Mulroy MF. *Regional Anesthesia: An Illustrated Procedural Guide,* 2nd ed. Little, Brown, 1995.

Plancarte R, Amescue C, Patt R. Superior hypogastric plexus block for pelvic cancer pain. *Anesthesiology* 73:236–239, 1990.

Zenz M, Panhaus C, Niesel H, Kreuschner H. *Regional Anesthesia.* Chicago: Yearbook Medical Publishers, 1988.

Patt. RB. *Cancer Pain.* J.B. Lippincott, 1993. Chaps. 22 and 23.

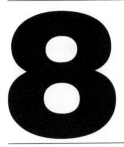

Treatment of Complications of Regional Anesthetic Blocks

David J. Wlody

I. Background. Properly performed regional anesthetic blocks are usually safe. Nevertheless, even a cursory examination of the literature will reveal a long list of reported complications. These complications have been classified in several ways: by the drug used; by the time of onset; by the organ system affected; and by the specific block performed. For the purpose of this review, **complications will be classified by the drug used—local anesthetic, narcotic, and neurolytic**—followed by a miscellaneous group of complications, some that are common to all pharmacologic agents, and others that are peculiar to a specific technique.

II. Complications of local anesthetics

A. Allergic reactions

1. Many patients report a history of allergic reactions to local anesthetics. It is important to obtain a **careful description of the symptoms** that occurred. For example, many of these episodes are associated with the intraoral injection of local anesthetics for dental procedures. In this setting an episode of lightheadedness, tachycardia, shortness of breath, or palpitations is almost certainly due to an accidental intravascular injection of epinephrine or local anesthetic, rather than a true local anesthetic allergy.

2. Nevertheless, the **amino-ester agents** have been shown to produce allergic reactions owing to their **structural similarity to para-aminobenzoic acid (PABA)**, which is known to be allergenic.

3. Because the amino-amide local anesthetics are not PABA derivatives, their allergenic potential is considerably less than that of the esters. It is important to realize that an apparent allergic reaction to an amide may be due to **methylparaben** (used as a preservative in multiple-dose vials), because it is structurally similar to PABA. Similarly, the antioxidant **metabisulfite** used in epinephrine can cause a reaction that may unfairly implicate an amide local anesthetic.

4. If time allows, **intradermal testing** of preservative-free local anesthetics can establish their allergenic activity. If such testing is unavailable, a patient with a reported history of allergic reaction can usually receive amide local anesthetics that are free of preservative and metabisulfite with minimal risk.

5. Treatment of allergic reactions is primarily supportive. **Urticaria** can be treated with **antihistamines,** such as diphenhydramine 25–50 mg IV. More severe symptoms such as **bronchospasm** should be treated with **epinephrine** (1:1000) 0.3 ml SQ q15 min prn. **Hydrocortisone** 100–200 mg IV is also useful. True anaphylaxis may require full resuscitative efforts, including the use of pressor agents and massive fluid replacement.

B. Intravascular injection

1. All the local anesthetics have **multiple systemic effects.** These are most clearly seen following the accidental intravascular injection of a large bolus of anesthetic.

2. **The primary manifestations** of systemic toxicity are within the CNS and the cardiovascular system. Initial symptoms of toxicity are **lightheadedness, dizziness,** and **circumoral paresthesias.** As the plasma level of local anesthetic increases, objective signs of CNS toxicity occur, such as **shivering** and **facial muscle twitching.** Eventually, generalized tonic-clonic seizures occur. If a sufficient dose of local anesthetic is given, this excitement stage is followed by **CNS depression, coma,** and **respiratory arrest.**

3. In general, **cardiovascular toxicity follows CNS toxicity,** and a higher level of drug in the plasma is required for cardiovascular system symptoms to occur.

Table 8-1. Recommended total anesthetic dose (mg/kg of body weight)

	Plain	Epinephrine containing
Procaine	6	9
Chloroprocaine	10	15
Lidocaine	5	7
Mepivacaine	5	7
Etidocaine	4	6
Bupivacaine	2.5	3
Tetracaine	1.5	3

   a. Levels of local anesthetic that produce seizures will cause increases in cardiac output that parallel the intensity of convulsive activity.
   b. As plasma levels increase further, the initial vasoconstrictive effect is followed by vasodilatation.
   c. Eventually, direct negative inotropic and chronotropic effects become manifest and, in combination with profound vasodilatation, will lead to circulatory collapse
4. Bupivacaine toxicity has a somewhat different presentation.
   a. Its ratio of cardiovascular collapse to CNS toxicity (CC/CNS) is lower than that of any other agent, which can lead to the almost simultaneous onset of seizures and cardiac arrest.
   b. Its toxicity is marked by severe ventricular arrhythmias.
   c. Its toxicity is considerably enhanced in pregnant women.
   d. Finally, resuscitation of a patient with bupivacaine cardiotoxicity is extremely difficult.
5. The prevention of systemic toxic reactions is obviously preferable to treating a reaction after it occurs.
   a. Careful, slow aspiration through the needle or catheter both before and during all injections is essential.
   b. When using **catheter techniques,** use an adequate test dose to rule out intravascular injection.
   c. Fractionate the total dose administered: e.g., 5 ml of agent given epidurally q3–5 min.
   d. Limit the total anesthetic dose to prevent absorption and delayed toxicity (Table 8-1).
6. The treatment of systemic toxicity should include
   a. Administration of **supplemental oxygen**
   b. Securing the airway, by endotracheal intubation if necessary
   c. Terminating the seizure. This can be accomplished with thiopental 50–100 mg IV. This drug has the advantages of immediate availability and a familiar pharmacologic profile. **Diazepam** 5–10 mg IV is also an effective choice. Although **succinylcholine** will terminate the peripheral manifestations of a seizure, it has no effect on the CNS. Therefore, when the neuromuscular blockade wears off, it will be necessary to administer thiopental or diazepam if seizure activity has not spontaneously stopped.
   d. Support of the cardiovascular system includes
      (1) Correction of hypoxia
      (2) Rapid fluid administration
      (3) Administration of ephedrine 5–10 mg IV to support the BP
      (4) Administration of atropine 0.4 mg to treat bradycardia
   e. Treatment of ventricular arrhythmias. There is evidence that large doses of **epinephrine** (5–10 mg) may be necessary in the resuscitation of patients with bupivacaine cardiotoxicity.[1] There are also experimental data that **bretylium** may be the antiarrhythmic drug of choice for bupivacaine-induced ventricular fibrillation.[2]
C. Arterial hypotension after neuraxial blockade
   1. Both spinal and epidural anesthesia produce **sympathetic blockade** through their action on preganglionic sympathetic fibers.

    a. A sympathetic block to T10 will cause vasodilatation in the lower extremities, leading to venous pooling and decreased venous return to the heart.

    b. Extension of the block to T6 will cause splanchnic vasodilatation and a further reduction in venous return.

    c. Block to T2 will cause vasodilatation in the arms, thereby removing the final compensatory mechanism for lower limb sympathetic blockade. This level of blockade can interrupt sympathetic output from cardiac accelerator fibers, which occasionally leads to an inappropriate bradycardia.[3]

    d. Any of these sympathetic blockade levels can lead to hypotension.

  2. Acute hypovolemia will accentuate the above-mentioned response and therefore is **a contraindication to neuraxial blockade.**

  3. Prevention of hypotension depends on **adequate hydration,** e.g., 500–1500 ml of crystalloid administered immediately before initiation of the block.

  4. A patient with a **pharmacologic sympathectomy** is extremely **sensitive to position changes,** because the body's vascular space behaves like a "bag of fluid." Any head-up position can lead to marked venous pooling in the gut and lower extremities, and should be avoided.

  5. Should hypotension occur, **treatment** should include

    a. Elevation of the legs, to improve venous return

    b. Intravenous fluid infusion

    c. Ephedrine 5–10 mg IV. Its mixed alpha- and beta-adrenergic agonist properties cause increased cardiac output through enhanced venous return and increased cardiac contractility.

  6. Bradycardia should be treated with atropine 0.4 mg if it is severe enough to cause hypotension.

D. Exaggerated spread of neuraxial block

  1. Three mechanisms for a high block

    a. Intrathecal injection of excessive local anesthetic. This will be marked by rapid loss of consciousness and apnea. This is probably not caused by direct phrenic paralysis but rather arterial hypotension, which leads to ischemia of the medullary respiratory center.

    b. Epidural injection of excessive local anesthetic. Again, direct motor paralysis of the diaphragm is unlikely to be the cause of respiratory arrest. Compared with a total spinal, the onset of apnea will be delayed considerably.

    c. Subdural injection is a rare complication of attempted epidural cannulation, in which patchy and sometimes extensive anesthesia follows the injection of small amounts of total anesthetic. It is usually distinguishable from a total spinal by its delayed onset.

  2. Whatever the cause of an exaggerated level of anesthesia, the **treatment is the same:**

    a. Support ventilation

    b. Protect the airway, by intubation if necessary

    c. Support the cardiovascular system

III. Complications of neuraxial narcotics

A. Pruritus

  1. The incidence of pruritus **following the use of spinal narcotics** is generally reported to be in the range of 60% to 90%. Many of these patients report pruritus only on careful questioning, and far fewer require treatment. Although there have been reports of pruritus following the spinal administration of most narcotics, there is some evidence that the more highly lipid-soluble agents have a somewhat lower incidence.

  2. The cause of pruritus is unknown. **Antihistamines** have been used with some success, although there is no evidence that histamine release is involved.

  3. Naloxone 0.04–0.10 mg IV typically gives good relief without reversing the analgesic effects of the narcotic. If pruritus recurs, a continuous infusion of 3–5 μg/kg/hr can give prolonged relief.

B. Urinary retention

  1. Urinary retention is a poorly understood complication of spinal narcotics that occurs especially in young male patients. It is generally unresponsive to cholinomimetics, but does respond to **naloxone,** indicating that this complication is in part mediated by opiate receptors.[4]

  2. Unfortunately, the doses of naloxone needed to reverse urinary retention are frequently high enough to reverse analgesia as well. As a result, the treatment of choice is **intermittent catheterization** as required.

3. Several reports have demonstrated that the use of epidural narcotics for chronic pain is usually not associated with this complication.

C. Nausea and vomiting

1. The use of spinal narcotics is associated with a 20% to 30% incidence of nausea and vomiting. The incidence of this complication appears to be agent specific, as there is a lower incidence with more highly lipid-soluble agents. The routine use of parenteral narcotics (IV or IM) is associated with an incidence rate of nausea and vomiting as high as 30%. The cause is unknown, although rostral spread via the cerebrospinal fluid (CSF) to the chemoreceptor trigger zone has been invoked.

2. Treatment consists of metoclopramide 5–10 mg IV or droperidol 0.625 mg IV. Low-dose naloxone (as in **Section III.A.3**) has also been effective.[5]

3. As with urinary retention, this complication occurs less frequently in patients treated with long-term narcotics for chronic pain.

D. Respiratory depression

1. The **most worrisome complication** of spinal narcotics is delayed respiratory depression, which is probably due to rostral spread of narcotics via the CSF to the medullary respiratory center.

2. Because they are rapidly absorbed by the spinal cord at the site of injection, highly lipophilic narcotics such as **fentanyl** and **methadone** are less likely to produce delayed respiratory depression than morphine, which is poorly lipid soluble.

3. Although all patients receiving spinal narcotics are at risk, certain patient groups are more likely to have respiratory depression, such as **the elderly, those with significant systemic illness, and those who have received large doses of parenteral narcotics.**

4. The prevention of respiratory depression depends on **adequate monitoring.** Ready and Wild have noted that the respiratory rate is a poor indicator of subsequent respiratory depression.[6] They recommend that the level of sedation be monitored hourly, because respiratory depression is invariably preceded by increasing somnolence over a period of several hours.

5. Respiratory depression can be managed by **naloxone** 0.1–0.4 mg, followed by a continuous infusion of 3–5 μg/kg/hr, which should not interfere with spinal narcotic analgesia.

IV. Complications of neurolytic agents

A. Specific agents

1. **Alcohol** is used in concentrations of 50% to 100% for neurolytic blocks. Because of its tissue-irritant effect, injection is very painful. The result of an accidental intravascular injection is usually entirely benign, although thrombosis of the vessel is possible.

2. **Phenol** has anesthetic activity, and its injection is therefore painless. This local anesthetic action provides a rapid indication of the extent of the block obtained. Although phenol can cause systemic toxicity (8–15 g), this is unlikely owing to the small doses used for neurolytic block (500–1000 mg).

3. The main risk of neurolytic block is **the spillover of the agent to adjacent neural structures.** Although eventual recovery of function will usually occur, there may be prolonged or even permanent debilitating injury. For this reason, the use of neurolytic blockade is best reserved for patients with limited life expectancy. It is essential, therefore, to perform an initial block with local anesthetic, both to ensure the efficacy of neurolytic block and to rule out injury to adjacent structures. The use of a radiopaque solution and fluoroscopic guidance can also help reduce injury to nearby structures.

   a. **Gasserian ganglion block** can lead to serious complications should injection be made into the CSF within Meckel's cave.

   (1) The third, fourth, and sixth cranial nerves can be affected, causing disturbances of ocular motility.

   (2) Permanent blindness may occur if the second nerve is blocked. In fact, any of the cranial nerves may be affected. Even a block whose effects are limited to the fifth nerve can have serious side effects.

   (3) Blockade of the motor fibers of the fifth nerve can interfere with mastication.

   (4) Loss of corneal sensation can lead to corneal ulceration, so the eye must be protected.

   b. **Stellate ganglion neurolysis** can be complicated by injury to the brachial plexus, causing persistent disability in the ipsilateral limb. A block of the phrenic nerve can cause **significant respiratory compromise** in a patient with preexisting pulmonary disease. The neurolytic drug in this procedure can also reach the subarachnoid space via an enlarged dural root sleeve.

c. **Neurolytic block** of the celiac plexus is commonly followed by hypotension owing to vasodilatation in the splanchnic bed. Compensatory vasoconstriction may be impaired in elderly patients, who would then require abdominal binders and elastic stockings to stimulate venous return. An accidental subarachnoid puncture may occur, causing significant direct neurologic damage. Indirect damage to the cord is possible through damage of vascular structures supplying the cord. **Hemothorax, pneumothorax,** and **renal injury** have all been reported.

d. **Lumbar paravertebral sympathetic block,** like celiac block, can be complicated by intrathecal injection, renal injury, and pneumothorax. Bilateral block will cause failure of ejaculation, but impotence does not occur.

V. Miscellaneous complications

A. Pneumothorax

1. **Pneumothorax** is not uncommon **after a supraclavicular brachial plexus block.** It generally develops hours after the procedure and therefore might not be immediately recognized. This complication can be life-threatening if the bilateral blocks have been performed in an outpatient.

2. Similarly, institution of **mechanical ventilation** after a failed block can produce a **tension pneumothorax.** For this reason, great caution is suggested during this procedure.

3. If **bilateral blocks** are performed, use of an **axillary block** on one side will eliminate the potential for bilateral pneumothorax.

B. Hematoma formation can cause neural compression and potentially irreversible injury. For this reason, **coagulopathy is a contraindication** to most regional techniques. Prolonged block of motor or sensory function should raise the concern of nerve compression and lead to rapid evaluation and, if needed, surgical decompression.

C. An **epidural catheter may break** during attempted removal, leaving a catheter segment within the epidural space. Surgical removal is seldom necessary given the nonirritating characteristics of the material used. It is essential, however, to inform the patient that this complication has occurred.

D. Postdural puncture headache

1. Postdural puncture headache is seldom dangerous, but frequently a nuisance to the physician and a source of severe discomfort for the patient. Conservative treatment of **hydration, bed rest,** and **analgesics** is seldom satisfactory.

2. It is the author's opinion that a debilitating headache that has not resolved in 48 hours is an indication for an **epidural blood patch** (EBP), which is safe and 95% effective and usually gives permanent relief.

3. **Technique**

a. With the patient in the lateral position, the epidural space is identified at a level close to the initial dural procedure.

b. When the loss of resistance is achieved, 20 ml of autologous blood is obtained under sterile conditions. Of this blood, 10–20 ml is injected through the epidural needle.

c. The patient is allowed to remain supine for 30 minutes. Ambulation with assistance is then permitted.

d. Complete relief is usually obtained within 2 hours.

e. The patient is urged to avoid heavy lifting or straining for 72 hours, because the Valsalva maneuver can disrupt the patch.

4. **Fever is a contraindication to EBP** because of the risk of introducing bacteremic blood in the neuraxis.

References

1. Kasten GW, Martin ST. Successful resuscitation after massive intravenous bupivacaine overdose in the hypoxic dog. *Anesthesiology* 61:A206, 1984.
2. Kasten GW, Martin ST. Bupavacaine cardiovascular toxicity: comparison of treatment with bretylium and lidocaine. *Anesth Analg* 64:911–916, 1985.

3. Cousins MJ, Bromage PR. Epidural neural blockade. In Cousins MJ, Bridenbaugh PO (eds.), *Neural Blockade* (2nd ed.). Philadelphia: J.B. Lippincott, 1988.
4. Gregg R. Spinal analgesia. *Anesthesiol Clin North Am* 7:79, 1989.
5. Lopez KA, Ready LB, Dorman BH. Prophpylatic transdermal scopolamine patches reduce nausea in postoperative patients receiving epidural morphine. *Anesth Analg* 68:144, 1989.
6. Ready LB, Wild LM. Organization of an acute pain service. *Anesthesiol Clin North Am* 7:229, 1989.

Neuraxial Approaches to the Treatment of Chronic Pain

David J. Wlody

I. **Background.** Neural blockade is a major modality in the management of chronic pain. Two of the more useful techniques are **subarachnoid and epidural block.** In this chapter the diagnostic, prognostic, and therapeutic use of neuraxial blockade, as well as the use of epidural steroids, intrathecal baclofen, and epidural spinal stimulation, is described.

II. **Diagnostic blockade**

A. **Preparation**

1. **A careful history and physical examination** are essential before undertaking diagnostic neural blockade. Boas and Cousins indicate that a careful psychological evaluation may provide a diagnosis without resorting to neural blockade.[1] The practice of utilizing a pain clinic solely as a nerve block service is mentioned here only to be condemned.

2. **Patients should fast** prior to a diagnostic block, as if they were to receive an anesthetic in the operating room. Intravenous access must be obtained before initiating the block, and full resuscitative equipment must be immediately available.

3. It is essential to **ensure** that **an adequate block** was performed before evaluating the patient's response. The use of **radiopaque local anesthetic solutions and fluoroscopy** will demonstrate whether the correct anatomic compartment was reached. Some objective measure of blockade, such as increased skin temperature or loss of deep tendon reflexes, should be elicited.

4. The patient's **response** to a diagnostic block **should be quantitated** as accurately as possible. This can be done through the use of a visual analogue pain scale. To obtain the most accurate measure of pain relief, the patient's level of pain intensity should be assessed before performing the block. In addition, the patient should be free of any systemic analgesics or sedatives at the time of the block.

B. **Differential subarachnoid block**

1. Differential subarachnoid block is based on the principle that **increasing concentrations of local anesthetic** will progressively block sympathetic, somatic sensory, and motor fibers. The solutions used are 5 ml of normal saline (placebo), 0.25% procaine, 0.50% procaine, and 1% procaine. If the saline solution gives relief, this represents either a placebo response or true psychogenic pain. If 0.25% procaine is effective, the pain is sympathetically mediated. If 0.50% procaine is effective, the pain is therefore somatic in origin. If 1% procaine gives no pain relief, it is assumed that the pain is central (e.g., due to a lesion above the level of the spinal cord) or there is encephalization of chronic pain.[2]

2. With the traditional differential spinal, the patient must remain motionless in the lateral position, with a spinal needle in situ while awaiting onset of the sequential blocks. This may be intolerable for a patient with severe pain. Raj and Ramamurthy describe a modification of this technique in which only two solutions are used, 2 ml of saline and 2 ml of 5% procaine dissolved in cerebrospinal fluid (CSF).[3] After determining the response to saline injection, the procaine is injected, the needle is removed, and the patient is observed. The rationale of this technique is that **motor, sensory, and sympathetic function will return in sequence** as the block wears off. Thus, if there is no relief immediately after the block is placed, the mechanism is central. If pain relief initially occurs but disappears after sensory block regresses, the pain mechanism is somatic. Finally, if pain relief persists after the block has receded, the pain is thought to be sympathetic in origin. The advantage of this technique is that it permits

the patient to perform those movements that ordinarily cause pain. This technique is also considerably less time-consuming than a classic differential spinal.

3. Differential subarachnoid block can also be performed with a 32-gauge **indwelling catheter.**[4] As with the modified differential spinal, this permits maximum patient movement during the study.

4. However, there is **some question** of whether a discrete sympathetic subarachnoid block can be performed without producing any **somatic block;** what appears to be sympathetically mediated pain may have a somatic component. For this reason, some have argued that a differential spinal is of limited utility in the diagnosis of sympathetically mediated pain.[5] Nevertheless, a differential spinal block can usually localize the segmental level of somatic pain, and it clearly demonstrates a central pain mechanism if a motor block with 1% procaine produces no relief.

C. **Differential epidural block**

1. **Continuous epidural anesthesia** can be used in a similar fashion to help determine the etiology of pain. As in a classic differential spinal, progressively increasing concentrations of local anesthetic such as lidocaine 0.5%, 1%, and 2% are injected, and the response to each is noted. Response to saline demonstrates psychogenic pain or placebo response; a response to 0.5% lidocaine suggests sympathetically mediated pain; a response to 1% lidocaine suggests a somatic mechanism; and a lack of response to 2% lidocaine suggests a central source.[2]

2. **A retrograde technique** can also be used, noting the return of pain during the regression of a block produced with 2% lidocaine.[2]

3. Advantages of this technique include **avoidance of dural puncture** and the **ability to titrate** the sensory block **to a precise dermatome level** in order to identify the segmental level of pain.

4. As with the differential spinal, a disadvantage of the differential epidural block is that **some sensory block may occur** even at very low concentrations of local anesthetics. In addition, there is clear evidence that systemically administered local anesthetics produce pain relief. The amount of lidocaine used in a differential epidural block can produce blood levels of the drug comparable to those produced after intravenous injection.[4] Thus, any pain relief produced may conceivably be influenced by the levels of local anesthetic present in the plasma.

III. **Prognostic neuraxial blockade**

A. **Rationale**

1. Permanent surgical or neurolytic lesions for the treatment of chronic pain clearly have risks. For this reason, it is desirable to **determine the response to a local anesthetic block** before performing an irreversible destructive procedure.

2. A similar **determination of the response to neuraxial opioids** should be made before the implantation of a permanent infusion pump.

B. **Drawbacks**

1. **A greater degree of pain relief may be obtained after local anesthetic block** than with surgical or neurolytic lesions. This may be a consequence of greater spread of local anesthetic, affecting structures that are not surgically sectioned.[1]

2. Although a patient may not be disturbed by the temporary sensory loss seen with local anesthetic block, **permanent anesthesia may be a source of considerable distress** and may, in fact, lead to neuralgia secondary to a deafferentation syndrome.

3. Despite initial pain relief, surgical section of a nerve **can lead to fibrosis and neuroma formation** that may eventually produce pain that is equally as distressing as the initial painful condition, despite initial pain relief.

4. Nevertheless, prognostic blockade is **useful to the extent that it can avoid unnecessary procedures,** because a lack of response to a prognostic procedure rules out further invasive interventions.

IV. **Therapeutic neuraxial blockade**

A. **Narcotics**

1. Before initiating long-term infusion of spinal narcotics, it is necessary to determine whether a therapeutic response to this technique can be obtained. Cousins et al. point out that deep, constant somatic pain shows the best response

to spinal narcotics, whereas intermittent somatic or visceral pain shows a less consistent response.[6] They recommend a **trial of epidural opioid** via a standard percutaneously placed catheter before considering a more invasive technique.

2. Once a therapeutic response is demonstrated, the **catheter system** will need to be **modified to minimize the risk of epidural abscess** formation during chronic use. This is most easily done by forming a subcutaneous tunnel and externalizing the injection port at the anterolateral chest wall. A chronic inflammatory response will occur at the exit site, but it is highly unlikely that an infection will track along the catheter into the epidural space.

3. Because an externalized catheter may interfere with daily activities such as bathing, it may be desirable in some patients to utilize a **totally implanted system.** There are two basic types of implanted systems.

   a. One type is a **portal system,** in which bolus injections of narcotic are made into a subcutaneously implanted reservoir that is joined to the epidural catheter. This system may require three or more injections per day, and it has the advantages of low cost and relatively fail-safe operation.

   b. The other type of implanted system is an **infusion pump,** in which a bladder containing pressurized gas produces a constant flow of drug from a fairly large reservoir. Such systems are expensive, but they have the pharmacokinetic advantage of producing a fairly constant level of analgesia. In addition, their reservoirs are large enough that they may need to be refilled only every 2 to 3 weeks, depending on dose requirements.

4. There are **theoretical advantages to both the epidural and intrathecal routes** for chronic opioid administration. The small doses used intrathecally are less likely to have any significant systemic effect. The avoidance of a dural puncture with the epidural route, though, will decrease the risk of spinal headache. In addition, an intact dura probably represents a significant barrier to infection. It may be reasonable to utilize the intrathecal route if an implanted reservoir pump is used, because the relative infrequency of reinjections minimizes the risk of bacterial contamination.

B. Local anesthetics

1. The therapeutic use of local anesthetic neuraxial blockade is primarily for the treatment of **acute pain.** There are **several chronic pain states,** however, that can respond favorably to a brief period of local anesthetic blockade. Such disorders include **reflex sympathetic dystrophy, causalgia, phantom limb pain, and postherpetic neuralgia.**

2. The **mechanism** behind the therapeutic response seen in these painful conditions **is unclear.** Interruption of the pain pathway is presumed to disrupt the vicious circle that perpetuates the pain.

3. A crucial aspect of this technique is the use of **aggressive physical therapy and patient mobilization** during the pain-free interval. Either a series of blocks can be performed or a continuous local anesthetic infusion via an indwelling epidural catheter can be used. If sufficiently low concentrations of local anesthetics are infused, minimal motor impairment will occur, and the patient will be able to undergo aggressive rehabilitative therapy.

4. If the block is not permitted to wear off, tachyphylaxis does not appear to be a significant problem. In fact, the **intensity** of the block **may increase over time,** necessitating careful monitoring for increasing muscle weakness and hypotension.

V. Miscellaneous techniques

A. Epidural steroids

1. The use of epidural steroids for the treatment of sciatica was first described in 1952. Bogduk has pointed out that the rationale for epidural steroids (i.e., an anti-inflammatory effect in irritated nerve roots) has never been established.[7] Nevertheless, there is a developing consensus that there is a significant **inflammatory component** in at least the early stages **of radicular pain.** Thus, administration of the anti-inflammatory agent directly to the affected root should have maximum effect.

2. **Intrathecal steroids** have been recommended in the past. However, meningitis, adhesive arachnoiditis, and other complications have been reported. As intrathecal steroids have no apparent advantage over the epidural route, their use is **not recommended.**[8]

3. The patient is placed in a **lateral decubitus position** with the painful side down. **Methylprednisolone acetate** (Depo-Medrol) 80 mg is suspended in 10

Table 9-1. Pain syndromes effectively treated with dorsal column stimulation

Causalgia and reflex sympathetic dystrophy
Stump pain
Phantom pain
Diabetic neuropathy
Plexus injuries (not avulsions)
Multiple sclerosis
Postherpetic neuralgia

ml of 0.25% **bupivacaine** and injected into the epidural space. The patient is maintained in the lateral position for 10 minutes.

4. The patient is reevaluated at 2 and 4 weeks. If relief was obtained but not sustained after the initial injection, the treatment is repeated. Most authorities recommend a maximum of three injections.

5. **Complications** are primarily related to the epidural puncture itself, such as a **headache** after accidental dural puncture. Transient **exacerbation of pain** has been reported. Although **depression of plasma cortisol levels** can occur, this appears to be clinically insignificant.

6. Although most studies show very good initial success rates, there is considerable **drop-off over time.** It appears that the best long-term results are seen in patients with recent onset of pain. Patients with long histories of back pain, and particularly those with sensory or motor deficits due to nerve root compression, are unlikely to obtain prolonged relief.[7]

B. **Epidural dorsal column stimulation**

1. **Spinal cord stimulation** was first described in 1967. Its use is explained by the gate-control theory of pain: A nonnoxious input to the spinal cord can modify the perception of a noxious stimulus.

2. Meyerson summarizes the **pain syndromes** that have been **effectively treated with dorsal column stimulation** (Table 9-1).[9] These syndromes are chiefly **neuropathic,** in that pain arises from injury to the nervous system itself. Pain arising from injury to nonnervous tissue is less likely to respond to this technique.

3. Most patients benefiting from dorsal column stimulation show some response to **transcutaneous electrical nerve stimulation (TENS).** Some patients, however, do not respond to TENS but achieve significant relief with dorsal column stimulation. This may be due to the inability to produce a paresthesia in the entire painful area with TENS.

4. The most common technique utilizes the percutaneous **placement of the stimulating electrode into the epidural space via a Tuohy needle.** Correct placement of the electrode is confirmed by production of a paresthesia throughout the painful area. The stimulating electrode is connected to a lead, which is tunneled subcutaneously and externalized. After a successful trial of stimulation is performed, the entire system can be internalized to minimize the risk of infection.

5. The patient is instructed to **activate the system when the pain is severe.** Typically, 20 to 30 minutes of stimulation will produce 2 to 4 hours of pain relief.

6. Successful use of this modality requires **careful patient selection.** As stated previously, neuropathic pain is more effectively treated than pain arising in nonnervous tissue. Patients with preexisting emotional disturbances are poor candidates for dorsal column stimulation. Finally, patients must accept that they will be dependent on this technique on a daily basis for many years.

7. Long-term **complications include** failure of pain relief due to **displacement of the electrode tip.** This can be corrected with the percutaneous technique. Should repositioning be required several times, placement of a multipolar electrode via a laminectomy is recommended, because these electrodes maintain a stable position over a prolonged period.

C. **Intrathecal baclofen**

1. One of the major manifestations of spinal cord injury is **lower extremity spasticity.** The standard treatment for this disorder is oral baclofen, a gamma-aminobutyric acid agonist that acts presynaptically to reduce motor neuron

excitability. Unfortunately, **large oral doses** are required for a therapeutic effect, because baclofen penetrates the blood-brain barrier poorly. These large doses are frequently associated with **unwanted side effects**, particularly somnolence.

2. **Intrathecal baclofen** has been shown to have considerable advantages over the oral route.[10] First, because the drug is perfusing the cord directly, the therapeutic response is usually greater than that seen with oral administration. Second, while central side effects can be seen with this technique, they appear to be less troublesome than those seen with high-dose oral therapy.

3. Patients are selected for this technique if standard oral doses are ineffective or cause intolerable side effects. Once the effective intrathecal bolus dose is determined (25, 50, or 75 μg), an **implantable pump** is programmed to deliver 1.5 to 2.0 times that dose over 24 hours. The rate can be adjusted to patient response if an externally programmable pump is used.

4. This technique is potentially useful in spasticity due to **demyelinating disease**.

5. Although Lazorthes et al failed to show the **development of tolerance** over an 18-month follow-up period,[11] it **remains to be seen** whether tolerance develops with chronic use.

References

1. Boas RA, Cousins MJ. Diagnostic neural blockade. In Cousins MJ, Bridenbaugh PA (eds.), *Neural Blockade* (2nd ed.). Philadelphia: J.B. Lippincott, 1988.
2. Raj PP, Ramamurthy S. Differential nerve block studies. In Raj PP (ed.), *Practical Management of Pain*. Chicago: Year Book Medical Publishers, 1986.
3. Raj PP, Ramamurthy S. Differential nerve block studies. In Raj PP (ed.), *Practical Management of Pain* (2nd ed.). St. Louis: Mosby–Year Book, 1992.
4. Bonica JJ, Buckley FP. Regional analgesia with local anesthetics. In Bonica JJ (ed.), *The Management of Pain* (2nd ed.). Philadelphia: Lea & Febiger, 1990.
5. Wilson PR, Lamer TJ. Pain mechanisms: anatomy and physiology. In Raj PP (ed.), *Practical Management of Pain* (2nd ed.). St. Louis: Mosby–Year Book, 1992.
6. Cousins MJ, Cherry DA, Gourlay GK. Acute and chronic pain: use of spinal opioids. In Cousins MJ, Bridenbaugh PA (eds.), *Neural Blockade* (2nd ed.). Philadelphia: J.B. Lippincott, 1988.
7. Bogduk N. Back pain: zygapophysial blocks and epidural steroids. In Cousins MJ, Bridenbaugh PA (eds.), *Neural Blockade* (2nd ed.). Philadelphia: J.B. Lippincott, 1988.
8. Benzon H. Epidural steroids. In Raj PP (ed.), *Practical Management of Pain* (2nd ed.). St. Louis: Mosby–Year Book, 1992.
9. Meyerson BA. Electrical stimulation of the spinal cord and brain. In Bonica JJ (ed.), *The Management of Pain* (2nd ed.). Philadelphia: Lea & Febiger, 1990.
10. Penn RD, Savoy SM, Corcos D, et al. Intrathecal baclofen for severe spinal spasticity. *N Engl J Med* 320:1517, 1989.
11. Lazorthes Y, Sallerin-Caute B, Verdie J-C, et al. Chronic intrathecal baclofen administration for control of severe spasticity. *Neurosurg* 72:393, 1990.

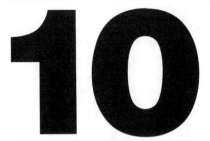

Neurolytic Procedures for Cancer Pain Management
Subhash Jain

I. Background. Nerve blocks, including subarachnoid, epidural, and local injection of neurolytic agents, are part of an armamentarium available to the physician in the fight against intractable cancer pain. The initial use of neurolytic nerve blocks was plagued by problems of asepsis, inexperience, and difficulty in limiting the spread of the injected agent to the nerves responsible for the pain without compromising other structures. As a result, such nerve blocks were long militated against as viable options for the treatment of cancer pain.

A. Neural blockade

1. Although the application of neurolytic substances to provide relief of pain for patients with cancer has been **practiced for many years,** neither the methods of blockade nor the useful pharmacologic agents have undergone marked change. Contemporary applications of these techniques represent an advance in care.

   a. Increased experience and the availability of additional alternatives permit more sophisticated decision-making with regard to screening patients and selecting the proper procedure.

   b. Recognition of the problem of "total pain" and integration of anesthetic care into a multidisciplinary matrix promise improved overall results.

   c. An increase in the dissemination of knowledge, number of skilled practitioners, and frequency of evaluations and procedures performed translates into greater benefit to more patients.

2. **Recent enhancements** of neurolytic techniques include

   a. The application of more sophisticated techniques with radiologic guidance, as in **CT-assisted localization of the celiac axis**

   b. Pituitary ablation

   c. The epidural application of phenol

B. General considerations

1. Despite limited revision in the principles and techniques of neurolytic blocks, **guidelines** for their use in clinical practice are presented to define their role in the context of comprehensive cancer pain management and by virtue of their unique utility to the anesthesiologist involved in managing cancer pain. Standard sources are recommended for the practitioner interested in technical details of individual procedures.[1,2]

2. Consideration for neurolytic intervention in patients with **cancer-related pain** is indicated when

   a. Symptoms cannot be controlled adequately with medications and other conservative therapy

   b. Life expectancy is limited

   c. Patients are extremely ill and weak and are poor candidates for surgical operations such as cordotomy

   d. Patients are suffering from **localized cancer pain** that involves visceral, somatic, traumatic, or peripheral neuralgias **not primarily associated with the central neuraxis**

3. Patients must undergo a **full medical examination** before they are considered for a neurolytic block. **Relative contraindications** to nerve blocks in the back include

   a. A history of trauma

   b. Infection

   c. Congenital anomalies

   d. Anticoagulant therapy

4. Initially, **aggressive narcotic and nonnarcotic medication** should be used to

achieve pain relief. Fears of addiction and tolerance should not lead to the premature use of more invasive and irreversible therapies. Only after other modalities prove unsatisfactory, because of either inadequate pain control or complications from the therapy itself (i.e., nausea, constipation, sedation), should neurolytic nerve blocks be considered.

5. Neurolytic blocks should always be preceded by a **temporary diagnostic block using local anesthetics** since
   a. Such injections are useful in **confirming the neurologic component** of the pain
   b. Various degrees of **relief** can be obtained **from repeated blocks with local anesthetics** alone

C. Physiologic considerations

1. Normal sensation is transmitted to the posterior horn of the spinal cord segment via peripheral somatic and visceral nerves. These are composed of various **nerve fiber types:**
   a. **A fibers** (further classified into alpha, beta, gamma, and delta) **are myelinated fibers** of various diameters (1–20 μm) and conduction velocities (12–120 m/sec).
   b. **B fibers are myelinated preganglionic sympathetic neurons** with diameters of 1 to 3 μm and conduction velocities of 14 m/sec.
   c. **C fibers are small unmyelinated nerves** with diameters of 0.5 to 1.0 μm with slow conduction velocities of 1.1 to 2.0 m/sec.
2. **Pain sensation is conveyed primarily by the A delta and the C fibers.** The former carry the fast, sharp, shooting pain sensations, and the latter carry the dull, aching, burning pains often associated with tumors.
3. **Susceptibility** of nerves to instilled solutions is **inversely proportional to their diameter and the presence or absence of myelin.** Differential nerve blocks are therefore possible. One can block the sensation of pain and temperature, mediated by the small, thin, unmyelinated C fibers, without sacrificing the other modalities of sensation and motor control carried by the thicker, myelinated fibers. This has been demonstrated with both hypotonic and hypertonic solutions, ammonium salt mixtures, and phenol.

D. Neurophysiologic aspects of impulse conduction

1. **A nerve membrane** is composed of a semipermeable double-thickness wall of lipid molecules with globular protein molecules interspaced throughout. Some of these proteins span the entire thickness of the membrane creating channels that permit ions to pass through the membrane. Sodium is actively removed out of the inner axoplasm environment, while potassium remains internally and a high sodium concentration remains externally. The membrane is less permeable to sodium than to potassium, allowing some potassium to diffuse down its concentration gradient to the outside of the cell. This generates a relative electrical imbalance of -70 to -90 mV.
2. **Depolarization** occurs when, as a result of an electrical stimulation, the membrane becomes more permeable to sodium, allowing a sudden, massive influx internally. Depolarization continues along the nerve as the impulse is carried along. This impulse propagation can be blocked by both local anesthetics and neurolytic agents. Local anesthetics produce a transient block by impeding the flow of sodium through the membrane channels. This prevents depolarization from occurring. Neurolytic solutions produce a permanent block through the disruption and destruction of nerve tissue. Such a block remains until the nerve tissue regenerates.

E. Neurolytic drugs

1. **Alcohol** is commercially available in 1-ml ampules as a colorless solution that can be injected readily through small-bore needles; it is hypobaric with respect to cerebrospinal fluid. Depending on the site of injection and the concentration of alcohol, administration is accompanied by a variable degree of discomfort that, at its extreme, is excruciating but transient. It is generally used undiluted (absolute or 100% alcohol) and, if left exposed to the atmosphere, will be diluted by absorbed moisture. Denervation and pain relief sometimes accrue over a few days following injection.
2. **Injectable phenol** requires preparation by a pharmacist, the process for which has been described by Raj.[3] Various concentrations of phenol prepared with saline, water, glycerine, and different radiologic dyes have been advocated. Phenol is relatively insoluble in water, and at room temperature concentrations

in excess of 6.7% cannot be obtained without the addition of glycerine. Phenol mixed in glycerine is hyperbaric with respect to cerebrospinal fluid but is so viscous that, even when warmed, injection is difficult through needles smaller than 20 gauge. Shelf life exceeds 1 year when preparations are refrigerated and are not exposed to light. Clinically, a biphasic action has been observed, characterized by an initial local anesthetic effect producing subjective warmth and numbness, which gives way to chronic denervation. The quality and extent of analgesia may fade slightly within the first 24 hours of administration.

3. **Ammonium sulfate** and **chlorocresol** are used less commonly to produce neurolysis.

F. **Effects of neurolytic agents on nerve tissue**

1. The neurolytic action of **alcohol** is through a dehydration action on the nerve tissue, with the extraction of cholesterol, phospholipids, and cerebrosides and the precipitation of mucoproteins. This results in **sclerosis of the nerve fibers and myelin sheath destruction.**[4]

2. **Phenol** acts by protein denaturation and, like ethyl alcohol, **is an extremely potent neurolytic agent.** There is a direct relationship between phenol concentrations and extended nerve destruction in the resultant block.[5-9] Maher noted that varied phenol concentrations in glycerine between 3.3% and 10% produced mostly sensory block with subarachnoid injection of less than 5%, whereas a higher concentration created motor blockades as well.[10] Initial observations described 5% phenol in Ringer's solution or oil contrast material as producing selective blocks of smaller nerve fibers.[7,11] Low phenol concentrations have also been described as having properties similar to those of local anesthetics.[7]

G. **Peripheral blockade**

1. Peripheral neurolysis has a definite, although limited, role in the management of **pain of malignant origin.** To ensure effective analgesia, neural interruption is planned proximal to the source of irritation. In technically difficult cases, such as blockade of upper intercostal nerves (where the overlying scapula and muscle increase the risk of a pneumothorax), a more proximal paravertebral or subarachnoid blockade should be elected. Anatomic landmarks tend to be more obvious in the presence of cachexia and weight loss. Because the sensory distribution of peripheral nerves overlaps, blockade of neighboring segments is recommended. Many peripheral nerves are of mixed function. A pretherapeutic prognostic block with local anesthetic is essential to evaluate the impact of concomitant motor deficit. In performing a peripheral neurolytic block, accuracy is essential for good results and to avoid damage to nontargeted structures. This is particularly true in the cervicofacial region, where abundant neural and vascular structures are closely spaced, and when alcohol or phenol is used because the diffusibility of each in biologic tissue is less than that of local anesthetics.

2. Regeneration of peripheral nerves is sometimes accompanied by the development of **neuritis or neuroma formation.** Alcoholic neuritis is related to incomplete destruction of somatic nerves, and its incidence is less when a solid, prolonged block has been obtained.[1] Alcohol seems to have more of a propensity to produce local irritation than does phenol, and local reaction seems to be less common in cranial nerves than in other peripheral nerves. CNS maladaptation to deafferentation, as well as local phenomena, may result in burning pain that has a potential to be even more objectionable than the original complaint of pain. The threat of postablative dysesthesia is of limited consequence when life expectancy is limited or intractable pain already exceeds tolerance levels.

H. **Subarachnoid versus epidural neurolysis**

1. **Subarachnoid neurolysis offers the following potential advantages** over classic epidural techniques:

a. Return of cerebrospinal fluid **verifies subarachnoid needle placement,** whereas localization of the epidural space must be inferred from the results of epidurograms and test doses of local anesthetic.

b. Subarachnoid neurolysis generally results in **more profound analgesia,** and, as a consequence, reinjection is required less often.

c. Subarachnoid injection is readily **performed on an outpatient basis.** Epidural neurolysis is accomplished by repeated administration of phenol through an indwelling catheter that requires inpatient hospitalization.

d. Gravity and position can be utilized to exert more precise control with subarachnoid injection than with epidural block.

e. The excessive viscosity of pure phenol-glycerine preparations prevents injection through small-caliber tubing. If an epidural block is planned with the intention of reapplication through a catheter, the phenol-glycerine mixture must be diluted with water, saline, or dye, reducing baricity and introducing the potential for reduced control of spread. A newly designed epidural catheter made from spiral stainless steel coils coated with fluoropolymers has been introduced to facilitate radiologic localization, aspiration, and repositioning.[12]

2. **The main advantage of epidural neurolysis is** its applicability **for pain that occupies a wide distribution or is bilateral.** The most commonly recommended neurolytic agent for epidural use is still **phenol.** Despite reports of favorable results utilizing alcohol,[13] its instillation produces agonizing pain in awake patients,[14] unless preceded by injections of local anesthetic, which reduce predictability. Postinjection neuropathy and neuralgia have been observed after epidural alcohol.

II. Specific nerve blocks

A. Cranial nerve blocks

1. Pain related to **malignant neoplasm of the head and neck** poses one of the most challenging management problems.

   a. **Conventional analgesic therapy may prove inadequate,** in part **because of failure of physiologic splinting,** a normal coping strategy unavailable when pain is aggravated by relatively involuntary activities such as swallowing, eating, talking, and moving the head. Cephalic pain is rarely limited to the distribution of a single nerve because of overlapping sensory innervation (cranial nerves V, VII, IX, and X, dorsal roots of the second and third cervical nerves).

   b. **Major surgical intervention introduces considerable risks** of mortality and morbidity and is regarded by many neurosurgeons as a last resort. Surgery is often accompanied by prolonged hospitalization, additional functional deficit, and disfigurement.

   c. **When pain is intractable, nonsurgical treatment** (radiotherapy, systemic and regional chemotherapy) should be **aggressively pursued.**

   d. If conservative measures have been exhausted, consideration should be given to **analgesic methods that produce generalized effects** (epidural or intraventricular narcotics, deep brain stimulation).

2. In selected patients, **blockade of the involved cranial and upper cervical nerves** is of great value. When ablative blocks or surgery is being considered, local anesthetic blocks help to ascertain the relative contribution of individual nerves to the painful state. Lasting pain relief is difficult to achieve with discrete nerve blocks because of sensory overlap and technical difficulties such as the tendency for tumors in these regions to erode and destroy surrounding tissue.

3. Oncogenic pain limited to the distribution of the **trigeminal nerve** or one of its branches may be amenable to **thermal or chemical interruption** of the involved nerve. When feasible, thermocoagulation may be the treatment of choice because analgesia can frequently be obtained without sensory loss.

4. When chemical block of a branch of the **fifth nerve** is to be undertaken, consideration should be given to the likelihood of further tumor extension and prophylactically extending the field of analgesia by blocking the **gasserian ganglion.**[15] Keratitis and corneal ulcer are possible complications but are of limited consequence.

5. If **extension** of analgesia is necessary, consideration may be given to blocking the **second and third cervical roots or the ninth and tenth cranial nerves. Bilateral block of cranial nerves IX and X should not be attempted** because resulting paralysis of pharyngeal and laryngeal muscles impairs swallowing and phonation.

6. When **neural blockade** is planned to eliminate pain **over the occiput and neck** and there has been **extensive radiotherapy,** the paravertebral approach to the cervical nerves may be difficult, and the **epidural route should be considered.**

B. Sacral nerve block

1. Selective blockade of the sacral nerve roots via their dorsal foramina is a **useful**

alternative to subarachnoid or caudal block in patients with pain from **pelvic or rectal malignant neoplasm** in whom bowel and bladder function are still intact. Pain may be due to direct invasion, chronic infection, fistula formation, or postradiation cystitis.

2. Diagnostic blocks of the individual sacral roots with local anesthetics performed in succession will determine the pathways involved in the transmission of pain. The **second and third sacral roots** are most commonly implicated in maintenance of **bladder function.** Unilateral predominance of innervation of detrusor reflex activity has been observed,[16] so **treatment that avoids bilateral S2 and S3 blocks** is likely to preserve function.

C. **Subarachnoid and epidural neurolytic block**
   1. The reader is encouraged to consult the classic reports of these nerve block procedures for detailed descriptions of the techniques and to review technical aspects.[1,17,18] The **advantages** of neuraxial neurolysis are
      a. **A high proportion of good results** in properly selected cases
      b. **Ease of performance** with minimal requirements for equipment
      c. **Minimal requirements for hospitalization**
      d. **Duration of pain relief** that is **adequate for the preterminal state**
      e. **Ease of repetition** when necessary
      f. **Suitability for aged or debilitated patients**
      g. **A low complication rate** when proper technique is observed
   2. Lytic neuraxial block produces pain relief by **chemical rhizotomy.** Nerve fibers are affected indiscriminately by both alcohol and phenol.[19,20] The degree and extent of sensory loss depend on the actual number of fibers destroyed rather than the fiber type destroyed, which is, in turn, determined by the concentration and quantity of the neurolytic agent.[21] This relationship is supported by reports of higher success rates in patients with pelvic malignant neoplasms who were treated with 10% and 15% subarachnoid phenol than in those treated with a 7.5% preparation,[22] and in patients with a variety of neoplasms treated with 15% versus 10% subarachnoid phenol.[23] Neither agent offers a clear advantage, except insofar as variations in baricity facilitate positioning of the patient in selected cases.[18,24]
   3. Chemical rhizolysis can be performed at **any level up to the midcervical region,** above which the spread of caustic agent to medullary centers carries significant risk of cardiorespiratory collapse. Subarachnoid injections of phenol at the C3–4 interspace have been carried out without complications.[25] Access to the subarachnoid and epidural spaces above the lumbar region presents a technical challenge to the physician that decreases with experience.

D. **Cervical block**
   1. The **aggressive growth characteristics of lesions involving the brachial plexus and chest wall** may have a role in the fair results that have been reported when employing subarachnoid phenol rhizolysis for brachial and upper thoracic pain,[26] a phenomenon that has also been observed after neurosurgical procedures for brachiothoracic pain.[27,28]
   2. In carefully selected patients, cervicothoracic subarachnoid neurolysis and epidural neurolysis have been utilized for **relief of upper-extremity pain** with relative success.[17]
   3. These options are **not considered unless**
      a. **Pain is intractable** and so severe as to render the involved limb immobile and useless.
      b. **An early trial of stellate ganglion blocks** is used **to exclude sympathetically mediated pain** that could be permanently blocked without sacrificing function.[29,30]
      c. **Pain involves the whole extremity.**
   4. **Brachial plexus block with dilute phenol** has been reported in a small number of patients as being moderately effective, but it introduces the risk of spread to adjacent structures and may require frequent repetition.[31]
   5. **Neuraxial block** with phenol or alcohol will often provide effective relief when **pain is related** to infiltration of the brachial plexus with **tumor or radiation fibrosis.** Motor and proprioceptive deficits are anticipated, emphasizing the importance of careful patient selection.

E. **Thoracic block.** Patients with **radicular thoracic or upper abdominal pain** are ideal candidates for discrete chemical rhizotomy because medication can be introduced distant from the major limb plexuses and the origin of nerves subserving bladder and bowel function. Intercostal muscle paresis may occur despite meticulous positioning, but seldom produces increased respiratory compromise.

F. Lumbar block

1. When employing subarachnoid techniques for pain in regions subserved by the **lumber nerves,** instillation of a neurolytic substance should be planned at the **level at which the involved nerve roots exit from the spinal cord** rather than from the vertebral column. The more proximal site of injection is advantageous because

   a. It affords greater surface area for exposure of the targeted neural tissue to the neurolytic drug.[1]

   b. The terminal portions of distal nerves are less exposed to the neurolytic agent, and therefore more discrete analgesia can be expected.

   c. The incidence of complications will be reduced.

2. Access to lumbar nerve roots is gained through **dural puncture between the low thoracic vertebrae.**

3. **Precautions** undertaken to maximize efficacy and limit complications include

   a. The use of an **operating room–type table** that can be readily manipulated

   b. Careful attention to **maintenance of patient posture**

   c. Conservative selection of **dosage and rate of injection**

   d. Communication with the patient to verify the desired location and extent of blockade

   e. Exposing the patient to **repeated procedures or injecting small boluses** through multiple needles

4. Patients need to be cautioned in advance that though the actual puncture and injection ordinarily produce only minimal discomfort, **maintenance of optimal posture** for 15 to 30 minutes after the neurolytic has been instilled **may be distressing.**

5. **Bowel and bladder dysfunction** are among the most feared complications of neuraxial lytic block, although their actual incidence and severity are low when proper technique is observed, regardless of the agent utilized.

G. Saddle block. Perineal pain and pelvic pain are amenable to neuraxial lytic blockade by a number of routes.

1. A useful approach for unilateral pain involves placing the patient in a **lateral position** and injecting the neurolytic agent through a **low lumbar puncture.**

2. If pain is bilateral, the procedure can be repeated after a few days, with the patient's **position reversed.** It is not uncommon for bilateral pain to resolve significantly after a unilateral block, making a second procedure unnecessary.[32]

3. A **true saddle block** can be utilized for pain that crosses the midline.[40] Hyperbaric phenol is introduced through a **low lumbar puncture,** and the patient is maintained in the sitting position modified by a **45-degree posterior tilt** for 15 to 30 minutes.

4. The injection of small volumes of dilute phenol via the **caudal route** has been described in a series of 26 patients with perianal pain due to malignant neoplasm.[33] Pain relief persisted for a mean of just 12.7 days, but only one complication (transient urinary retention) was described. As temporary urinary or even anal dysfunction can be anticipated in many patients, these techniques should be **reserved for patients with indwelling catheters or patients who are bedridden and accept the risk of additional deficit.**

H. Sympathetic nerve block. Local anesthetic infiltration of the sympathetic nervous outflow can be performed for diagnostic, prognostic, or therapeutic purposes.

1. A **diagnostic nerve block** helps to establish the relative contribution of the autonomic versus somatic nervous system to pain transmission.

2. Response to local anesthetic blockade is **prognostic** in that it helps to determine whether repeated local anesthetic blocks, a neurolytic block, or surgery is likely to provide prolonged relief.

3. In carefully selected patients, a **therapeutic effect** may be obtained either by serial injections of a local anesthetic drug or by the injection of a neurolytic agent.

I. Cervicothoracic (stellate) ganglion block

1. Neurolytic stellate ganglion block is **hazardous** because

   a. The cervicothoracic ganglion is **difficult to locate** with precision.

   b. Spread to nontargeted structures may produce severe complications because of the close **proximity of major neurovascular structures.**

   c. Specific risks such as

       (1) **Erosion**
       (2) **Thrombosis or spasm of major vessels**
       (3) **Cerebral infarction** from intravascular injection
       (4) **Prolonged hoarseness** from spread to the recurrent laryngeal nerve
       (5) **Upper limb dysfunction** if elements of the brachial plexus are affected
       (6) **Sloughing of the superficial tissues**
  2. There are anecdotal reports of **stellate gangliolysis** performed with up to 10 ml of 6% aqueous phenol with good results and no complications.[29]
  3. Bonica[1] recommends
    a. Reserving neurolytic stellate block for **exceptional cases**
    b. **Limiting the injectate** to either a small volume of phenol or no more than 1.5 ml of absolute alcohol
  4. The following **precautions** should be observed:
    a. **A thorough trial** of local anesthetic blockade
    b. **Careful explanation** of the procedure and its possible sequelae
    c. **Radiologic visualization** of a characteristic spread of contrast medium
    d. **Meticulous aspiration and needle immobilization**
    e. **Evidence of sympathetic block** following the injection of 1 to 2 ml of local anesthetic solution
    f. Injection of 1 to 2 ml of **dilute neurolytic preparation** (3% to 6% phenol)
    g. **Flushing the needle before its removal**

J. Lumbar sympathetic block
  1. Neurolysis of the lumbar sympathetic ganglia may be undertaken providing trials of local anesthetic injections have been shown to provide pain relief. In the presence of malignant disease, the most common **indications** for lumbar sympatholysis are
    a. **Pelvic pain of urologic, gynecologic, or rectal origin**
    b. **Lower extremity pain from lymphedema**
    c. **Reflex sympathetic imbalance**
  2. **Technique**
    a. **Three needles are positioned** with their tips anterior to the psoas muscle, at the anterolateral aspect of the bodies of the second, third, and fourth lumbar vertebrae.
    b. It has become common practice to substitute a **single injection of a large volume of local anesthetic** solution (up to 20 to 30 ml) through a single needle positioned in the correct fascial plane near the second lumbar vertebra. Results are comparable, and patient discomfort is reduced.[34]
    c. Concern that **large columns of injectate may spread** outside the correct fascial compartment to involve lumbar somatic nerves still influences **most practitioners to rely on two or three needles when a neurolytic agent is used.**

K. Celiac plexus block
  1. **Neurolytic celiac plexus block** has received widespread attention because of its excellent potential to relieve upper abdominal and referred back pain secondary to malignant neoplasm involving structures derived from the foregut. The most common **indications** for celiac plexus block are
    a. **Pancreatic cancer**
    b. **Neoplasms involving** the
      (1) **Distal esophagus**
      (2) **Stomach**
      (3) **Liver and bile ducts**
      (4) **Small bowel**
      (5) **Proximal colon**
      (6) **Adrenals**
      (7) **Kidneys**
  2. **Neurolytic celiac plexus block approaches**
    a. **The posterior percutaneous approach,** using two needles (6-in., 20-gauge), is most commonly advocated.
    b. **The anterior approach,** which has had renewed interest as radiologists have become more experienced with this route for biopsy and drainage procedures.
    c. **A transaortic technique,** which is similar to conventional approaches, except that the needle is deliberately passed through the aorta, in a manner resembling the transarterial method of brachial plexus blockade.

d. The deliberate perforation of both diaphragmatic crura under CT guidance to ensure the spread of injectate anterior to the aorta.

e. Injection under direct vision by the surgeon **at the time of laparotomy.** At times this may not be possible because diagnosis is made on a nonsurgical basis or because of the presence of diffuse intra-abdominal disease.

3. An 85% to 94% incidence of **good to excellent pain relief** has been obtained in several large series of patients undergoing neurolytic celiac plexus blocks for pain from pancreatic cancer itself,[35] or from a variety of intra-abdominal conditions,[36,37] although repetition is required in some patients. In a series of 136 patients, analgesia was present until the time of death in 102 patients (75%), and in another 17 patients (12.5%), pain relief was maintained for more than 50% of survival time.[35]

4. The **location of the celiac plexus** deep within the retroperitoneum near the vertebral column and in close proximity to major vessels (aorta, vena cava, and their branches) and viscera (kidneys, pleura) provides the **potential for complications of devastating proportions:**
   a. Pneumothorax
   b. Chylothorax
   c. Pleural effusion
   d. Convulsions
   e. Paraplegia

5. Nevertheless, the results of several large series indicate that, given sufficient attention to detail, the **incidence of complications should be minimal.** In a series of 136 patients, the only complication of any significance was pneumothorax, which occurred in 2 patients, neither of whom required tube thoracotomy.[35] Also, of 114 blocks performed in another group of 100 patients, the only significant complication was partial unilateral lower extremity paralysis in an obese patient who could not be positioned properly.[36] Postural hypotension and diarrhea occur frequently but are usually self-limiting.

6. **To produce optimal results**[37,38]
   a. At the level of the **inferior border of the twelfth rib, an insertion site no greater than 7.0 to 7.5 cm lateral** to the corresponding spinous process is desirable to avoid renal puncture.
   b. Two needles should be utilized.
   c. Through each needle **25 ml of solution** should be injected.
   d. Proper **depth of insertion** may slightly exceed that which has been traditionally taught.
   e. The **left-sided needle tip should be placed at the junction of the lower and middle thirds of the first lumbar vertebral body,** and the **right-sided needle tip 1 cm higher.**
   f. When the **celiac artery** can be identified, **injection** should be planned **0.5 to 1.0 cm below its origin.**

7. When neurolytic solutions are to be injected, **radiographic verification is desirable** from medicolegal and technical standpoints. The use of a CT scan adds to the cost, procedure time, and logistic difficulties but provides improved documentation of the spread of injectate and relationships between needle trajectory, viscera, and vasculature.

L. **Superior hypogastric block**
   1. Pelvic pain can be caused by **malignancy of a pelvic organ** and is often somatic, visceral, or both. The pelvic organs are innervated by both somatic and sympathetic fibers. In advanced pelvic malignancy, the incidence of pain can be as high as 95%.
   2. **A select group of patients require neuroablative and neurolytic procedures** when other modalities fail to relieve intractable pain. The technique requires adequate support of biplanar radiologic facilities as well as a well-trained physician, as injury to sacral nerve fibers or to hollow viscus (i.e., rectum, bladder, or ureter) can occur.

III. **Conclusion**
   A. **Patient selection and education are essential,** as there are very real limitations, complications, and side effects that must be accepted before the placement of such a block. Such preliminary discussions are also helpful in avoiding legal proceedings by an already litigious population.
   B. **Neurolytic nerve blocks offer an excellent option for the physician in the fight**

to control cancer pain. Their success is mostly dependent on the individual patient, the patient's understanding and cooperation, and the experience of the physician. With proper training and experience, such blocks can be easily utilized to help provide relief.

References

1. Bonica JJ. *Management of Pain.* Philadelphia: Lea & Febiger, 1954. Pp. 672–701.
2. Cousins MJ, Bridenbaugh PO (eds.). *Neural Blockade* (2nd ed.). Philadelphia: J.B. Lippincott, 1988.
3. Raj PP (ed.). *Practical Management of Pain.* Chicago: Year Book Medical Publishers, 1986. Pp. 857–858.
4. Cousins MJ, Bridenbaugh PO. *Neural Blockade in Clinical Anesthesia and Management of Pain.* Philadelphia: J.B. Lippincott, 1980.
5. Gallagher HS, Yonezawa T, Hoy RC, Derrick WS. Subarachnoid alcohol block: II. Histologic changes in the central nervous system. *Am J Pathol* 38:679–693, 1961.
6. Nathan PW, Scott TG. Intrathecal phenol for intractable pain. Safety and dangers of method. *Lancet* 1:76–80, 1958.
7. Nathan PW, Sears TA, Smith MC. Effects of phenol solution on the serve roots of the cats: an electrophysiological and histological study. *J Neurol Sci* 2:7–29, 1965.
8. Nourj Eldin F. Preliminary report uptake of phenol by vascular and brain tissue. *Microvasc Res* 2:224–225, 1970.
9. Pappo I, Visca A. Phenol rhizotomy in the treatment of cancer pain. *Anesth Analg* 53:6, 1974.
10. Maher RM. Neurone selection in relief of pain. Further experiences with intrathecal injection. *Lancet* 1:6–19, 1957.
11. Iggo A, Walsh EG. Selective block of small fibers in the spinal roots by phenol. *Brain* 83:701–708, 1960.
12. Racz GB, Sabonghy M, Gintautas J. Intractable pain therapy using a new epidural catheter. *JAMA* 24B:579–581, 1982.
13. Korevaar WC, Kline MT, Donnelly CC. Thoracic epidural neurolysis using alcohol. *Pain* S4:T33, 1987.
14. Holland AJC, Youssef M. A complication of subarachnoid phenol blockade. *Anaesthesia* 34:260–262, 1979.
15. Madrid JL, Bonica JJ. Cranial nerve blocks. *Adv Pain Res Ther* 2:347–355, 1979.
16. Simon DL, Carron H, Rowlingson JC. Treatment of bladder pain with transsacral nerve block. *Anesth Analg* 61:46–48, 1983.
17. Bonica JJ. The management of pain of malignant disease with nerve blocks. *Anesthesiology* 15:280–301, 1954.
18. Swerdlow M. Intrathecal neurolysis. *Anaesthesia* 33:733–740, 1978.
19. Smith MC. Histological findings following intrathecal injections of phenol solutions for relief of pain. *Br J Anaesth* 36:387–406, 1963.
20. Peyton WT, Semansky EJ, Baker AB. Subarachnoid injection of alcohol for relief of intractable pain with discussion of cord changes found at autopsy. *Am J Cancer* 30:709, 1937.
21. Stewart WA, Lourie H. An experimental evaluation of the effects of subarachnoid injections of phenol-pantopaque in cats: a histological study. *J Neurosurg* 20:64–72, 1963.
22. Ischia S, Luzzani A, Ischia A, et al. Subarachnoid neurolytic block (L5–T) and unilateral percutaneous cervical cordotomy in the treatment of pain secondary to pelvic malignant disease. *Pain* 20:139–149, 1984.
23. Takagi Y, Koyama T, Yamamoto Y. Subarachnoid neurolytic block with 15% phenol glycerine in the treatment of cancer pain. *Pain* S4:T33, 1987.
24. Katz J. Current role of neurolytic agents. *Adv Neurol* 4:471–476, 1974.
25. Stovner J, Endresen R. Intrathecal phenol for cancer pain. *Acta Anaesth Scand* 16:17–21, 1972.
26. Swerdlow M. Spinal and peripheral neurolysis for managing Pancoast syndrome. *Adv Pain Res Ther* 4:135–144, 1982.
27. Pagni CA. Neurosurgical treatment: status of the problem. *Adv Pain Res Ther* 4:165–182, 1982.
28. White JC, Sweet WHL. *Pain and the Neurosurgeon: A 40-Year Experience.* Springfield, IL: Charles C. Thomas, 1969.

29. DeBacker LJ, Kienzle WK, Keasling HH. A study of stellate ganglion block for pain relief. *Anesthesiology* 20:618–623, 1959.
30. Warfield CA, Crews DA. Use of stellate ganglion blocks in the treatment of intractable limb pain in lung cancer. *Clin J Pain* 3:13–15, 1987.
31. Mullin V. Brachial plexus block with phenol for painful arm associated with Pancoast's syndrome. *Anesthesiology* 53:431–433, 1980.
32. Watson CPN, Evans RJ. Intractable pain with cancer of the rectum. *Pain Clin* 1:29–34, 1986.
33. Rohde J, Hankeimeier U. Neurolytic caudal blocks for the relief of perianal cancer pain. *Pain* S4:T32, 1987.
34. Lofstrom JB, Cousins MJ. Sympathetic neural blockade of upper and lower extremity. In Cousins MJ, Bridenbaugh PO (eds.), *Neural Blockade* (2nd ed.). Philadelphia: J.B. Lippincott, 1988. Pp. 461–500.
35. Brown DL, Bulley CK, Quiel EC. Neurolytic celiac plexus block for pancreatic cancer pain. *Anesth Analg* 66:869–873, 1987.
36. Thompson GE, Moore DC, Bridenbaugh PO, et al. Abdominal pain and alcohol celiac plexus nerve block. *Anesth Analg* 56:1–5, 1977.
37. Moore DC, Bush WH, Burnett LL. Celiac plexus block: a roentgenographic, anatomic study of technique and spread of solution in patients and corpses. *Anesth Analg* 60:369–379, 1981.
38. Ward EM, Rorie DK, Nauss LA, et al. The celiac ganglia in man: normal anatomic variations. *Anesth Analg* 58:461–465, 1979.

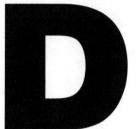

Psychological Approaches

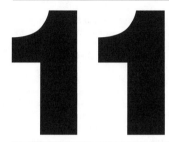

Psychological Assessment in Chronic Pain Syndrome

N. Timothy Lynch
Douglas R. Lyman

I. **Background.** Psychological assessment of patients with chronic pain is extremely important both for its diagnostic value and for treatment planning.[1] At the first visit, every patient should be evaluated by a clinical psychologist and should complete a psychological data-base profile.[2] The psychologist is an important part of the multidisciplinary approach that characterizes successful chronic pain management.

   A. **Psychological models** and approaches to the treatment of chronic pain have gained increased popularity since the 1940s. Co-evolving with innovative treatment approaches, psychological evaluation has improved the clinical and scientific understanding of the chronic pain syndrome. Several factors have contributed to the rise of the psychological contribution in evaluation and treatment of patients with persistent pain:

   1. The **failure of purely somatic etiologic treatment** to manage chronic pain
   2. The contribution of psychology in the **development of innovative treatments**
   3. The **increasing acceptance of various psychological models** such as operant conditioning and cognitive-behavioral modification in explaining adjustment to chronic pain

   B. **The definition of psychological assessment** is the application of various standardized and nonstandardized tests, clinical interviews, observations of patient behavior, a review of social systems, and available medical records to help treating staff and the patient attain mastery of persistent pain and reach patient-defined goals.

   C. **Objectives of psychological evaluation**
   1. **To identify the patient's responses** to persistent pain and evaluate the consequences of each response
   2. **To identify environmental factors** that have shaped and maintained inappropriate or nonadaptive antalgic behavior
   3. **To identify personality factors** contributing to the acquisition and maintenance of antalgic behavior such as affect, motivation, and cognition
   4. **To assess goals** of the patient and factors influencing goal attainment
   5. **To establish an appropriate plan of treatment**
   6. **To continually assess** the patient's **improvement** in treatment and determine additional treatment if necessary
   7. **To determine future needs** and challenges to generalization of acquired skills

   D. **When to consider a psychological assessment.** Pain clinics should routinely provide a psychological evaluation as a standard part of the initial clinic visit. Psychological evaluation should include assessment of the following:
   1. Evidence of significant **lifestyle change,** including disruption within vocational, avocational, and social functions
   2. Evidence of **medication mismanagement,** misuse, abuse, and addiction
   3. **Medical noncompliance,** including failed therapy appointments, inordinate demands on medical services, or difficulty communicating with caregivers, employers, and family
   4. **Antalgic behavior** beyond what objective findings would suggest is reasonable
   5. **Significant change in mood** with the presence of psychological distress, including depression, anxiety, excessive irritability, fear, and anger
   6. The existence of **secondary gain,** including litigation and monetary payments **for ongoing pain and disability**

   E. **Differentiation between types of pain**
   1. **Acute pain,** frequently the result of injury, disease, or surgery, is a biologic signal typically leading to activities promoting healing and the elimination of

pain. When the individual combines various approaches such as rest, seeking medical advice, worry, and eliciting sympathy, healing begins to take place. The intensity of pain eventually begins to subside and continues to subside until it stops altogether and a healing plateau is reached. Pain in the acute phase is a symptom of underlying pathology and physical duress.

2. **Chronic pain,** however, may become a disease entity unto itself. Symptoms associated with persistent pain include depression, avoidance behavior, dependency, medication abuse, sleep disruption, and physical deconditioning. Chronic pain syndrome cannot be treated effectively unless the psychological and vocational issues are addressed. Unlike acute pain, the motivational, behavioral, affective, social, sensory, and cognitive aspects of each patient with chronic pain need to be understood to develop and determine the most appropriate course of treatment. Psychological evaluation is a critical first step in achieving these ends.

3. **Cancer pain.** There is growing recognition of the psychological sequelae of cancer pain and the need for increased use of narcotic analgesics to manage cancer pain appropriately.

4. **AIDS-related pain.** Patients with AIDS and HIV have specific pain treatment requirements and should be treated differently from patients with acute, chronic, or cancer pain. Psychological treatment is more complex owing to the involvement, for example, of subcortical dementia.[3]

II. **Spheres of psychological functioning**
   A. **Sensory sphere.** The patient's sensory experience is frequently an indicator of adjustment to persistent pain. However, because pain is a private experience, assessment strategies are always subjective and unique to each individual. It is difficult to determine whether patients responding similarly to sensory questions are experiencing comparable pain feelings. The location, subjective experience of pain, reasons for pain increase, and methods of pain relief are most commonly assessed.

   B. **Cognitive sphere.** Recent concepts of pain, most noticeably the gate-control theory, view the experience of pain as a function of motivational and cognitive influences.[4] For example, effective coping strategies and skills have been associated with positive patient outcome. A patient's use of self-control strategies seems to be considerably influenced by beliefs regarding effectiveness and outcome.[5]

   C. **Emotive sphere.** Depression and anxiety are universally observed among those with persistent pain. While anxiety, for instance, may motivate an individual to seek medical attention for acute pain, anxiety associated with persistent pain may lead to increased muscle tension exacerbating painful symptoms. Depression adversely affects motivation, sleep quality, and the frequency of antalgic behavior. Excessive anger isolates the patient and has adverse social implications.

   D. **Behavioral and social sphere.** Fordyce suggests that the chronic pain syndrome should be viewed in the same fashion as other acquired behaviors.[6] Antalgic behaviors, initially performed to minimize discomfort, are selectively shaped by environmental contingencies and maintained by various schedules of reinforcement in ways described by B.F. Skinner and other behaviorists. Furthermore, the environment provides antecedents that serve as cues for various types of pain behavior. Behavioral techniques such as extinction of inappropriate behaviors and reinforcement of adaptive behaviors are an essential part of the pain rehabilitation protocol. Possible pain reinforcers to be considered are compensation, avoidance of responsibilities through pain behavior, attention from spouse and other family members, time off from an unpleasant job, and drug misuse or addiction.

   Furthermore, the patient's past history of adjustment in medical, family, vocational, and educational settings provides meaningful insight into how the patient has dealt with challenges in the past, including any previous compensable injuries.

III. **Psychological assessment techniques.** A psychologist evaluating a patient with chronic pain should be aware that the patient may believe that the referring source thinks the pain is imaginary and must be prepared to answer questions and respond to patient concerns. Failure to do so may further enhance the level of suspiciousness many pain patients already harbor. **As a general rule, it is reasonable to believe that the patient has real pain** and sincerely convey that belief at the time of the initial contact.

   A. **Review of the available medical history** prior to the evaluation is as important with patients with chronic pain as with any other type of patient. An expeditious approach is to send the patient a structured questionnaire to be completed before the interview. A questionnaire helps to prepare a logical sequence of questions regarding patients' pain problems, but also suggests to patients that an effort has been made to understand their problems and challenges. Many patients are reluctant to repeat their entire medical history, and a structured questionnaire may reduce the emotionally trying task of repeating the nature of their pain. A structured questionnaire should minimally contain the following information:

1. The referral source
2. Demographics such as age, marital status, and educational experience
3. The location, duration, and etiology of the pain
4. A brief review of prior interventions (surgery, physical therapy modalities, psychotherapy, work-hardening)
5. Medication use
6. Litigation status
7. Short-term as well as long-term goals for treatment

B. **The clinical interview** is a good opportunity to
   1. **Assess the subjective nature of the pain experience**
   2. **Observe antalgic behavior**
   3. **Assess patients'** own **beliefs** regarding their condition
   4. **Assess** the **premorbid functioning** of the individual:
      a. An inconsistent work record
      b. History of drug abuse
      c. Psychiatric history
      d. Functioning in the family
      e. Employment, educational and avocational background
      f. Level of cognitive functioning and intelligence
   5. **Review contingencies** for pain behavior
   6. **Evaluate symptoms** of chronic pain:
      a. **Sleep disturbance**
         (1) Ability to initiate sleep
         (2) Ability to maintain sleep
         (3) Early awakening
         (4) Quality of sleep including restfulness and any disruption of REM sleep
      b. **Review medication use**
      c. **Review mood changes**
      d. **Note evidence of posttraumatic stress syndrome** in cases of traumatic accident
   7. **Determine an appropriate treatment protocol:**
      a. Inpatient or outpatient pain management program
      b. A work-hardening program, typically with the focused goal of returning to the previous job after extensive reconditioning
      c. Physical therapy
      d. Occupational therapy
      e. Vocational counseling
      f. Psychotherapy
      g. Psychiatric consultation
      h. Family counseling
      i. Treatment for alcoholism or abuse of licit and illicit drugs
      j. No treatment

C. **Observation of antalgic behavior**
   1. Patients convey pain to others through various behaviors. In acute stages of pain, these behaviors may serve to lessen discomfort and promote healing. As pain progresses for months and possibly years, antalgic behaviors are likely to come under control of **environmental contingencies.** A careful observer may be able to notice the presence of such behaviors within the clinical interview. If possible, observation should be conducted under varying conditions to assess the reliability of antalgic behaviors and the antecedents of such behavior. Frequently, antalgic behavior may be more pronounced in the presence of a spouse or when discussing litigation. Fordyce suggests that operant factors may influence pain behavior in three distinct ways:[7]
      a. **Positive reinforcement** of pain and disability behavior
      b. **Negative reinforcement** of avoidant behavior
      c. **Extinction of adaptive well behavior**

2. Examples of pain behavior include
  a. Unsolicited **verbal complaints** of pain
  b. Vocal intonations—moaning, gasping, sighing
  c. Nonverbal presentations of pain
    (1) Gait that is unusually slow or guarded or inappropriate use of assistive devices such as canes and crutches
    (2) Inability to sit for more than 30 minutes—frequently patients will estimate their sitting tolerance as much less than the time they spent sitting in the interview
    (3) Unusual standing posture and excessive muscle tension
    (4) Facial expression, including grimacing and wincing
    (5) Excessive muscle tension
    (6) Palliative pain behavior—such as rubbing, holding, and bracing. Many patients have kinesophobia or specific fears of movement. They are motivated to avoid behaviors that are believed to increase discomfort. The patient enters into an endless cycle of avoidance and deconditioning, which can increase pain, leading to further avoidance.
D. Specific assessment questionnaires. Objective tests are being increasingly utilized in the assessment of the chronic pain patient. Many techniques have been designed specifically with the persistent pain population in mind. Other questionnaires have been standardized on dissimilar populations and have been extended to those with chronic pain.
1. Subjective pain reports
  a. The McGill Pain Questionnaire (MPQ) has found considerable popularity among clinicians and researchers in the area of pain. Unlike the Minnesota Multiphasic Personality Inventory and the SCL-90-R, the relationship to pain is readily identified by the patient. The MPQ consists of 102 words related specifically to the experience of pain. These words have been categorized into three major classes: sensory, affective, and evaluative qualities. Adjectives in each of 20 subgroups are ranked such that the first word implies the least discomfort and the last word in a group represents the most discomfort. Derived measures are the pain-rating index, the number of words chosen, and the present pain intensity.
  The MPQ has been found to discriminate successfully between various painful conditions, as well as between those patients with objective and no objective findings for pain. Elevated affective scores, which have been associated with increased suffering, correlate with greater sickness impact, hostility, anxiety,[8] and emotional disturbance independent of pain intensity.[9] The senior author (N.T.L.) has found that those with an elevated sensory score have a less favorable response to treatment. The MPQ is easy to administer, and most patients have few complaints. It is also an effective tool to monitor progress of treatment.
  b. The Dartmouth Pain Questionnaire (DPQ) was initially introduced as an adjunct to the MPQ.[10] This scale consists of four objective measures including the number of pain complaints, types of somatic interventions, extent of impaired functioning, and level of adaptive functioning, as well as a subjective measure assessing changes in mood secondary to persistent pain. The DPQ is relatively easy to administer and yields a ratio score comparing adaptive to nonadaptive pain behaviors. Although receiving little attention in the pain literature, the DPQ has very good reliability and validity, is an acceptable predictor of pain clinic outcome, and has utility as a research tool.
  c. Numerical and visual analogue scales. Two strategies to assess the strength of pain are the numerical scales and the visual analogue scale (VAS).[11]
    (1) The numerical scale is a unidimensional scale in which patients assign a number value to their pain. Typically the scale extends from 0 to 10 or from 0 to 100, where 0 is no pain and 10 or 100 is the maximal pain one can experience.
    (2) With the VAS the patient is presented with a 10-cm line that represents the pain experience. The anchor "no pain" is at the far left; the anchor "unbearable" is on the far right. Both measures are easy to use from the clinician's and patient's perspective and can be used as a state measurement of discomfort.
  d. Pain drawings have a diagnostic utility in that they may reveal dermatomal, sclerotomal, and myotomal distributions. Unusual distributions within the

pain drawing may have psychological significance. A number of studies have found an association between atypical distributions and magnification of pain symptoms on the drawings associated with distress on other psychological tests.

2. **Cognitive-behavioral sphere.** Several questionnaires have been developed to objectively assess cognitive strategies such as distraction, instructional self-talk, imagery, and education.

   a. **Coping Strategies Questionnaire (CSQ).** Rosenstiel and Keefe developed a Likert-type scale to assess the types of strategies pain patients use to tolerate pain.[5] Those patients employing active skills such as diverting attention, reinterpreting sensations, and using appropriate self-statements make better adjustments to their situations and endorse fewer catastrophizing statements. The strategies are

      (1) Diverting attention
      (2) Reinterpreting pain sensations
      (3) Calming self-statements
      (4) Ignoring pain sensations
      (5) Praying and hoping
      (6) Catastrophizing
      (7) Increasing activity

   b. **Vanderbilt Multidimensional Pain Inventory (VMPI).** Nicassio et al reported the results of a 27-item self-report questionnaire that assesses the frequency with which patients use various active or passive coping strategies.[12] Those scoring higher on the **active scale** reported less depression, greater self-efficacy, and less physical impairment. Those with elevated scores on the **passive scale** reported increased depression, increased pain, and higher functional impairment.

   c. **Health locus of control.** Based on the original work of Rotter,[13] Wallston and his coworkers have suggested that the locus of control is an effective concept in understanding how patients attempt to control their response to health-related problems. Wallston suggests three orthogonal dimensions reflecting an internal or external approach. The **multidimensional health locus of control (MHLC) scales** are internality, chance or luck, and powerful others. Several studies suggest that increases on the chance and powerful others scales are associated with depression, the presence of compensation, and the belief that luck is the predominant factor in achieving good health. Lyman failed to find a substantial difference on the MHLC scales between pain patients with successful and unsuccessful outcome.[14] Attitudes toward health may not reflect attitudes toward pain control. Lyman rewrote the items of the MHLC to reflect an orientation toward self-control of pain and found that increased internal scores were associated with more frequent use of distraction and affirmative self-statements in response to pain. Patients with increased chance scores were more likely to catastrophize and demonstrate more incidents of pain behavior. Addressing the assumptions and expectation of control are important factors in outcome of treatment.

   d. **The Multidimensional Pain Inventory (MPI)** was designed as a broad-spectrum assessment device based on cognitive-behavioral theory that includes subjective, behavioral, and psychophysiological scales:[15]

      (1) Section I
         (a) Interference—the degree to which pain interferes with normal daily activities
         (b) Support—the amount of attention the spouse directs toward the pain behavior of the patient
         (c) Pain severity—the subjective severity of the pain as well the reported level of suffering associated with pain
         (d) Life control—the extent to which the patient is able to deal with problems in the immediate past
         (e) Affective distress—the immediate mood state

      (2) Section II
         (a) Punishing responses—the frequency with which the patient's pain behavior is met with irritation, frustration, or anger by the spouse or significant other
         (b) Soliciting responses—the degree to which the spouse is encouraging of antalgic behavior

        (c) Distracting responses—the distractive techniques the spouse invokes to assist the patient to be less attentive to pain

   (3) Section III, a sampling of the patient's reports of activities at and away from home

        (a) Household chores

        (b) Outdoor work

        (c) Activities away from the home

        (d) Social activities

        (e) General activity level

   (4) The MPI is a valid and reliable instrument that correlates well with such affective measures as the Beck Depression Inventory, Depression Adjective Checklist, and State-Trait Anxiety Inventory. **Strengths** of the MPI are that

        (a) It is easily administered.

        (b) The relationship to pain is obvious for the patient.

        (c) It is a multidimensional tool that combines patient beliefs, environmental contingencies, and their effects on behavior.

3. Emotive sphere. Researchers have suggested that pain tolerance is an important aspect of coping with pain. Pain tolerance appears to be mainly influenced by the psychological state of the individual. Tolerance is increased by diminished affective arousal, distraction, and motivation. A careful evaluation of the emotional state of the patient is important to understand the pain experience.

  a. The Beck Depression Inventory (BDI) is a 21-item questionnaire yielding an overall depression index. Items reflect psychomotor retardation, disruption in social, sexual, and daily routines, the presence of depressed affect, and suicidal ideation. The BDI is relatively easy to administer and can be used to assess response to antidepressant medication and treatment.

  b. The State-Trait Anxiety Inventory (STAI) is a psychological test that measures both state and trait aspects of anxiety.[16] State anxiety refers to levels of anxious arousal that fluctuate over time. Trait anxiety is a more stable dimension of anxiety that is relatively consistent over time. State anxiety appears to increase as the patient completes pain clinic treatment but typically falls below pretreatment levels 1 or 2 months after treatment. Many patients, as discharge nears, become uncertain of their ability to use acquired skills outside a supportive environment. Tests such as the STAI can help in identifying individuals who may need further support as the time for discharge approaches.

  c. SCL-90-R is a commercially available 90-item questionnaire that generally takes approximately 25 minutes to complete.[17] Scales include obsessiveness, interpersonal sensitivity, depression, anxiety, hostility, phobic anxiety, paranoid ideation, and psychoticism. The SCL-90-R also may be helpful in uncovering a number of unmentioned symptoms, including headaches, hyperventilation, and suicidal ideation.

    (1) Generally, the SCL-90-R is more palatable to the patient than the longer, more probing Minnesota Multiphasic Personality Inventory.

    (2) Patients are given a choice of five responses, which gives an indication of strength of behavior.

    (3) It is a state-oriented questionnaire and may be used to measure change as a result of treatment.

  d. The Minnesota Multiphasic Personality Inventory (MMPI and MMPI-2) remains one of the most frequently used questionnaires among pain clinics.[18] Recent scoring techniques offer specific interpretative reports that address issues important to understanding the pain patient. Several studies have found that the MMPI is **not a strong tool in predicting pain treatment outcome;** nevertheless, it can be **immensely helpful in assessing emotional distress and personality factors** influencing treatment. Unlike many other personality questionnaires, the MMPI has several validity scales that indicate potential motivations of the patient.

    Clinical scales of the MMPI include hypochondriasis, depression, hysteria, psychopathic deviate, masculine/feminine, paranoia, psychasthenia, schizophrenia, hypomania, and social introversion. The MMPI can be interpreted clinically or by using actuarial techniques. Clinical interpretation can usually be done by an experienced clinician who uses past experiences and knowledge to draw a clinical picture. The actuarial method is bound by statistical profiles and is frequently labeled as a "cookbook" approach. A limitation of the actuarial method is that an elevation of a single score may be a false-positive result. Many patients will yield a profile with an elevated schizophrenic score, which does not suggest the presence of psychosis, but rather signifies alienation and confusion. This can be explained by the patient's having lost a job, experienced role reversal in the family, or taking large amounts of narcotic pain medication.

The most common configuration of the original MMPI is the elevation of the hypochondriasis, depression, and hysteria scales, frequently referred to as the "conversion V." This does not imply that the nature of the pain is nonorganic, but may forewarn of the aptness of the patient to demonstrate antalgic behaviors. **Several problems** have been experienced with the use of the MMPI.

(1) The **original MMPI** in its full form is **567 questions long,** which can take up to 3 hours to complete. Many patients who cannot sit longer than 30 minutes balk considerably at the length of the test. The **shorter version of 399 questions** does not allow for the scoring of specialty scales such as the low back pain scale and the manifest anxiety scale. We have not found the 168-question version to be helpful.

(2) Many questions of the original MMPI suggest to the patient an underlying **assumption of imaginary pain, malingering, or psychopathology.** This has been somewhat reduced with the MMPI-2, but nevertheless continues. We have found that administration of the MMPI is best reserved for selected patients after inclusion into the pain management program. Frustration is frequently registered regarding the redundancy of many of the items.

(3) Many patients have difficulties responding comfortably in the **true/false format** and leave many items without a response. Furthermore, the true/false format may have limitations in measuring change before and after treatment.

(4) **Misinterpretation** of the MMPI is quite problematic, especially if the clinician is unfamiliar with the content of each scale or is unfamiliar with chronic pain and typical chronic pain patient profiles. For example, a study reported by Ahern et al suggested a higher rate of neuroticism among pain patients with headaches.[19] In their sample, headache patients had higher hypochondriasis, depression, and hysteria scales than a nonheadache group. Each of these scales, however, has at least several items reflecting headache activity. When the headache items are removed from analysis, there does not appear to be an appreciable difference after all.

4. Vocational sphere: Career Assessment Inventory (CAI). It is important to assess how individuals relate to their work environment. Frequently a mismatch exists in which patients have little in common with their jobs. This factor may have significant implications for return-to-work issues and motivation. The CAI has 370 items using a Likert-type response format in which the patient can respond "like a lot," "like somewhat," "indifferent," "dislike somewhat," or "dislike a lot" to areas of interest that include activities, school subjects, and occupations.[20] The CAI determines the strength of interest in six major groups:

a. Realistic—reflects an interest in working tools, with little social interaction

b. Investigative—indicates an interest in science and mathematics, with solving problems as a central interest

c. Artistic—indicates interest in self-expression through artistic media

d. Social—indicates that the person is good at solving problems of a personal nature and helping others and is comfortable working in groups

e. Enterprising—suggests an appeal for sales and business

f. Conventional—indicates a person who prefers jobs in which novelty is minimal and feels most comfortable in nonleadership roles

E. Psychophysiologic responses. Biofeedback is an adjunct treatment and assessment procedure that has been utilized extensively in pain rehabilitation treatment programs.[21,22] The types of biofeedback that have been most frequently utilized are

1. Electromyography

2. Thermal biofeedback
3. Electrodermal response
4. The purpose of these measurements has been pedagogic (instructing a patient in electromyographic muscle relaxation) and clinical (observing the patient's electrodermal response to emotionally latent topics). The global measures of thermal biofeedback have been useful in an introductory biofeedback intervention because of its ease of interpretation and patient comprehension (measurement units such as temperature versus microvolts) and ease of demonstrable control.

IV. **Diagnosis.** DSM-IV provides a number of diagnostic categories that include pain among the decision criteria or as an adjunct symptom.

A. **Somatoform disorders** are typified by a constellation of symptoms that suggest a physical disorder without demonstrable organic objective findings.

1. **Conversion disorder (300.11)** is associated with the loss or alteration of motor or sensory function. The physical manifestation is preceded by stressors or conflict. The symptoms are not under willful control as seen in malingering. Social, family, and vocational spheres are disrupted.

2. **Hypochondriasis (300.7)** is characterized by fear of disease with physical symptoms. Frequently, the preoccupation will continue despite contrary and objective evidence and reassurance that the condition does not exist. Impairment in social and occupational function is noted.

3. **Somatization disorder (300.81)** is characterized by a frequent number of unintentionally produced somatic complaints beginning before age 30. Most are vague, dramatic, resistant to medical intervention, and without organic pathology. Impairment is grossly in excess of what the physical findings would suggest.

4. **Pain disorder (307.80)** is characterized by unintentionally produced pain causing significant distress. Psychological factors are involved in onset as well as maintenance of pain.

B. **Factitious disorder (300.16)** represents an intentional production of physical symptoms that are under the control of the patient. Unlike malingering, symptoms are clearly not produced for financial gain or to avoid specific activities. These activities are frequently of a compulsive nature; the patient may have a need to assume the sick role.

C. **Psychological factors affecting a medical condition (316.00).** In this condition, an actual demonstrable physical condition exists. However, psychological and environmental conditions contribute to the severity of the problem. Stress-related physiologic responses cause symptoms of the medical condition. Tension headaches are an example of this diagnostic entity.

D. **Adjustment disorder (309.00)** characterizes the response many patients have to a persistent and unresolved physical condition. The reaction to pain may include impairment in the various spheres of functioning with an overreaction to pain or stress. Frequently, this disorder is accompanied by depressed or anxious mood, which differentiates this disorder from psychological factors affecting a physical condition.

E. **Malingering (V65.2).** In this condition, the patient has intentionally produced deceptive or grossly exaggerated symptoms. Motivation is determined by various incentives in which the patient either avoids responsibility or gains benefits from the sick role. Identification of incentives differentiates malingering from factitious disorder.

V. **Conclusions.** A battery of tests is the most common approach in the complete assessment of the often complex chronic pain syndrome. Several questionnaires, such as the MPQ and DPQ, have validity in the classification of pain and may be used in both predictive and outcome studies but do not offer insight to the extent of depression or thought disorder, as does the MMPI. Other questionnaires such as the CSQ and the MPI can be helpful in determining direction of treatment, the need for family intervention, and education. The STAI assists in discovering contributing factors such as posttraumatic stress syndrome and measuring resolution.

The most accurate and indispensable assessment, however, is the judgment of the experienced clinician, along with behavioral observation, record review, and appropriate, selected diagnostics. Treatment of these complex patients is equally dependent on accurate perception, judgment, and sensitive clinical skill in utilizing information gathered during the assessment.

References

1. Stanton-Hicks M. Upper and lower extremity pain. In Raj PP (ed.), *Practical Management of Pain*. Chicago: Mosby–Year Book, 1992. P. 320.
2. Tollison CD. *Handbook of Chronic Pain Management*. Baltimore: Williams & Wilkins, 1989. P. 657.
3. Lynch NT, Addison RA, Manning B, Glare P. Nonpharmacologic control of pain in HIV. In Carr D (ed.), *La Douleur du SIDA*. Chicago: Robert G. Addison, 1994.
4. Tan SY. Cognitive and cognitive-behavioral methods for pain control: a selective review. *Pain* 12:201–228, 1982.
5. Rosenstiel AK, Keefe FJ. The use of coping strategies in chronic low back pain patients: relationship to patient characteristics and current adjustment. *Pain* 17:33–44, 1983.
6. Fordyce WE. Pain viewed as a learned behavior. In Bonica JJ (ed.), *Advances in Neurology*, Vol. 4. New York: Raven, 1974.
7. Fordyce WE. *Behavioral Methods for Chronic Pain and Illness*. St. Louis: C.V. Mosby, 1976.
8. Kremer E, Atkinson JH. Pain measurement: construct validity of the affective dimension of the McGill Pain Questionnaire with chronic benign pain patients. *Pain* 11:93–100, 1981.
9. McCreary C, Turner J, Dawson E. Principal dimensions of the pain experience and psychological disturbance in chronic low back pain patients. *Pain* 11:85–92, 1981.
10. Corson JA, Schneider MJ. The Darmouth Pain Questionnaire: an adjunct to the McGill Pain Questionnaire. *Pain* 19:56–69, 1984.
11. Reading AE. Testing pain mechanisms in persons with pain. In Wall PD, Melzack R (eds.), *Textbook of Pain*. New York: Churchill Livingstone, 1984.
12. Nicassio PM, Brown GK, Wallston KA, et al. Predictors of pain coping strategies in patients with rheumatoid arthritis. Presented at the Society of Behavioral Medicine Annual Meeting, Vanderbilt University, Nashville, TN, 1987.
13. Rotter JB. *Social Learning and Clinical Psychology*. Engelwood Cliffs, NJ: Prentice-Hall, 1954.
14. Lyman DR. Prediction of chronic pain clinic outcome using psychometric and demographic predictors. Doctoral dissertation, Marquette University, 1988.
15. Turk DC, Rudy TE. Toward an empirically derived taxonomy of chronic pain patients: integration of psychological assessment data. *J Consult Clin Psychol* 56:233–238, 1988.
16. Spielbeger CD. *Manual for the State-Trait Anxiety Inventory*. Palo Alto, CA: Consulting Psychologists Press, 1983.
17. DeRogatis L. *SCL-90-R Administration, Scoring and Procedures Manual* (revised version). Townson, MD: Clinical Psychometric Research, 1983.
18. Butcher NB, Dahlstrom WG, Graham JR, et al. *MMPI-2, Manual for Administration and Scoring*. Minneapolis: University of Minnesota Press, 1989.
19. Ahern DK, Lezzi A, Hursey K, Follick MJ. The co-occurrence of chronic low back pain and headache: prevalence, neuroticism, and treatment outcome. *Clin J Pain* 4:27–31, 1988.
20. Johansson CB. *Career Assessment Inventory*. Minneapolis: National Computer Systems, 1986.
21. Cram J. EMG scanning in the diagnosis of chronic pain. *Biofeedback Self Regul* 2:229–241, 1983.
22. Lynch NT, et al. Persistent pain. Boston: Kluwer Academic, 1988.

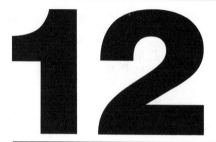

Psychological Aspects of Chronic Pain Management

Allen H. Lebovits
Lynette E. Bassman

I. Background

A. Pain is one of the most complex of human experiences, and it is the most **common symptom** for which people seek medical attention.[1]

B. Pain is defined by the International Association for the Study of Pain as **"an unpleasant sensory and emotional experience associated with actual or potential tissue damage."**[2] Accordingly, the perception of pain is not exclusively reliant on tissue damage or organic dysfunction but, rather, is strongly influenced by psychological, societal, and cultural factors.

C. Chronic pain patients may be difficult to work with because they can be manipulative, noncompliant, and hostile.[3] Pain may be intractable as well, and is associated with depression in many patients.[4,5] A variety of **psychological intervention techniques** have been developed and shown to be efficacious. With proper assessment, these tools can be used to help patients decrease or eliminate their pain, or cope with it more effectively.

D. The **multidisciplinary team approach** is common and advisable because of the complexity of chronic pain.[6,7] Such a team typically consists of an anesthesiologist, a psychologist, a physiatrist, nurses, and a social worker as a minimum; in large pain centers, the team also might include acupuncturists, vocational rehabilitation specialists, neurologists, orthopedists, and neurosurgeons. To receive accreditation from the Commission on Accreditation of Rehabilitation Facilities (CARF), all chronic pain programs must be interdisciplinary and have as part of the core team a psychologist or psychiatrist.

II. Basic concepts of chronic pain

A. Biopsychosocial model. Chronic pain is the end product of physiologic, psychological, and social processes.[1] These biopsychosocial determinants of chronic pain interact with one another: Neurophysiologic responses to noxious stimuli can trigger psychological responses, while psychological states can affect the neurophysiologic system by enhancing or inhibiting the transmission of noxious signals. Environmental influences such as stress, secondary gain, and financial compensation can greatly affect the patient's perceived level of pain intensity. Stress and trauma are often substantially related to pain perception and exacerbation.[8]

B. Acute pain. It is important to recognize the differences between acute pain and chronic pain. The therapeutic management of chronic pain with acute pain therapies not only is inappropriate but also can lead to iatrogenic injury. The distinction between acute and chronic pain is not simply a matter of duration of the symptom.

1. Acute pain most often **leads to anxiety,** which serves as a signal that something is wrong, causing the individual to act to treat the problem and to avoid further damage. When pain becomes chronic, it is often associated with depression.

2. Acute pain **is biologically useful,** while chronic pain loses this function.

3. Acute pain **is a symptom of an underlying medical condition,** but when it is chronic, the pain itself becomes the disease.

4. **The etiology** of acute pain **is almost always known,** while chronic pain is often based on a complex interaction of physical and psychological factors.

5. **Narcotics are often effective** for acute pain, but with chronicity comes the risk of drug addiction. Narcotics are usually contraindicated for chronic benign pain.

6. **Cure and relief are almost always attainable** in acute pain but may not be possible with chronic pain. This is an important therapeutic principle that is often difficult for chronic pain patients to comprehend. Rehabilitation, coping,

and a return to an optimal level of functioning are important goals in chronic pain management.

C. **Chronic pain syndrome (CPS).** The chronic pain patient often loses the motivation to do anything about the pain and to continue his or her normal activities. This is clearly maladaptive with respect to the organism's healing process. In many cases, patients with chronic pain become overly dependent on others; they derive rewards from their pain in the form of increased attention and affection, increased leisure time, and decreased responsibilities. This serves as a disincentive to recovery and further subverts the healing process. Other features of CPS include

1. Constantly **focusing on the pain**
2. **Complaining about the pain**
3. **Dramatic** and observable pain and illness **behavior** (grimacing, groaning, bracing, limping, etc.)
4. **Overuse of medications**
5. **Increased health care utilization**
6. **Family dysfunction.** The spouses of CPS patients also display clinically significant levels of depression and anxiety.[9,10]

D. **Depression.** The most prevalent psychological characteristic of chronic pain patients is depression.[4,5] Depression and chronic pain occur together so frequently that chronic pain has been described as a variant of depressive disorder.[11] It is often difficult to distinguish whether the depression is a precipitant of the pain or a result of living with long-term pain.

E. **Real versus imagined pain**
1. In the chronic pain population, there are patients with pain for which **no physical etiology can be found** or for which multiple diagnostic procedures and consultations are negative, yet the pain does not subside. Alternatively, the pain may follow a distribution not consistent with respect to the underlying anatomic structures. Such pain may respond well to placebo treatments. Given such data, pain specialists often conclude that the pain is "all in the patient's head," and subtly or not so subtly alter their approach to the patient. This often causes the patient to feel angry and threatened, and can also lead to an increase in the severity of the pain.
2. It is important to understand that even though no physical cause can be found for the pain, **the pain is just as real to the patient** as is pain with a known etiology. It is always possible that there is a physical cause that even the most thorough workup has failed to reveal. If the patient reports perceiving pain, we believe the patient and treat the patient as if there were a known discernible cause. The one exception to this is in the case of **factitious disease, or Munchausen syndrome.** In this relatively unusual presentation the patient reports pain perception when none is present, or self-inflicts injury in order to be admitted to hospitals.

III. **Psychological intervention.** The general goal of most psychological interventions with chronic pain patients, particularly with cognitive-behavioral treatment strategies, is to reconceptualize the patient's view of pain from the belief that it is an uncontrollable medical symptom to a belief that the pain is subject to the patient's control.[12]

A. **Relaxation training,** one of the most commonly used psychological interventions with chronic pain patients, can be accomplished in several ways.
1. **Diaphragmatic breathing** is based on the idea that when breathing is calm and slow, thoughts will also tend to slow down and become less troublesome. Focusing attention on the breath distracts the patient from troubling thoughts, unpleasant situations, and pain.
2. In **progressive muscular relaxation** attention is focused on individual muscle groups, which are alternately tensed and relaxed. Patients learn to recognize and differentiate feelings of tension and relaxation. With practice, voluntary relaxation can become nearly automatic and can be achieved quickly. This technique is particularly helpful for patients whose pain prevents them from falling asleep.
3. In **imagery,** the patient concentrates on a multisensory imaginary experience. Relaxation through imagery can be greatly facilitated through hypnosis.

B. **Behavioral therapy** is one of the primary modes of psychological intervention with chronic pain patients.[13] The operant view of pain acquisition is that pain behaviors are often directly and positively reinforced (by well-meaning family

members, friends, or coworkers) and indirectly reinforced by the avoidance of aversive contingencies (negative reinforcers) such as work or marital conflict.
1. The **main objectives** of behavioral therapy for pain management are to
   a. **Reduce the frequency of pain behaviors** such as grimacing, limping, complaining, moaning, clutching, holding, or rubbing the affected area, teeth-clenching, rigid posturing, and requests for pain medications
   b. **Increase functional capabilities**
   c. **Reduce health care utilization**
2. One way that this goal is accomplished is to withdraw reinforcement for pain behaviors and increase rewards for "well" behaviors. A neutral response is given when pain behaviors are exhibited, rather than the increase of attention and nurturance that are so often present in the home. **Rewarding responses** (such as increased attention) are given only when the patient has engaged in healthy behaviors. Very **specific schedules of gradually increasing activity** levels as well as physical exercise are established.
3. **The family of the patient is taught to apply these principles consistently at home** and their resistance to applying these techniques is addressed. Some family members will feel that it is cruel to treat the patient this way, or they may feel that their own role as caretakers is in danger as the patient regains normal healthy functioning.
C. **Cognitive restructuring**
   1. In cognitive restructuring patients are taught to **identify maladaptive themes** that pervade their thinking **and to replace them with more adaptive thoughts.** The maladaptive thoughts often take the form of statements about oneself or the illness that are negative, overgeneralizing, and catastrophizing:
      a. "The pain will never go away."
      b. "Something is terribly wrong with me."
      c. "The pain will lead to hospitalization and surgery."
      d. "My husband hates me because I can't do the things I used to do."
   2. The idiosyncratic thoughts associated with the patient's pain experience are identified, and **alternative positive thoughts** are acknowledged. A list of accurate statements about the pain is generated and rehearsed:
      a. "There are things I can still do."
      b. "Sometimes my pain is not so bad."
D. **Psychotherapy** is an important part of the treatment of many chronic pain patients. Whatever the etiology of the pain, the life of the patient is affected by the pain, and psychological maladjustment often occurs.
   1. In **supportive therapy**, the therapist identifies and reinforces existing coping abilities and encourages the patient to utilize all available social supports.
   2. In **group therapy** patients meet on a weekly basis, with a psychologist as group facilitator, with the following goals:[14]
      a. Help each other develop coping strategies
      b. Provide support
      c. Promote the concept of universality
      d. Be a forum for shared catharsis
   3. **Marital therapy** is indicated when chronic pain serves to "rescue" a failing marriage by providing a new focus to distract the couple from the real conflicts between them. In some couples, the relationship is based on one partner's need to dominate and control and the other partner's need to be dependent. If the pain no longer exists, the relationship is threatened by the equality of roles that then becomes possible. Through marital therapy, the couple can be helped to identify these maladaptive patterns and to develop alternative strategies for balancing their relationship.
   4. **Family therapy** can be useful when the entire family system is affected by the person's pain and is involved in helping maintain the invalid role. Pain can be the symptom of the ills of the entire family system; treating the symptom without treating the roots of the problem—the family dysfunction—will be fruitless.
   5. **Psychoanalytic psychotherapy** can be helpful in cases of pain that is created or maintained by the patient's conscious or unconscious psychological needs. The aim of such therapy is to bring to the patient's awareness the needs that are being fulfilled by the pain and discuss alternative ways of filling those needs.

IV. Complicating factors
 A. Disincentives to recovery
  1. Secondary gain factors include
   a. Avoidance of work and household responsibilities
   b. Interpersonal conflicts
   c. Sexual interactions
  2. Financial disincentives
   a. Worker's compensation due to an injury on the job may lead some individuals to prolong the period of paid unemployment by maintenance of symptoms. When the work is not pleasant and satisfying enough to serve as a powerful reinforcer, and when compensation compares favorably with that available through work, the lure of an extended paid vacation may be difficult to resist.
   b. Patients in **litigation** may feel encouraged to maintain their symptoms until the trial is settled.
 B. Drug addiction. Because potentially addictive drugs are used in the management of pain, patients can become addicted to prescription medications, such as acetaminophen (Tylenol) with codeine, or butalbital (Fiorinal). A careful assessment is necessary to determine whether the patient is manipulating the system to secure medication. It may be necessary to refer the patient to a drug treatment program or to gradually taper the medication while working with the patient to overcome issues of dependency.
 C. Physician–patient interaction
  1. Good communication between the physician and the patient can enhance the rate of compliance with prescribed treatment regimens and strengthen desirable placebo effects. However, the chronic pain patient is particularly frustrating and difficult to treat, not only because of the refractory nature of the pain, but also because of the passive-aggressive, noncompliant, manipulative, and sometimes hostile behavior that can occur.[3]
  2. Intervention in a difficult physician–patient relationship can take the form of
   a. Monitoring the patient's ongoing reactions to the health care provider
   b. Formal educational presentations to the staff or the clinic about negotiating the potential pitfalls involved in maladaptive interactions with chronic pain patients
   c. Individual consultations by the psychologist and **case conferences** with physicians about particularly difficult patients to sort through personal reactions to the patient

References

1. Chapman CR, Bonica JJ. *Chronic Pain.* Kalamazoo, MI: Upjohn Company, 1985.
2. Merskey H. Classification of chronic pain, descriptions of chronic pain syndrome and definitions of pain terms. *Pain* S217 (Suppl 3), 1986.
3. Lebovits AH, Richlin DM. Chronic pain and Crohn's disease: treatment difficulties. *Clin J Pain* 3:31–37, 1987.
4. Romano JM, Turner JA. Chronic pain and depression: does the evidence support a relationship? *Psychol Bull* 97:18–34, 1985.
5. Turk DC, Okifuji A, Scharff L. Chronic pain and depression: role of perceived impact and perceived control in different age cohorts. *Pain* 61:93–101, 1995.
6. Lebovits AH. Chronic pain: the multidisciplinary approach. *Int Anesthesiol Clin* 29:1–7, 1991.
7. Flor H, Fydrich T, Turk DC. Efficacy of multidisciplinary pain treatment centers: a meta-analytic review. *Pain* 49:221–230, 1992.
8. Lebovits AH, Yarmush J, Lefkowitz M. Reflex sympathetic dystrophy and posttraumatic stress disorder: multidisciplinary evaluation and treatment. *Clin J Pain* 6:153–157, 1990.
9. Ahern DK, Adams AE, Follick MJ. Emotional distress and marital disturbance in spouses of chronic low back pain patients. *Clin J Pain* 1:69–74, 1985.
10. Schwartz L, Slater MA, Birchler GR, Atkinson JH. Depression in spouses of chronic pain patients: the role of patient pain and anger, and marital satisfaction. *Pain* 44:61–67, 1991.

11. Blumer D, Heilbronn M. Chronic pain as a variant of depressive disease, the pain prone disorder. *J Nerv Ment Dis* 170:381–406, 1982.
12. Holzman AD, Turk DC, Kerns RD. The cognitive-behavioral approach to the management of chronic pain. In Holzman AD, Turk DC (eds.), *Pain Management—A Handbook of Psychological Treatment Approaches*. New York: Pergamon, 1986. Pp. 31–50.
13. Keefe FJ, Dunsmore J, Burnett R. Behavioral and cognitive-behavioral approaches to chronic pain: recent advances and future directions. *J Consult Clin Psychol* 60:528–536, 1992.
14. Gentry WD, Owens D. Pain groups. In Holzman AD, Turk DC (eds.), *Pain Management—A Handbook of Psychological Treatment Approaches*. New York: Pergamon, 1986. Pp. 100–112.

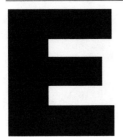

Physical Techniques

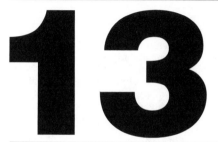

Physical Modalities in Chronic Pain
Rajka Soric

I. **Background.** Pain is often considered a useful physiologic feedback mechanism that enables people to curtail further injury to a particular tissue or part of the body. It serves little other purpose beyond this and ultimately leads to disability and psychosocial strain.

In an acute pain syndrome in which the etiology is usually well established, management can be aimed at the cure of the painful condition by eradicating its cause.[1] In **chronic pain syndromes** in which the cause of the pain as well as the underlying pathophysiologic processes are either not known or not curable, **symptomatic treatment** of pain is resorted to. Treatments should be started with the most benign modalities progressing to those with more serious side effects to ensure that the treatment does not result in a condition worse than the illness itself.

To provide the maximum benefit and restore the patient to optimal function, **each indicated modality should be given a fair trial,** in which two or more modalities should never be simultaneously used, as it will be difficult to know which one is providing the relief. On the other hand, simultaneous therapy with more than one therapeutic modality may ultimately be required. Physical modalities should be used with caution and carefully assessed at regular intervals so that the efficacy of the treatment may be evaluated.

II. **Therapeutic heat**

A. **Effects.** The therapeutic effects of heat may be local or distant. At the cellular level, heat increases the metabolic rate, nerve conduction velocity, and muscle contractility.[2] Because heat also stimulates inflammation, it will enhance pain when applied to superficial inflamed tissue, as when a patient with severe sunburn takes a hot shower.[2] On the other hand, if pain occurs as a result of accumulated metabolites in a poorly perfused area, applied heat will cause vasodilatation and rapid removal of the pain-producing substances.

Heat is also used as an adjunct to other physical modalities. For example, heating a stiff joint decreases the viscosity of the synovial fluid, thereby facilitating therapeutic stretching.

The **optimal therapeutic effect** of heat is achieved when the tissue temperature is **between 41°C and 45°C** during the treatment session.[3] If the temperature is allowed to rise above 45°C, permanent structural changes in the tissue can occur. Before this happens, however, patients usually experience pain and the modality can be removed before tissue damage occurs.

The distant effects of heat include the consensual vascular response, causing the heat applied to one part of the body to reflexively dilate the vessels in a distant part of the body. The relaxing and sedating effect of heat is also a distant therapeutic effect. The response to heat is influenced by the rate of the temperature change, as well as the temperature itself. In general, vigorous heating is used in more chronic conditions such as stretching out of contractures.[1]

B. **Contraindications.** Because of the theoretical possibility of a burn, patients with **mental confusion** or **grossly impaired sensation** should not be using heat. Further contraindications include **ischemic areas,** acutely inflamed areas, and fresh bleeds. Tissues overlying **malignant growths** should also never be heated for fear of enhanced metabolic activity.

C. **Heating modalities**

1. **Superficial devices** result in a temperature rise of the skin, subcutaneous tissue, and, in some instances, superficial musculature. These include the heating pad, hot water bottle, hydrocollator pack, paraffin wax bath, and heating lamp.

2. **Deep-heating devices** result in a temperature rise in muscles, bones, and deep joints by converting a primary form of energy into heat. The most common clinical indications for the use of deep-heating modalities are chronic or acute inflammatory conditions and soft-tissue shortening. Caution must be exercised not to apply deep-heating modalities over malignant growths or around the eyes, testes, or pregnant uterus, as the heat enhances tissue metabolism.

    a. **Short-wave diathermy.** Radio waves of predetermined frequency are converted into electrical current. Particular attention must be paid to screen the patients who have metallic implants, as these may selectively heat and cause deep burns.[4]

    b. **Ultrasound** utilizes sonic energy that is converted into heat. The ultrasound is applied via a sound head or an applicator that is rhythmically moved over the treatment field, which is either immersed in water or covered with gel.[1] This is the only modality that allows precise dosimetry. If pulsed ultrasound is applied, temperature elevation is minimal and the mechanical effect of the ultrasound is used to loosen adhesions and help resolve edema in inflammatory tissue.

    c. **Microwave diathermy** is the conversion of electromagnetic waves into heat.

III. **Therapeutic cold (cryotherapy)** is a relatively safe, inexpensive, and simple-to-use modality whose physiologic effects are opposite to those produced by heat.[5] Because it also acts as a counterirritant utilizing the gating mechanism, it is often used in chronic conditions as well as in acute inflammatory or traumatic conditions. Ice cubes in plastic bags and massage with ice cubes mounted on a wooden stick are the most commonly used ways of applying cold to the affected areas.[5] Vapocoolant sprays are also used in stretch-and-spray techniques when treating myofascial pain syndromes.

IV. **Transcutaneous electrical nerve stimulation (TENS)** has become a major therapeutic tool and is still gaining in popularity.[1] TENS is discussed more extensively in Chapter 14. The mechanism of its action is still not fully understood. It appears to depend on stimulation frequency, pulse width, and intensity.[6] The analgesic effect of TENS may be achieved through peripheral mechanisms or by altering the level of circulating endorphins and enkephalins. Low-frequency TENS is associated with the central and the peripheral actions of endogenous endorphins, leading to gradual onset of pain relief and elevation of the pain threshold. The rapid onset of analgesia with high-frequency TENS, on the other hand, is most likely achieved through the gating mechanism in the substantia gelatinosa.[7] Sites of electrode placements are most often chosen by trial and error. One usually starts by applying electrodes over the dermatomes, along the course of the peripheral nerve, or simply over the painful area. The efficacy of TENS in chronic pain is less than in acute, shorter-lasting pain.[8] The complicating fact is perhaps the phenomenon of adaptation, which can occasionally be solved by changing the stimulation parameters. TENS is probably **one of the safest modalities** used. Although cardiac arrythmias are not a contraindication for the use of TENS, the presence of **a cardiac pacemaker usually is a contraindication.** Other than minor and transient skin irritations and occasional allergic reactions to the conductive gel or adhesive tape, adverse reactions are exceedingly rare.

V. **Biofeedback** is a process that enables the patient to monitor and influence his or her own bodily function by becoming aware of the degree of muscle contraction. The principle of action is to influence the motor activity, which can be monitored by either visual or auditory output on the electromyograph. Headaches, particularly of migrainous or tension type, have often been treated with biofeedback, and some authors have reported up to a 20% success rate in controlling the latter.[9,10]

VI. **Therapeutic exercise** is underutilized as a treatment modality for chronic pain. It is defined as a prescribed movement of the body or isolated body parts.[2] In many chronic pain patients, the level of activity is severely reduced, which eventually leads to deconditioning. This process is often accompanied by a sense of general fatigue, depression, and poor self-image. To counteract these problems, a set of low-load, rhythmical, and repetitive exercises should be prescribed. The best examples of such activities are walking, swimming, calisthenics, and bicycling. The other type of exercise is the so-called goal-specific exercise that eventually leads to improved strength, endurance, and posture and an increase in generalized mobility.

    A. **Strengthening exercises**

        1. **Isometric exercises** in which the joint does not move are achieved by simultane-

ous contraction of the agonist and the antagonist muscles or by the use of an external force.[2]

   2. **Isotonic exercises,** the most commonly prescribed, are associated with joint movement. They may be achieved either with gravity eliminated or against gravity, and resistance and can be done by the patient alone.
   3. **Isokinetic exercises** are performed through the full range of motion and against constant speed and constant resistance. Muscle is strengthened at all lengths rather than just one. Unfortunately, expensive equipment is required that is not readily available in outpatient clinics.
   B. **Range of motion (stretching) exercises** are used when there is altered joint mobility. An example would be the patient with a marked hip joint contracture who, as a result, develops hyperextension of the lumbar spine. Unless the hip joint contracture is reduced, the patient will inevitably suffer from low back pain because of the stress transmitted through the facet joints as a result of hyperextension. Application of heat prior to stretching will decrease the viscosity of the connective tissue and make stretching easier. Subsequent cooling, on the other hand, will provide a good analgesic effect. Stretching exercises involve a slow, prolonged stretch of a muscle, allowing it to elongate and eventually relax. This is particularly important in spastic patients whose abnormal muscle tone causes pain; however, the effect of these exercises in these patients is often temporary.
   C. **Postural exercises** are beneficial in patients with chronic pain due to abnormal posture, especially those with neck and low back pain. With exaggerated cervical lordosis, shoulders are protracted and the trapezii remain in spasm. In an attempt to restore the posture, visual biofeedback may be used. Patients are instructed to stand in front of the mirror and do the exercises. Unfortunately, only a small percentage of patients are compliant with these exercises on a regular basis.
   D. **Relaxation exercises** are a hypnosis-based tool utilized when chronic muscle contraction is contributing to a patient's pain.[11] The patient is made aware of what it feels like to have the muscles relaxed.
VII. **Laser therapy.** Lasers (light amplification by stimulated emission of radiation) are divided into cold, soft lasers and high-powered, hot lasers depending on the optical energy of the device. The therapeutic effect of the hot laser is based on the properties of light, which when absorbed are transferred into heat.[12] Such thermal effects are lacking in low-powered, cold lasers, which provide energy in the red visible spectrum.
     Laser treatments in patients with chronic pain produce symptomatic analgesia, reduction of edema, enhancement of collagen deposition, and peripheral nerve regeneration. Although the exact mechanism by which these effects are achieved is still unknown, the most frequently cited hypotheses are relief of arterial spasm, excitation of the mitochondrial membranes, and enhanced levels of serum serotonin.[13]
VIII. **Acupuncture.** Although acupuncture originated some 4000 years ago in China, it became an acceptable therapeutic modality in the Western world relatively recently after studies of the neurochemical mechanisms became available, providing scientific explanations for its effects. It is presumed that insertion of the acupuncture needles and their electrical and mechanical stimulation stimulates the inhibitory center for pain in the ventral gray matter, resulting in the release of endorphins.[14]
IX. **Mobilization techniques** are passive exercises directed toward restoration of joint mobility, tissue extensibility, and perfusion.[2]
   A. **Traction** is a distractive force applied to tissue in an attempt to stretch the soft tissues or to distract articulating surfaces. It is used primarily for the cervical and lumbar spine,[2] and it may alleviate radicular pain by decreasing the pressure and irritation of the spinal roots. Although the weights necessary to actually distract the vertebral bodies exceed the weight usually used in practice, many patients obtain relief. It is believed that this relief is a result of stretching the muscles, which leads to their relaxation, thus improving local circulation and achieving an analgesic effect. Another reported benefit of spinal traction is the separation of the facet joints.[14]
     Careful clinical and radiologic assessment of the patient is mandatory before applying traction. **Specific contraindications are spinal malignancy, osteomyelitis of the spine, a bleeding diathesis, severe osteoporosis, vertebrobasilar or carotid artery insufficiency, and severe rheumatoid arthritis of the spine.**[15]
     Cervical traction may be delivered as either a constant or intermittent force.

It may be manual or mechanical and should be applied with the neck in flexion, as this will enhance the vertical diameter of the intervertebral foramina.

Lumbar traction, on the other hand, can only be delivered by an apparatus with special split tables used to minimize friction.[16]

B. **Manipulation** is a forced passive movement, carrying the articular elements beyond the usual physiologic range of motion, which secondarily relieves muscle spasm. This muscle spasm is believed to result from a reversible minor interarticular derangement.[17]

Manipulation may be direct or indirect.[18] In direct manipulation, thrust is applied directly to the structure involved, whereas in indirect manipulation the patient's body is used as a lever. The **same contraindications as** outlined above **for traction** apply for manipulation. Patients usually experience a substantial immediate relief of pain after the manipulation, which reoccurs after 24 hours. In addition to treating the cervical and lumbar spine, manipulation is often beneficial for coccygodynia.[19]

C. **Massage** is the most frequently used mobilization technique. It is recognized in Europe as a therapeutic modality, but not so across the North American continent. Massage has a definitive soothing and relaxing effect, although only temporary. Many believe that its effects include improved tissue perfusion, stretching of shortened soft tissues, resolution of edema, and enhanced removal of metabolic waste products.[16]

Several different massage techniques have been described. In **petrissage,** small areas of the skin and subcutaneous tissue are lifted and pressure is applied by the masseuse's fingers. **Kneading** consists of the same technique, but larger areas of the skin are treated.[17] **Effleurage,** or stroking, which is done with the palm of the hand, may increase the circulation by applying pressure centripetally. **Friction massage,** the most painful of the techniques, is probably the most effective because it loosens adhesions. It entails application of a significant force over a small area of contact between the thumb and finger and the patient's skin, with oil or powder being employed to minimize friction. Certain conditions are considered **contraindications,** such as **open skin areas, suspected deep vein thrombosis, and acute inflammatory processes.**

X. **Hydrotherapy.** Therapeutic water may be heated or cooled, agitated or not. When heated, it brings about relaxation and a sense of well-being. Its buoyancy effects reduce the weight-bearing stresses across the joint. The most often used modes of hydrotherapy are therapeutic pools, Hubbard tanks, and whirlpools.

XI. **Orthotics and assistive devices.** Orthotics can improve the alignment of a particular body part, reduce weight-bearing stresses, and limit painful movement. The most frequently prescribed and used orthotics are the cervical and lumbar supports. Neck braces do not provide pain relief by immobilization but, rather, serve as a reminder to the wearer to maintain proper posture with the added benefit of warmth. Lumbosacral corsets limit the mobility of the spinal segment and unload the axial skeleton by increasing intra-abdominal pressure. Neither of the two is recommended for the chronic pain patient, however, unless very specific indications exist.

In patients who suffer from chronic inflammatory arthritis of the wrist, wrist orthoses are particularly beneficial in reducing movement and thereby decreasing pain.[20]

Assistive devices, such as canes, crutches, walkers, and long-handled reachers, are used when patients are unable to manage their activities of daily living because of pain, or when structural abnormalities present a mechanical barrier in managing a particular function.

References

1. Myers SJ. Psychiatric management of chronic benign pain. In Brisman R (ed.), *Neurosurgical and Medical Management of Pain: Triguinal Neuralgia, Chronic Pain and Cancer Pain.* Boston: Kluwer Academic, 1989. Pp. 113–124.
2. Soric R, Devlin M. Role of physical medicine. In Tollison D (ed.), *Handbook of Chronic Pain Management.* Baltimore: Williams & Wilkins, 1989. Pp. 147–162.
3. Lehman JF, Masock AJ, et al. Effect of therapeutic temperatures on tendon extensibility. *Arch Phys Med Rehabil* 51:481–487, 1970.
4. Lehman JF, DeLateur BJ. Therapeutic heat. In Lehman JF (ed.), *Therapeutic Heat and Cold* (3rd ed.). Baltimore: Williams & Wilkins, 1982. Pp. 404–562.

5. Lehman JF, DeLateur BJ. Cryotherapy. In Lehman JF (ed.), *Therapeutic Heat and Cold* (3rd ed.). Baltimore: Williams & Wilkins, 1982. Pp. 563–602.

6. Graff-Redford SB, Reeves JL, Baker RL, Chin D. Effects of transcutaneous nerve stimulation on myofascial pain and trigger point sensitivity. *Pain* 37:1–5, 1989.

7. Fischer E, Solomon S. Physiological responses to heat and cold. In Licht S (ed.), *Therapeutic Heat and Cold* (2nd ed.). Baltimore: Williams & Wilkins, 1965. Pp. 126–169.

8. Gersh MR, Wolf SL. Application of electrical nerve stimulator in the management of patients with pain. *Phys Ther* 65:314–322, 1985.

9. Peck CL, Kraft SM. Electromyographic biofeedback for pain related to muscle tension: a study of tension headache, back and jaw pain. *Arch Surg* 112:889–895, 1977.

10. Health and Public Policy Committee, American College of Physicians: Biofeedback for Headaches. *Ann Intern Med* 102:128–131, 1985.

11. *EMG J33 Handbook.* Boston: Cyborg Corporation, 1977.

12. Stillwell GK. *Therapeutic Electricity and Ultraviolet Radiation* (3rd ed.). Baltimore: Williams & Wilkins, 1983.

13. Waylonis GW, Wilke S, O'Toole D, et al. Chronic myofascial pain: management by low-output helium–neon laser therapy. *Arch Phys Med Rehabil* 69:1017–1020, 1988.

14. Bishop B. Pain: its physiology and rationale for management. *Phys Ther* 60:24–37, 1980.

15. Yates DAH. Indications and contraindications for spinal traction. *Physiotherapy* 4:55, 1972.

16. Halsted LS, Grabois M. Physical modalities of treatment. In Halstead LS, Grabois M (eds.), *Medical Rehabilitation.* New York: Raven, 1985.

17. Mennel J. *Back Pain: Diagnosis and Treatment Using Manipulative Technique.* Boston: Little, Brown, 1960.

18. Maigne R. The concept of painlessness and opposite motion in spinal manipulation. *Am J Phys Med* 44:55, 1965.

19. Greenmann PE. Manipulative therapy in relation to total health care. In Korr J (ed.), *The Neurologic Mechanisms in Manipulative Therapy.* London: Plenum, 1978.

20. Malaick MM. Functional restoration—upper extremity orthotics. In Hopkins HL, Smith HD (eds.), *Willard and Spackspan Occupational Therapy* (6th ed.). Philadelphia: J.B. Lippincott, 1983. Pp. 453–640.

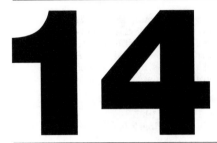

Transcutaneous Electrical Nerve Stimulation
Ronald E. Wilson

I. **Background.** Transcutaneous electrical nerve stimulation (TENS) is the application of electrical stimulation to the skin for pain reduction. TENS is among the earliest forms of patient-controlled analgesia, and active and intelligent participation by the patient is needed to achieve a good result. Initial TENS training can be accomplished in the first office visit, with several follow-up visits required to develop proper technique.

II. **Mechanism of action.** In 1965, Melzack and Wall proposed the **gate theory** of pain, which hypothesized that nonnociceptive nerve fibers can, via inhibitory collateral nerve fibers, antagonize the firing of second-order ascending pain neurons in the dorsal horn of the spinal cord.[1] TENS units were therefore developed to provide a patterned electrical stimulation to the skin over peripheral afferent nerves, which would, it was believed, directly stimulate the nonnociceptive fibers. This would block the transmission of pain impulses and prevent the sensation of pain from ascending to the brain.

Basbaum and Fields proposed a **model of endogenous pain control** to explain the effects of TENS.[2] Their data support the existence of supraspinal descending pain control systems that use inhibitory neurotransmitters and endorphins. They propose that neurons in either the brain stem periaqueductal gray matter or the medulla send inhibitory messages down to the dorsal horn of the spinal cord. One of several relay connections between the afferent sensory system and the endogenous pain control system might be activated by TENS. Related to this is the fact that naloxone has been shown to reduce the effect of TENS.

The **information-processing theory** has also been proposed to explain the neurophysiology of TENS action. This theory considers that sensation is associated with defined neuroanatomic pathways and neurotransmitters and sensory information is encoded by trains of electrochemical impulses that pass through these pathways. Because these codes can be "scrambled" by inserting extraneous pulses into the signal, it is believed that TENS may thereby reduce central pain perception.

Besides reducing pain perceptions, there are other physiologic and psychological effects of TENS: It increases skin blood flow, modulates sympathetic and reflex tone, acts as a placebo, and as an external device may satisfy unfulfilled dependency needs.

None of the above hypotheses, however, clarifies which type of stimulation is clinically most effective. The best choice of electrical patterns is based on clinical observations. Stimulation should feel pleasant and permit the patient to improve his or her functional status. According to the gate theory, TENS may be effective by stimulating large sensory afferents that hold the pain gate closed. Stimulation should feel like the sensory modalities that these fibers mediate: light touch, pressure, or vibration. In order to "scramble" the pain code, TENS should approximate the endogenous pain signal. TENS based on the information-processing model therefore would mimic the character of the patient's pain. Sharp, intense stimuli would be appropriate for sharp pain, whereas constant low-intensity stimulation would be better for steady, dull, aching pain. As there is not a single best pattern of stimulation, patients must use trial and error to find which pattern best helps their problem.

III. **Indications.** Although many different types of pain have been treated with TENS (Table 14-1) the most common indication is **localized musculoskeletal pain**, unrelieved by nonsteroidal anti-inflammatory drugs or mild analgesics. In this context, TENS is more frequently used to treat chronic pain than acute pain owing to the amount of time needed to teach TENS utilization.

Table 14-1. Pain treated with transcutaneous electrical nerve stimulation

Muscle contraction pain
Amputation/phantom limb pain
Psychogenic pain
Neuralgia
Radicular pain
Headache
Burn pain
Ischemic pain
Dermatologic pain
Myofascial pain
Arthritis pain
Reflex sympathetic dystrophy
Labor pain
Postsurgical pain
Cancer pain
Visceral pain

Unpredictable, brief, intermittent pain such as tic douloureux is difficult to treat because the patient cannot time treatment schedules. Deafferentation dysesthesia and central pain also respond poorly to TENS.[3]

IV. Contraindications

A. Cardiac pacemakers. In patients with cardiac pacemakers there are no reports of deaths from TENS application on the extremities, back, or neck.[4] TENS electrodes should not be placed directly over the pacer or the chest.

B. Skin. Electrodes should not be placed on broken or insensate skin.

C. Psychological history. Demented or psychotic patients may inadvertently misuse TENS units. In patients with a history of electrical misadventure, including former prisoners of war, TENS may evoke anxiety and symptoms of posttraumatic stress syndrome.

V. Side effects and adverse reactions

A. Contact dermatitis. If this occurs, electrode components should be changed.

B. Burns. Electricity can cause skin burns if electrode resistance is high or unevenly distributed. Skin with decreased sensation should not be stimulated.

C. Painful muscle contraction. Stimulation should not be allowed to produce muscle contraction, which could cause soreness and spasm.

VI. Drug interactions. Some practitioners think that TENS, especially acupuncture-like TENS, which may be mediated by endorphins, is ineffective in patients taking narcotics. Although the net effect of TENS may be limited in these patients, TENS can add pain relief in a well-managed medication program. Cancer patients on high-dose narcotics can have significant augmentation of pain relief with TENS. The therapist trying to help a patient design a treatment schedule must consider the kinetics of the pain medications that the patient is taking.

The use of drugs that potentiate the action of endogenous pain-suppressing neurotransmitters in the spinal cord may improve TENS and should be used appropriately. In an ideal clinical practice, the prescription of TENS should follow the use of mild analgesics, be used concurrently with neurotransmitter reuptake inhibitors, and precede the use of narcotics.

VII. Dosage and administration. The three dosage components to TENS therapy are **electrode placement, stimulus parameters, and treatment schedule.**

A. Electrode placement is empiric and based on the therapist's experience and observation of the patient's response. Dermatome and peripheral nerve distributions are usually the targets of TENS. The user places one of a pair of electrodes at the painful area and the other closer to the spinal cord along the distribution of the appropriate nerve or dermatome. The next pair of electrodes can be placed at a second site along the nerve or dermatome or over a second painful site.

The principle for choosing the sites of electrodes varies with the theory applied. With the information-processing theory, for example, "scrambling" would be

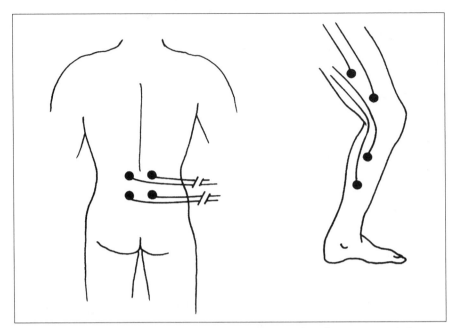

Fig. 14-1. Typical electrode placements for lumbar pain and saphenous nerve pain. Placement of electrodes on the back can be difficult for the elderly patient with arthritis. Longer electrode leads may be needed when electrodes are placed on the distal part of the leg.

optimized if the nerve fibers transmitting the pain are stimulated above the pain receptor, thereby inserting extra impulses into the impulse code. Because afferent nerve fibers have overlapping distributions into adjacent spinal segments, TENS is also effective if stimulation is applied to nerves or dermatomes adjacent to the level of the pain. Figure 14-1 shows typical electrode placement for lumbar back pain and saphenous nerve pain. Although electrode placement charts are available, they are only starting points, as the most efficacious placements must be found by trial and error.

Electrodes should be placed away from motor nerves when possible to prevent muscle contractions. Unfortunately, this may prevent stimulation of the muscle afferents involved in deep muscle pain. The therapist will show the patient how, by systematically varying the sites of stimulation, distances between electrodes, and the polarity of the stimulation (by switching the leads), to optimize pain relief.

Prior to electrode placement the skin should be clean, dry, and free of lotions or insulating oils. Good electrode application with a thin even coat of conductive gel results in low resistance and provides a stronger intensity of stimulation for a given stimulator output. Low resistance also allows the unit to be operated at lower-amplitude settings, thereby conserving batteries. The electrodes must not touch, nor should the conductive gel be spread across the skin between them. This will short-circuit the electrodes, and patients will report little sensation at full-amplitude settings. Loose, uneven application will result in unsettling variation in stimulation when the patient moves. Electrodes not firmly held against the skin are uneven conductors and may have areas of high current densities. These hot spots produce heating and skin burns.

B. Stimulus parameters
   1. Intensity is the sensation felt by the patient, which is a function of pulse amplitude (voltage or amperage) and duration. Placement of electrodes close to afferent nerves and achievement of low resistance at the electrode-gel-skin interface will increase intensity. Peak voltages are between 0 and 150 V. For comparison, static electric shocks, commonly experienced at home, have amplitudes of thousands of volts.

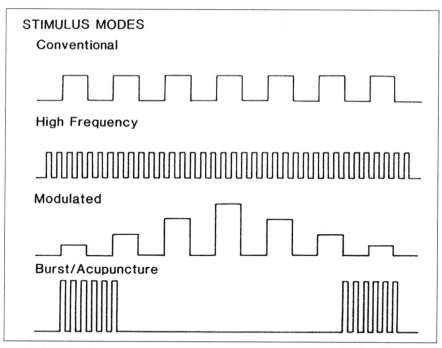

Fig. 14-2. Modes of transcutaneous electrical nerve stimulation (TENS). Each square-wave impulse has an amplitude (height) and duration (width). The number of impulses occurring in 1 second is the frequency. Modulated amplitude is shown, but frequency or duration can be modulated on some units. Baseline end is 0.375 seconds.

Intensity can be adjusted by varying the voltage setting or the pulse duration. The latter adjustment is not critical and is not available on all units. The stimulation should be clearly felt but not unpleasant. Most of the sensation will be under the electrode, but when the electrodes are over a superficial sensory nerve, the user will note paresthesia in that nerve distribution. If muscle twitches are noted, patients should be instructed to reduce stimulus intensity or move the electrodes.

2. Modes of stimulation. For units, see Figure 14-2.
   a. Conventional (most popular mode)—a repeated square-wave impulse at a rate of 10–30 Hz, which feels like a gentle tap or throb at slow rates and a buzz or tickle at higher rates.
   b. High frequency—conventional TENS at rates of approximately 100 Hz, which feels like a sharp vibration or tingle.
   c. Modulated—resembles a wavelike oscillation and has been compared to a soothing massage. Some clinicians recommend periodically lowering the intensity to prevent physiologic accommodation. The user should be careful to avoid muscle stimulation at the peaks.
   d. Burst/acupuncture (second most popular mode)—a brief train of high-intensity, high-frequency stimulation repeated at regular intervals, which feels like recurrent pinches or needle sticks. In theory, this mode may induce release of endorphins or other long-acting neurotransmitters in the endogenous pain control pathways.

   Initially, conventional TENS is usually used. The patient is told to adjust the stimulus to a comfortable amplitude slightly above sensory threshold and dial in a pleasant frequency. After the patient has become well oriented to conventional TENS, other modes of stimulation can be demonstrated and the patient can be instructed to perform sequential trials of each mode. Low-intensity burst mode (acupuncture-like) is our next choice for low back pain, and modulated modes are favored by patients with extremity pain.

C. Treatment schedules. TENS is advantageous over other forms of analgesia for variable pain because it **can be adjusted frequently.** Good TENS users make intensity adjustments every 15 to 30 minutes and average a total of 3 to 5 hours of treatment a day. The unit can and should be turned off when pain is tolerable. This conserves batteries, and off periods may prevent conditioning of the nervous system. Pain diaries can be helpful in organizing a schedule. Experienced users will use TENS during activities to achieve functional goals such as taking a longer walk, doing household chores, or maintaining work performance by activating the unit shortly before periods of predictable pain.

Electrodes should not be left in place overnight to ensure good skin hygiene. Falling asleep with an activated TENS unit involves the risk of burns and shocks. Patients with occasional night pains should get out of bed and apply TENS for 15 to 30 minutes, then return to bed. Chronic night pain requires careful assessment of sleep disturbance and appropriate treatment.

VIII. The TENS trial

   A. Avoid pain medication the morning of the trial. The patient must have some pain so that the professional can observe the behavioral response to TENS. Before demonstrating the stimulus, the clinician should carefully note baseline pain behavior and examine the patient with attention to any objective functional limitations due to pain (limited range of motion, difficulty walking, etc.).

   B. Place one electrode directly over the point where the patient indicates that he or she has pain. Place the other electrode in the cutaneous distribution of the nerve supplying the painful area proximal to the first electrode. Another pair of electrodes can be placed more proximally along the same nerve or dermatome supplying the painful area also.

   C. Ask the patient to rate the pain on a pain scale. Carefully activate the unit (after notifying the patient that a small buzzing will be felt) and have the patient indicate when the tingle is first felt. This is the sensory threshold. Increase the amplitude slightly so that the patient is plainly aware of the stimulation but avoid discomfort.

   D. Demonstrate how to operate the unit. Point out any muscle contraction to the user and reduce the amplitude or move the electrodes if this occurs. If contractions are permitted unabated, muscle soreness will occur.

   E. Stimulate the patient for several seconds at a low frequency, then for several seconds at a higher frequency, and adjust the unit until the patient finds the best setting. Keep the unit on at the selected frequency and intensity and instruct the patient to turn it off if it becomes uncomfortable.

   F. Send the patient to a waiting area with the activated TENS unit for 30 to 60 minutes. During this time the patient should remain active and not take any pain medicine. Afterward the patient is interviewed and reexamined.

   G. Patients with good responses are given a treatment schedule and instructed how to operate the unit and how to care for the electrodes. Patients are also instructed in proper skin care, which includes removing the electrodes every night or, if the skin becomes irritated, cleaning residual gel from the skin with plain soap and water, and avoiding lotions and oily soaps that interfere with skin conductivity. If minor irritation develops at one site, the patient should relocate the electrodes. If the irritation persists, the affected skin should be examined to determine if there is contact dermatitis or a burn. The patient is warned against falling asleep with the unit on.

   H. The patient should return to the clinic in 1 to 2 weeks for follow-up with the unit in place and operational. A clinical evaluation is repeated, and the unit and electrodes are inspected. The patient's technique is observed and critiqued in order to optimize treatment. Other stimulation modes can be demonstrated, which the patient can then try.

   I. Special technical concerns. Patients with impaired dexterity due to arthritis will have difficulty adjusting small controls, so a unit with larger controls should be provided. If the stimulation is disturbingly irregular or hard to maintain at a comfortable level, this is probably the result of poor electrode application and not electronic malfunction. To avoid skin problems, electrodes should not be left in place for long periods and the same stimulating sites should not be used every day. Patients should be encouraged to rotate electrode placement.

   Battery life is a good indicator of how much the patient is using the TENS unit. When a conventional battery only lasts 1 or 2 days, the unit is being used at an excessively high intensity or with improper electrode application. Conventional alkaline batteries should last about 1 week with moderate use and

1 month with light use. A rechargeable battery should last at least 1 day without noticeable fade even with heavy use. Rechargeable batteries will short cycle if not fully discharged with each use. Most users exchange a pair of rechargeable batteries between the unit and the recharger for economy. A spare conventional battery should be kept by the patient who cannot always remember to recharge.

IX. Equipment
A. Units
1. **Disposable sterile integrated TENS and electrode packages** are applied in the operating room for postsurgical therapy.
2. **Large console units** are used for physical therapy departments.
3. **Shirt-pocket-sized** units have two independently controlled channels for stimulating two sites with controls for mode, frequency rate, and intensity (amplitude or amplitude and duration).
4. **Knobs and dials are easier to manage** for most patients than digital pushbutton controls. Controls, especially that for amplitude, should be readily accessible. Frequency control from 0 to 100 Hz should be available. Most units, including conventional TENS, will have two patterns of stimulation.
5. **Most TENS units** supplied by reputable dealers **are sturdy and durable.** Maintenance is minimal. Good-quality batteries should be used and removed when the unit is stored to avoid damage if the batteries leak. After repeated use, the electrode sockets on the unit can loosen and make poor contact. As most units are not reparable, this is usually a terminal condition for the TENS unit. Patients can avoid this problem by being careful when inserting the electrode pins and avoiding tension on the wires.

B. Electrodes and gel.
The most practical electrodes are simple carbon black rubber disks with plugs to attach to pin electrodes. The 2-in.-diameter carbon black electrode can be cut to any convenient shape. Special TENS gels are available, but electrophysiologic gels such as Red Dot or Aquasonic are adequate and can be purchased in bulk.

A particularly useful specialized gel is Tensive Conductive Adhesive Gel, made by Parker Laboratories (Orange, NJ). This relatively inexpensive gel conducts well and is designed to be the primary adhesive for carbon black electrodes. The patient applies a thin layer of this gel to the carbon black electrodes and presses it to the skin. Tensive will hold electrodes on most sites in place for the day. Paper tape on the edges of the disk will increase the stability of electrodes held down with Tensive gel over sites that are prone to movement. One 60-g tube lasts 1 to 2 months and can be another index of TENS usage. At night the electrodes are rinsed clean. With good care no other maintenance is required. Some venders recommend periodically regenerating carbon black electrodes by gentle boiling.

Disposable pregelled electrodes are available in a variety of forms that may be used one or more times. Again, electrodes approximately 1 to 2 in. in diameter are most appropriate. Large electrodes, which are supposed to disperse the current density over a larger surface, may be useful for some patients with back pain, but the added expense is rarely justified. Some of these electrodes are left in place by patients for a week, but this is not advisable. Although convenient, the use of pregelled electrodes can become expensive. Patients who discard TENS because of cost may reconsider if offered a less-expensive electrode.

References

1. Melzack R, Wall PD. Pain mechanisms: a new theory. *Science* 150:971, 1965.
2. Basbaum AT, Fields HL. Endogenous pain control systems: brainstem spinal pathways and endorphin circuitry. *Annu Rev Neurosci* 7:309, 1984.
3. Meyler WJ, de Jongste MJ, Rolf CA. Clinical evaluation of pain treatment with electrostimulation: a study on TENS in patients with different pain syndromes. *Clin J Pain* 10:22, 1994.
4. Rasmussen MJ, Hayes DL, Vlietstra RE, Thorsteinsson G. Can transcutaneous electrical nerve stimulation be safely used in patients with permanent cardiac pacemakers? *Mayo Clin Proc* 63:443, 1988.

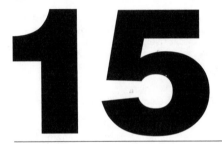

Electrodiagnosis in the Evaluation and Management of Low Back Pain

Arlene M. Braker
Sridhar V. Vasudevan

I. Background. Patients with low back pain often have involvement of their peripheral or central nervous system. To evaluate and treat such patients, physicians frequently request electrodiagnostic examinations. Often performed by neurologists and physiatrists, electrodiagnosis should be considered an extension of the history and physical examination.

Electrodiagnostic testing includes electromyography (EMG), which studies the electrical activity of muscle; nerve conduction studies, which investigate the action potentials of peripheral nerves; and evoked potential studies, which involve the analysis of electric waveforms elicited by an electrical stimulus generated in the peripheral nervous system and recorded over the CNS.

II. Indications

A. To define the location of a nerve fiber lesion, for example, at the root or plexus level

B. To determine the severity and chronicity of the lesion

C. To rule out an underlying neuromuscular disorder: i.e., myopathy when there is clinical weakness, or peripheral polyneuropathy when sensory symptoms predominate

D. To evaluate nerve damage (axonal degeneration) or regrowth even before it is clinically evident

E. To provide objective evidence for a lesion when history or physical examination is equivocal

F. To correlate electrophysiologic data studies: CT and MRI scans show significant pathology in 30% to 60% of normal persons, although EMG rarely does. Conversely, EMG may be sensitive to disk herniation in the 10% found surgically that CT and MRI failed to confirm.

III. The motor unit. The anatomic unit of study in electrodiagnosis—the motor unit—is formed from an anterior horn cell, its axon, the terminal branches of the axon, neuromuscular junctions, and all the muscle fibers supplied by the anterior horn cell. When the pathways of the motor units from a spinal cord level are disrupted by compression of a nerve, for example, EMG or nerve conduction study changes may result.

IV. Electrodiagnostic studies. When a patient with low back pain is referred for electrodiagnostic studies, the process begins with the physician obtaining the patient's medical history and performing an appropriate and relevant physical examination, especially of the muscles innervated by the nerve roots, plexus, or peripheral nerves in question.

A. Electromyography is performed by inserting a needle electrode into a muscle. In EMG studies, the electrical properties of muscle cells are evaluated. Fitting the pattern of EMG abnormalities to a lesion that is anatomically and clinically consistent with patient presentation is essential to an adequate study. When radiculopathy, plexopathy, spinal stenosis, or paraspinal or spinal metastases are suspected, EMG may be an important diagnostic tool. Paraspinal examination may correlate with a postoperative "failed back syndrome." EMG may be used to rule out a suspicion of myopathy or peripheral polyneuropathy when physical examination or history dictates that this would be in the differential diagnosis. EMG also is helpful in providing prognostic implications, depending on the degree of axonal degeneration and regeneration findings.

1. Muscle at rest is usually electrically silent. Abnormal findings during rest include fibrillations or positive sharp waves. A fibrillation potential is the electrical activity associated with the contracting of a single muscle fiber,

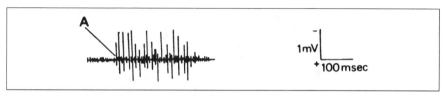

Fig. 15-1. Normal insertional activity (A = point of needle insertion or movement). (From Sethi RK, Thompson LL. *The Eletromyographer's Handbook* (2nd ed.). Published by Little, Brown and Company. Copyright © 1989.)

which may occur spontaneously or following needle advancement (Fig. 15-1). They are believed to represent increased excitability of the muscle membrane and occur in a wide variety of conditions, including muscle trauma, electrolyte disturbance, severance of nerve supply, and muscle disease.

2. **Insertional activity** is usually described as findings of fibrillation potentials or positive sharp waves initiated with needle advancement. Normally, electrical activity stops when needle advancement stops (Fig. 15-2). Postinsertional activity is abnormal. It may be produced by a variety of states, including trauma, inflammation, metabolic disorders, or nerve compression, leading to axonal degeneration. A decrease in insertional activity may be observed when the muscle has undergone fibrotic or atrophic changes, as in the case of a remote injury or underlying chronic neuromuscular disease.

3. **Minimal contraction.** Next, the **motor unit action potential (MUAP),** which reflects the electrical activity of a single anatomic motor unit, is examined. The summated electrical activity of muscle fibers innervated by a single anterior horn cell and within recording range of the electrode results in the electrical waveform of the MUAP (Fig. 15-3). With minimal contractions, the following characteristics are distinguished: amplitude, duration, phasicity, and the rate of recruitment of additional units (Fig. 15-4). These qualities allow the electromyographer to comment on the chronicity of a nerve compression. In the first 72 hours, a decreased number of motor units may be the only abnormality. Should an axon have undergone degeneration and, with time, regrown, the motor units may be observed as having a large amplitude, prolonged in duration and increased in polyphasicity.

4. **Maximal contraction.** The recruitment pattern in a maximal contraction reflects a combination of factors, including volition and the number of units available for recruitment. In the case of nerve compression, fewer motor units may be detectable owing to compressed axons undergoing a conduction block.

B. **Nerve conduction studies,** also known as electroneurography (ENG), can be performed on a number of peripheral motor and sensory nerves. They can help in determining the extent of a peripheral nerve lesion and in differentiating a nerve conduction block from a nerve that has been severed.

1. **Motor nerves.** To perform a motor nerve conduction study, a peripheral nerve is stimulated transcutaneously, causing a muscle contraction. Surface or needle electrodes are used to detect the evoked **compound muscle action potential (CMAP),** known as the motor response (Fig. 15-5). By stimulating at a distal location along the course of the nerve, a distal latency (the time interval between the onset of stimulus and onset of a resultant CMAP) is determined. Similarly, by stimulating at a more proximal site, the proximal motor latency may also be measured. A nerve conduction velocity can then be calculated by dividing the distance between the two points of stimulation by the differences between the proximal latency and the distal latency. A conduction delay or prolonged latency may be related to site-specific nerve compression. Diffuse slowing of nerve conduction velocity is more commonly related to a peripheral polyneuropathy secondary to a demyelinating process. The amplitude and shape of the responses can also be evaluated. If a low-amplitude response is found, this suggests reduction of conductive axons, implying an axonal compromise. Increased width (duration) of the CMAP response may be related to temporal dispersion or conduction at different speeds along various fibers being stimulated. This is also common in demyelinating disorders.

2. **Sensory nerves.** Electrodes are placed over the course of the sensory nerve

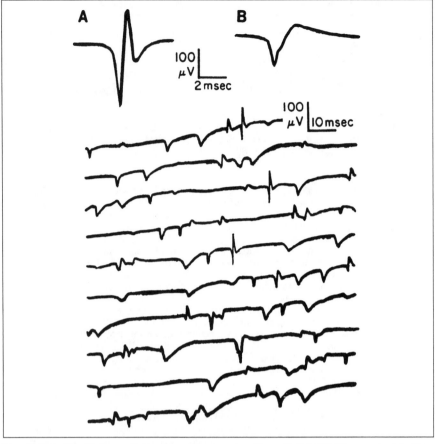

Fig. 15-2. A. Fibrillations. **B.** Positive sharp waves. (From Sethi RK, Thompson LL. *The Eletromyographer's Handbook* (2nd ed.). Published by Little, Brown and Company. Copyright © 1989.)

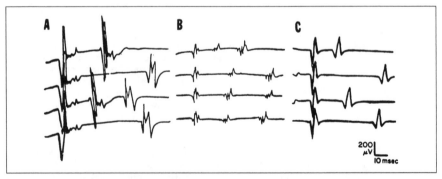

Fig. 15-3. Motor unit action potentials. **A.** Neuropathic—large, prolonged, polyphasic. **B.** Myopathic—small, short, polyphasic. **C.** Normal. (From Sethi RK, Thompson LL. *The Eletromyographer's Handbook* (2nd ed.). Published by Little, Brown and Company. Copyright © 1989.)

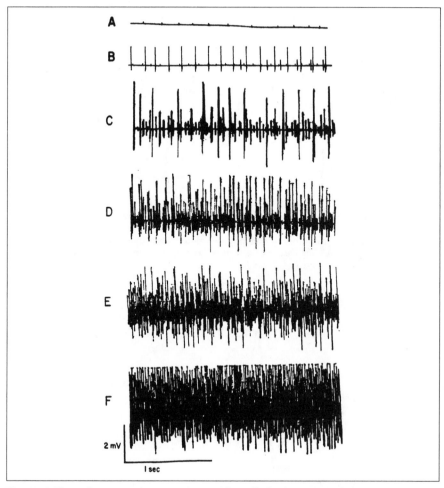

Fig. 15-4. Normal motor unit recruitment with graded voluntary contraction. **A.** Minimal effort with an onset frequency of 5/sec. **B.** Recruitment of a second motor unit with increased effort—recruitment frequency of 10/sec. **C–F.** Increasing motor unit recruitment with a graded increase in effort leading to a complete interference pattern with maximal effort **(F).** (From Sethi RK, Thompson LL. *The Eletromyographer's Handbook* (2nd ed.). Published by Little, Brown and Company. Copyright © 1989.)

rather than over a muscle belly. Frequently, the peak rather than the onset of the action potential is used for a latency measurement in sensory nerve conduction studies (Fig. 15-6). These tests are particularly useful to rule out a peripheral polyneuropathy or an isolated peripheral nerve lesion.
3. **"Late" responses** are potentials that have a longer latency than the CMAP, and actually evaluate motor nerve conduction proximal to the site of stimulation.
   a. **Hoffman reflex (H-reflex)** is used to evaluate S1 radiculopathy. This is a late CMAP having a consistent latency evoked by a submaximal stimulation of the tibial nerve. It is considered to be a neurophysiologic spinal reflex (electrophysiologic equivalent of the ankle jerk) resulting from stimulation of afferent fibers in the mixed nerve supplying the gastrocnemius and activation of motor neurons returning to the gastrocnemius through a monosynaptic reflex arc (Fig. 15-7). In acute S1 radiculopathy, the H-reflex may be absent or delayed in comparison with the contralateral extremity. When the

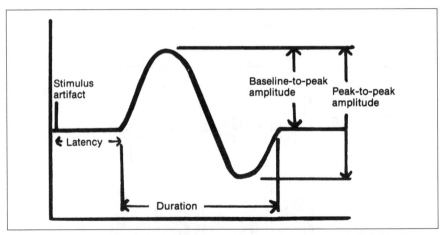

Fig. 15-5. Measured parameters of a compound motor action potential (CMAP). (From Sethi RK, Thompson LL. *The Eletromyographer's Handbook* (2nd ed.). Published by Little, Brown and Company. Copyright © 1989.)

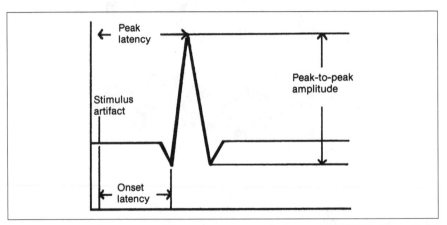

Fig. 15-6. Measured parameters of a sensory nerve action potential (SNAP). (From Sethi RK, Thompson LL. *The Eletromyographer's Handbook* (2nd ed.). Published by Little, Brown and Company. Copyright © 1989.)

H-reflex is bilaterally abnormal, this may implicate a midline disk or mass, lumbar spinal stenosis, or less likely, bilateral plexopathy or bilateral radiculopathy. H-reflex changes occur before EMG changes occur and in some situations may be the only abnormality if there is no axonal degeneration.

b. F wave, evoked intermittently from a muscle by a supramaximal stimulation of any motor nerve, is believed to result when a motor nerve fiber conducts an impulse in the reverse of its normal direction of conduction. The impulse rebounds off an anterior horn cell and returns to be recorded over the muscle. As various fibers may be responsible for the production of an F wave, the latencies and configuration of F waves vary with each stimulation. (Fig. 15-8). Since only motor fibers are needed to produce an F wave, posterior root (sensory fiber) disorders do not disrupt it. The F wave may be useful in evaluating a proximal-site lesion when a proximal-site stimulation is technically difficult—for example, in suspected intragluteal sciatic injuries.

C. Somatosensory evoked potentials. Electrical stimulation of peripheral sensory

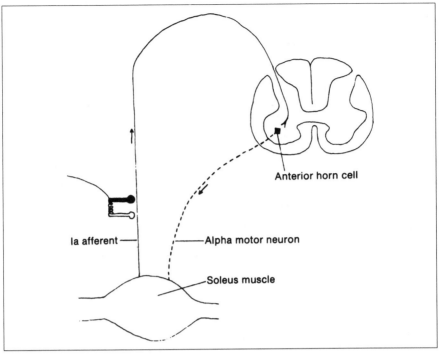

Fig. 15-7. Stimulation of the posterior tibial nerve to elicit the H-reflex. (From Sethi RK, Thompson LL. *The Eletromyographer's Handbook* (2nd ed.). Published by Little, Brown and Company. Copyright © 1989.)

nerve fibers elicits biologic electric waveforms of low amplitude called somatosensory evoked potentials. In practice, a mixed peripheral nerve of the extremity or a cutaneous nerve in the distribution of a dermatome is stimulated, and spinal and contralateral scalp recordings are obtained. Many repetitions are required to perform the study to eliminate baseline brain electrical activity. The stimulus is rarely uncomfortable for the patient, but an anxious patient may require more study time to reduce muscle artifact. Interruptions or delays in bilateral somatosensory evoked potentials in the patient with low back pain are significant when lumbar spinal stenosis is suspected. When a chronic lumbosacral radiculopathy is suspected, dermatomal stimulation studies may be indicated. A unilateral delay or absence may suggest a chronic radiculopathy in the absence of definite EMG changes. When a peripheral neuropathy is present, lumbar potentials may be absent, and a scalp response delay would then be nonspecific.

V. Limitations
  A. Lack of patient cooperation can limit the scope of the study.
  B. Axonal degeneration cannot be confirmed before 7 to 14 days.
  C. An area of interest may be inaccessible owing to a cast or open wound.
  D. A peripheral neuropathy, muscle trauma, or metabolic disturbance can limit the specificity of interpretation.
  E. Nerve root compression (seen on CT, MRI, or myelogram) not leading to axonal degeneration or significant conduction block may not be revealed as EMG abnormalities (EMG, however, may be abnormal when only a few fibers have undergone degeneration, without the presence of a significant anatomic or radiologic abnormality).
  F. It is operator dependent, and the areas examined must be properly determined by the differential diagnoses generated from the history and physical examination.

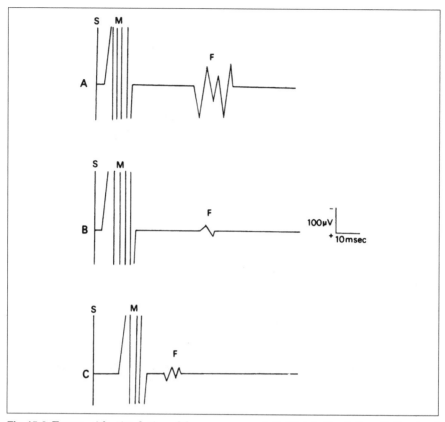

Fig. 15-8. F wave with stimulation of the same nerve. **A, B.** Distal stimulation. **C.** Proximal stimulation. Note variation of latency, amplitude, and configuration in **A** and **B**; more proximal stimulation results in a shorter F-wave latency **(C)**. Stimulus *(S)* and M-response *(M)* are off the vertical scale. (From Sethi RK, Thompson LL. *The Eletromyographer's Handbook* (2nd ed.). Published by Little, Brown and Company. Copyright © 1989.)

Selected Readings

Brown WF, Bolton CF (eds.). *Clinical Electromyography* (2nd ed.). Boston: Butterworth–Heinemann, 1993.

Johnson EW. *Practical Electromyography.* (2nd ed.). Baltimore: Williams & Wilkins, 1988.

Wilbourn AJ, Aminoff MJ. The electrophysiologic examination in patients with radiculopathies. *Muscle Nerve* 11:1011–1114, 1988.

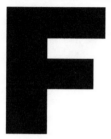

Other Approaches to Chronic Pain Management

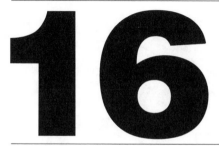

Neurosurgical Approaches to Chronic Pain Management

Bennett Blumenkopf

I. Background

A. Neurosurgeons are intimately involved with the **management of painful disorders.** This involvement may attempt to resolve the underlying mechanism for the pain, such as in the case of a radicular syndrome due to a ruptured lumbar disk through diskectomy. Often, however, the neurosurgical approach attempts to achieve palliation of the pain; hypophysectomy for the diffuse bone pain associated with metastatic cancer is an example.

B. This discussion reviews the **basic anatomy and physiology involved in pain** transmission, neurosurgical procedures performed to alleviate pain, and neurogenic or deafferentation pain. This type of pain is less well understood scientifically and certainly more difficult to manage clinically. A new neurosurgical approach to this problem will also be presented.

II. Neuroanatomy and neurophysiology of pain.
A basic appreciation of the anatomy and physiology of pain transmission is required to understand not only the many causes of pain but also the available procedures used to alleviate the pain.[1-3]

A. Anatomy

1. **The nervous system** involves the peripheral nerves, which convey the important sensory information about the organism to the central centers, the spinal cord, the brain stem, and the brain itself. In addition, the skin, mucous membranes, and periosteum may be considered the most peripheral expanse of the nervous system, for these structures contain the sensory receptors. These receptors, of which there are probably billions, are varied. Some receptors are specific for a single modality, while others are polymodal. When considering the perception of pain, **free nerve endings** in the integument, viscera, and periosteum are generally believed to represent the receptor (Fig. 16-1).

2. Among the various subtypes of peripheral nerve fibers, two appear especially concerned with pain transmission—the **nonmyelinated C fibers** and the **thinly myelinated A delta fibers,** the **primary nociceptive afferents.** The cell bodies or neurons of all the nociceptive afferent fibers are located within the dorsal root ganglia of each spinal root or the gasserian ganglia of the trigeminal roots. Two subpopulations of neurons, one large and one small, are related to each fiber type, the A delta fibers and C fibers, respectively. These neurons are bipolar with their central connections in the spinal cord or brain stem.

3. The spinal cord is topographically divided into the dorsal and ventral horns and, furthermore, into laminae (of Rexed) related to the cell types present. The central fibers of the primary nociceptive afferents, the A delta and C fibers, terminate in the superficial regions of the dorsal aspect of the spinal cord, specifically laminae I, II, and III. The first integration of pain information occurs in the **dorsal root entry zone (DREZ).** The neurons in laminae I and II, along with other cells more deeply situated in laminae IV and V, project their fibers, the **secondary nociceptive afferents,** to the thalamus. These fibers constitute the **spinothalamic tract.**

4. The spinothalamic tract decussates within a segment or two of its segmental level and traverses the anterolateral column of the spinal cord. Another pathway of secondary afferents projects to the brain reticular formation. Both the direct spinothalamic tract and the indirect **spinoreticulothalamic tract** terminate in the thalamus, especially the ventrobasal complex. From the thalamus, tertiary projections go to the cerebral cortex, specifically the primary and secondary somatosensory areas. The actual role of the thalamus and cortex in pain is more complex and certainly less clear.

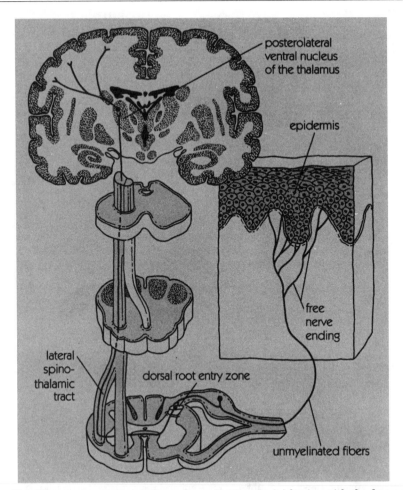

Fig. 16-1. The nervous system pathway for nociception (pain) begins with the free nerve endings as receptors, which are present in the skin, mucous membranes, and periosteum. The nociceptive afferent fibers, represented by the unmyelinated C-fibers and the thinly myelinated A-delta fibers with their cell bodies in the dorsal root ganglia, enter the dorsal root entry zone and synapse in the dorsal horn. Here, the first integration of pain occurs. The secondary nociceptive afferents decussate (cross) and then traverse the lateral spinothalamic tract to the rostral centers. Ultimately, pain is perceived at the cortical level.

B. Physiology

1. The impulses generated by the free nerve endings serve to inform the organism of a potentially noxious, damaging influence. These impulses are conveyed to the central structures by the two types of nociceptive afferents, which seem to subserve different types of pain experience. The **A delta fibers** are faster conducting and reflect a sharp, localized pain. The unmyelinated **C fibers**, being slower conducting fibers, convert a poorly localized dull, burning, or aching sensation.
2. Other neural systems exist that attempt to modify pain. In the peripheral nerves, the large myelinated **A alpha and A beta fibers** have an inhibitory effect on the spinothalamic neurons. This effect is probably mediated by inhibitory interneurons locally at each level of the dorsal horn laminae II and III. Also, the dorsal column nuclei and other brain stem locations project caudally to

Table 16-1. Neurosurgical pain procedures

Procedure	Studies (Ref. No.)
Peripheral	
Peripheral neurectomy	Dellon and Mackinnon, 1984, 1986 (4,5)
Rhizotomy	Loeser, 1972 (6); Onofrio and Campa, 1972 (7); Esposito et al, 1985 (8)
Selective posterior rhizotomy	Sindou and Goutelle, 1983 (9)
Ganglionectomy	Smith, 1970 (10)
Central, spinal cord	
Cordotomy	Spiller and Martin, 1912 (11)
Midline myelotomy	Sindou and Daher, 1988 (12)
Spinal stimulator	De La Porte and Siegfried, 1983 (13)
Intrathecal narcotic analgesia	Penn et al, 1984 (14); Auld et al, 1985 (15)
Dorsal root entry zone lesion	Nashold and Ostdahl, 1979 (16); De La Porte and Siegfried, 1983 (13)
Central, brain	
Mesencephalotomy	Basbaum and Fields, 1984 (2)
Brain stimulator	Adams et al, 1974 (17); Hosobuchi, 1986 (18)
Hypophysectomy	Levin et al, 1980 (19)

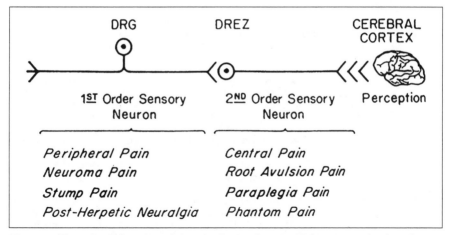

Fig. 16-2. The pain pathway involving the first-order neuron present in the dorsal root ganglion (DRG), the first-order synapse at the dorsal root entry zone (DREZ), the second-order neuron present in the spinothalamic tract, and ultimately the pathway to the cerebral cortex, where pain is perceived. The different types of pain and how they relate to their sites within this pathway are depicted.

lamina I or IV and V and with direct stimulation inhibit the activity in the nociceptive thalamic cells.

III. **Neurosurgical pain procedures.** Based on this knowledge of the anatomy and physiology, a variety of neurosurgical procedures divided into two broad categories can be performed: **peripheral** procedures and **central** procedures (Table 16-1 and Fig. 16-2). These categories are based on the region of the nervous system addressed by the operative management.

A. **Peripheral procedures**

1. **Peripheral nerve**

a. **Decompression.** Compression of peripheral nerves is often painful and a variety of decompression procedures are routinely done, including **carpal tunnel release** for the syndrome caused by median entrapment and **ulnar nerve transposition** at the elbow for tardy ulnar palsy.

b. Stimulation. Peripheral nerve stimulation has also been used in the management of chronic pain, particularly that following nerve injury. This approach attempts to selectively stimulate the large myelinated fibers that inhibit the pain pathway at the level of the dorsal horn. This may be performed with either a transcutaneous electrical nerve stimulation (TENS) device or an implanted device known as peripheral nerve stimulator (PNS).

c. Neurectomy. One may suppose that cutting a nerve, **peripheral neurectomy,** would abolish future pain impulses conveyed from the periphery, and thereby abolish pain. However, several problems with this approach limit its applicability.

(1) **Complications.** A significant overlap (both dermatomal and sclerotomal) exists in the distribution of innervation among the peripheral nerves. Thus, rarely is a pain limited to the zone of a single peripheral nerve. Furthermore, most peripheral nerves are mixed motor and sensory. A peripheral neurectomy procedure could, therefore, incur an **unacceptable motor deficit.** Finally, the development of **deafferentation pain** (as discussed below) is a major complication of peripheral nerve section. Accordingly, this procedure is rarely done for pain.

(2) **Indications.** An exception to the above concerns would be neurectomy performed for **pain following injury to the superficial radial nerve.**[4,5] This is often a difficult pain secondary to trauma, including the placement of peripheral intravenous catheters just above the radial aspect of the wrist. A variety of neurectomy approaches have been attempted, including absolute alcohol injection and neuroma resection with implantation into muscle or bone.

2. Nerve root

a. Decompression. The nerve roots are also sensitive to compression, such as occurs with intervertebral disk herniation or foraminal stenosis. Decompression of the root either through **diskectomy** or **foraminotomy** results in pain relief.

b. Rhizotomy

(1) **Technique.** The next most proximal approach involves sectioning of the sensory fibers that make up the peripheral nerves. This procedure, **rhizotomy,** may be performed extradurally or intradurally.[6–8] In the former, the entire dorsal root is sectioned, whereas in the latter, the multiple rootlets that make up the dorsal root are cut. **Selective posterior rhizotomy**[9] has also been described; this procedure limits the involvement to the ventrolateral aspect of the rootlet, where the small pain fibers (small myelinated and unmyelinated) are organized. In these procedures, a **segmental** region of analgesia will be created corresponding to the dermatomal levels included.

(2) **Indications.** Rhizotomy, including the selective procedure, has proved useful in the management of **pain due to malignant involvement of the brachial plexus** (Pancoast's syndrome), the **chest wall,** and occasionally the **pelvis;** its usefulness is limited in benign processes owing to the frequent development of a deafferentation syndrome, postrhizotomy dysesthesia.

3. Dorsal root ganglia: ganglionectomy

a. Technique. Excision of the sensory ganglia, ganglionectomy, removes the dorsal root ganglia at multiple levels.[10,18] There is a suggestion that this procedure is an advantage over sensory rhizotomy because up to 20% of the nociceptive afferents traverse the **ventral root.**

b. Indications. This procedure is also performed for **segmental-restricted pain,** such as postthoracotomy pain and postherpetic neuralgia. The results with regard to pain relief, however, are modest.

B. Central procedures are divided between those performed on the spinal cord and those performed on the brain stem and high centers.

1. Spinal cord. A number of procedures are performed on the spinal cord itself in an attempt to palliate pain; both ablation and stimulation have been done.

a. Cordotomy

(1) **Technique.** This procedure is designed to destroy the spinothalamic tract.[11] An anterolateral cordotomy may be accomplished either through a formal hemilaminectomy with sectioning of the ventral spinothalamic

tract, or more recently through a percutaneous approach using a radiofrequency electrode. This results in **contralateral analgesia** below the level of the procedure.

(2) **Indications.** An anterolateral cordotomy is remarkably effective in the situation of **malignant pain that is predominantly one sided,** such as a metastasis in the femur.

(3) Unfortunately, bilateral cordotomies are generally not performed because of **respiratory complications.** Furthermore, the deafferentation syndrome, **postcordotomy dysesthesia,** severely limits its usefulness in benign pain syndromes.

b. **Midline commissurotomy or myelotomy**

(1) **Technique.** This procedure simultaneously divides at the level of the anterior commissure the decussating pain fibers in both spinothalamic tracts originating from both sides of the body.[12] Accordingly, through a single cord incision, bilateral effects are produced, providing the site of the pain is limited and segmentally located.

(2) **Indications.** Commissurotomy at the lower lumbosacral spinal segments (conus medullaris) has been employed in cases of **midline perineal, pelvic, and rectal pain,** generally of **malignant etiologies.**

(3) **Complications.** This procedure does, however, have a significant morbidity risk owing to its technically difficult nature. Lower extremity paresis and visceral dysfunction result. Hence, it is not generally popular.

c. **Stimulation of the dorsal column or spinal cord** has been applied to cases of **chronic benign pain,** particularly the **failed back syndrome** following a ruptured intervertebral disk.[13] The stimulation current presumably activates the descending (bulbospinal) inhibitory pathways to provide pain relief. Paresthesia is perceived with the stimulation, which should also be in the distribution of the pain.

d. **Intrathecal pharmacotherapy**

(1) **Technique.** This approach to pain relief at a spinal level, which takes advantage of the basic neurochemistry of pain, **intrathecal narcotic analgesia (ITNA),** has gained popularity.[14,15] Small doses of preservative-free morphine, when instilled directly into the cerebrospinal fluid or into the epidural space, provide profound and prolonged analgesia in a number of circumstances. A variety of implanted pump devices have been designed for chronic therapy.

(2) **Indications.** ITNA has been employed mostly for cases of malignant pain due to **multiple metastases, particularly osseous** ones. More recently, cases of benign pain due to arachnoiditis and postherpetic neuralgia have been managed through this approach.

(3) **Complications.** Tolerance to the opiate remains a problem and a long-term concern.

2. **Brain.** As is the case at the spinal cord level, both stimulation and ablation procedures for pain have been described.

a. **Mesencephalotomy**

(1) **Technique.** Many regions in the mesencephalon and diencephalon are intimately involved with the processing of pain information. These regions of the brain stem are approached using stereotaxic techniques with precisely defined and determined targets (Fig. 16-3).

(2) **Indications. Stereotaxic mesencephalotomy** is indicated for **cephalobrachial pain due to carcinoma,** particularly nasopharyngeal cancer with base-of-the-skull involvement.[20] In addition, **thalamic syndrome pain** is managed by this approach. Interestingly, not only is the pain relieved by this procedure, but so is the suffering component of the pain experience.

b. **Stimulation**

(1) **Technique.** Stimulation of areas in the midbrain and thalamus, or **deep brain stimulation (DBS),** has been used in cases of chronic benign pain and malignant pain.[17,18] Currently, DBS is investigational and performed in only a limited number of neurosurgical centers. Several implantable devices are available for this technique.

(2) **Indications. A variety of chronic pain syndromes,** including cancer pain and pain due to benign etiologies, have been managed by DBS. The analgesia following midbrain stimulation appears to be opiate mediated,

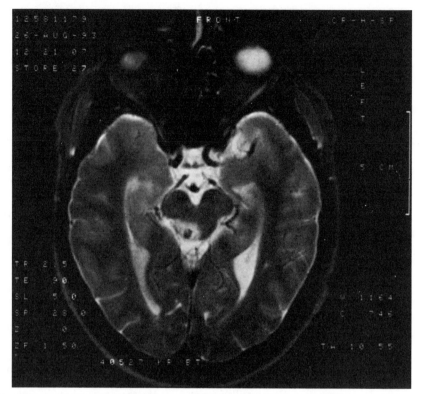

Fig. 16-3. Axial T2-weighted MRI scan showing right-sided mesencephalotomy lesion within the brain stem performed in a patient with brachial plexopathy pain from metastatic breast cancer.

while that following thalamic stimulation does not. Interestingly, tolerance to the former technique does seem to develop (i.e., "opiate tolerance").

   c. Hypophysectomy
      (1) Technique. The pituitary gland may be surgically excised by the transsphenoidal route or chemically ablated using absolute ethanol injections. The latter approach is particularly suited for the debilitated individual because it is relatively stress free (Fig. 16-4).
      (2) Indications. This procedure is particularly effective in palliating the pain of **metastatic cancer** (especially osseous metastases).[19] In cases of hormonally responsive malignancies, such as breast or prostate carcinoma, a remarkable, long-lasting pain relief (>90% response rate) is often achieved. In cancers that are not hormonally dependent, such as GI tract adenocarcinomas, pain relief is still often obtained, though to a lesser degree (approximately 70% response rate). The mechanisms responsible for this effect of hypophysectomy are not understood.
      (3) Complications. The development of diabetes insipidus and hypopituitarism frequently accompanies the analgesic result, owing to concurrent neurohypophyseal and adenohypophyseal damage. Thus, long-term patient management frequently includes supplemental hormonal replacements. Rarely, injury to structures surrounding the sella turcica can occur, such as to the optic or ocular motor nerves.

IV. Deafferentation pain
   A. This is a pain problem that is conceptually different from most pain and probably less familiar to most physicians.[21] In fact, deafferentation pain is common in

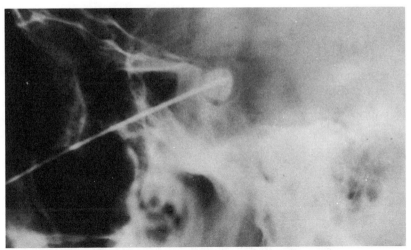

Fig. 16-4. Lateral skull radiograph showing placement of a spinal needle within the sella turcica for injection of absolute ethanol performed in a patient with metastatic prostate cancer and severe bony metastasis pain.

clinical medicine and very difficult to manage effectively. Deafferentation pain, or **neurogenic or central pain** as some refer to it, involves the perception of painful sensations, such as burning, tearing, or throbbing, in a region of the body that is partially or totally sensorially deprived. Thus, all or some of the peripheral nociceptors are physically disconnected from the central centers.

B. In cases of deafferentation pain, the pain does not result from an ongoing, peripheral noxious stimulus. Rather, this phenomenon results from **changes at the CNS level.** The mechanisms thought to explain this unusual phenomenon involve anatomy and physiology. The nervous system and the pain pathways, in particular, are arranged like a circuitry with positive or excitatory and negative or inhibitory influences. These actions are mediated by neurotransmitters or neuromodulators released by neurons to act on the receptors of other neurons. An analogous situation exists for hormonal actions on their target tissues.

C. Recent discoveries on the receptors in the nervous system have revealed a finding that may explain the phenomenon of deafferentation pain.[22] When the influence upon a receptor is removed (e.g., the loss of transmitter substance due to the sensory disconnection), the neuron attempts to compensate by increasing its number of receptor sites to ensure a response to even the most trivial amount of transmitter substance present. A situation of supersensitivity or **hypersensitivity** thus **develops.**

D. An example relates to the ineffectiveness of cutting nerve roots to relieve pain. By doing so, the primary afferent fibers are lost, and consequently, the afferent excitatory transmitters diminish. Those cells in the dorsal horn laminae responsive to these substances increase their receptor sites and become hypersensitive.[23] These central neurons become hyperirritable as demonstrated by single-cell recordings in the dorsal horn of the spinal cord following dorsal root section. This hyperirritability would then be transmitted throughout the nervous system circuitry to higher brain regions. Clinically, this may present as "deafferentation pain." The same may hold true if one attempts to cut a central pathway, e.g., cordotomy. Hypersensitivity in the brain stem or thalamus may create deafferentation pain. Interestingly, the **onset of deafferentation pain may be delayed.** Thus, rhizotomy or cordotomy for the treatment of malignant pain may be useful in a patient with limited life expectancy, generally less than 1 year.

E. Among the deafferentation pain syndromes are **amputation or phantom limb pain, root avulsion pain, peripheral nerve injury pain, quadriplegic and paraplegic pain, and postherpetic neuralgia.** The prevalence of deafferentation pain in these conditions is surprisingly high, and each of these situations is quite common.

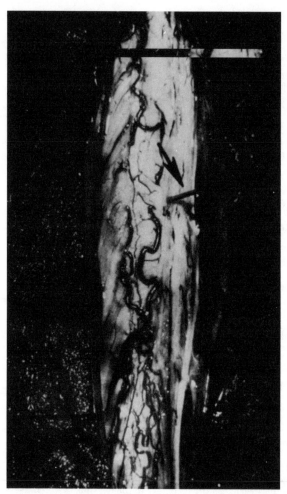

Fig. 16-5. Intraoperative photograph showing placement of the DREZ electrode (arrow) within the spinal cord for creation of the radiofrequency coagulation lesions performed in a patient with brachial plexus avulsion pain.

Some sort of deafferentation pain is suffered by 50% to 90% of amputees, 80% to 90% of patients with brachial plexus avulsions, and 10% to 20% of paraplegics.

F. The pain syndromes that develop in these situations may involve **similar mechanisms** and are **often disabling.** A procedure has been developed to attempt to deal with these pains and appears promising. Based on the hypothesis that the pain is due to hypersensitivity of neurons in the dorsal horn laminae, an attempt is made to diminish or silence the hyperirritability and relieve the pain.

1. **Technique. DREZ lesions** involve the placement of a very small needle electrode in the spinal cord dorsal horn for the destruction of those hyperactive, hyperirritable neurons (Fig. 16-5).[16,24]

2. **Indications.** The results are good, especially in patients with brachial plexus avulsion pain, paraplegia and quadriplegia pain, and phantom limb pain.

3. **Complications.** It is not clear why the creation of a DREZ lesion does not produce a deafferentation situation more distally in the circuitry. This may be because damage is limited to nerve cells and not to fiber tracts. However, deafferentation is a concern, and continued follow-up is required. For the moment, an encouraging new procedure exists for these difficult pain problems.

References

1. Albe-Fessard D, Berkley KJ, Kruger L, et al. Diencephalic mechanisms of pain sensation. *Brain Res Rev* 9:217–296, 1985.
2. Basbaum AI, Fields HL. Endogenous pain control systems: brainstem spinal pathways and endorphin circuitry. *Annu Rev Neurosci* 7:309–338, 1984.
3. Fields HL, Heinricher MM. Anatomy and physiology of a nociceptive modulatory system. *Philos Trans R Soc Lond B* 308:361–374, 1985.
4. Dellon AI, Mackinnon SE. Susceptibility of the superficial sensory branch of the radial nerve to form painful neuromas. *J Hand Surg* 9B:42–45, 1984.
5. Dellon AL, Mackinnon SE. Treatment of the painful neuroma by neuroma resection and muscle implantation. *Plast Reconstr Surg* 77:427–435, 1986.
6. Loeser JD. Dorsal rhizotomy for the relief of chronic pain. *J Neurosurg* 36:745–750, 1972.
7. Onofrio BM, Campa HK. Evaluation of rhizotomy. *J Neurosurg* 36:751–755, 1972.
8. Esposito S, Bruni P, Delitala A, et al. Therapeutic approach to the Pancoast pain syndrome. *Appl Neurophysiol* 48:262–266, 1985.
9. Sindou M, Goutelle A. Surgical posterior rhizotomies for the treatment of pain. In Krayenbuhl H (ed.), *Advances and Technical Standards in Neurosurgery,* Vol. 10. Wien: Springer-Verlag, 1983. Pp. 147–185.
10. Smith FP. Trans-spinal ganglionectomy for relief of intercostal pain. *J Neurosurg* 32:574–577, 1970.
11. Spiller WG, Martin E. The treatment of persistent pain of organic origin in the lower part of the body by division of the anterolateral column of the spinal cord. *JAMA* 58:1489–1490, 1912.
12. Sindou M, Daher A. Spinal cord ablation procedures for pain. In Dubner R, Gebhart GF, Bond MR (eds.), *Proceedings of the Vth Word Congress on Pain.* New York: Elsevier Science, 1988. Pp. 477–495.
13. De La Porte C, Siegfried J. Lumbosacral spinal fibrosis (spinal arachnoiditis). Its diagnosis and treatment by spinal cord stimulation. *Spine* 8:593–603, 1983.
14. Penn RD, Paice JA, Gottschalk W, Ivankovich AD. Cancer pain relief using chronic morphine infusion. *J Neurosurg* 61:302–306, 1984.
15. Auld AW, Maki-Jokela A, Murdoch DM. Intraspinal narcotic analgesia in the treatment of chronic pain. *Spine* 10:777–781, 1985.
16. Nashold BS Jr, Ostdahl RH. Dorsal root entry zone lesions for pain relief. *J Neurosurg* 51:59–69, 1979.
17. Adams JE, Hosobuchi Y, Fields HL. Stimulation of internal capsule for relief of chronic pain. *J Neurosurg* 41:740–744, 1974.
18. Hosobuchi Y. Subcortical electrical stimulation for control of intractable pain in humans. *J Neurosurg* 64:543–553, 1986.
19. Levin AB, Katz J, Benson RC, Jones AG. Treatment of pain of diffuse metastatic cancer by stereotactic chemical hypophysectomy: long term results and observations on mechanism of action. *Neurosurgery* 6:25B–262, 1980.
20. Nashold BS Jr. Brainstem stereotaxic procedures. In Schaltenbrand G, Walker AE (eds.), *Stereotaxy of the Human Brain.* New York: George Thieme Verlag, 1982. Pp. 475–483.
21. Nashold BS Jr. Deafferentation pain in man and animals as it relates to the DREZ operation. *Can J Neurosci* 15:5–9, 1988.
22. Blumenkopf B. Neurochemistry of the dorsal horn. *Appl Neurophysiol* 51:89–103, 1988.
23. Ovelmen-Levitt J, Johnson B, Bedenbaugh P, Nashold BS Jr. Dorsal root rhizotomy and avulsion in the cat: a comparison of long term effects on dorsal horn neuronal activity. *Neurosurgery* 15:921–927, 1984.
24. Nashold BS Jr, Higgins AC, Blumenkopf B. Dorsal root entry zone lesions for pain relief. In Wilkins RH, Rengachary SS (eds.), *Neurosurgery.* New York: McGraw-Hill, 1985. Pp. 2433–2437.

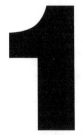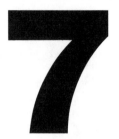

Epidural Adhenolysis and Dorsal Column Stimulation Analgesia

Yasin N. Khan
Mary M. Conaway

I. Epidural adhenolysis

A. Background. Epidural scarring or adhesions can cause persistent pain that presumably is produced by compression and irritation of inflamed nerves within the epidural space. A mixture of local anesthetic, corticosteroids, and hypertonic saline is used during lysis of adhesions, and after the procedure the patient is conventionally placed on a physical therapy program. Adhesions can occur from any of the following conditions:

1. Radiculopathies
2. Degenerative diseases (osteoarthritis or rheumatoid arthritis)
3. Vertebral body fractures
4. Metastatic disease of the vertebrae
5. Postsurgical epidural adhesions
6. Herniated nucleus propulsions
7. Chymopapain injections
8. Facet joint syndrome
9. Spinal stenosis
10. Whiplash injuries

B. Mechanism of action

1. **Local anesthetics** block the sodium channels at the membrane level, thus preventing depolarization of axons and thereby stopping the transmission of electrical signals along these structures. Blocks of different fibers produce paralysis.

2. **Anti-inflammatory corticosteroids.** Cortisol and its synthetic analogues prevent or suppress the development of local heat, erythema, swelling, and tenderness by which inflammation is recognized. They inhibit not only the early phenomenon of the inflammatory process (edema, fibrin deposition, capillary dilatation, leukocyte migration into the inflamed area, and phagocytic activity), but also the later manifestations (capillary proliferation, fibroblast proliferation, deposition of collagen, and still later cicatrization).

3. **Hypertonic saline** may have two beneficial actions:

   a. The reduction of cellular edema by causing water to migrate out of cells (i.e., an osmotically induced fluid shift), which reduces the pressure on the nerve

   b. A local anesthetic-like effect on intact dorsal rootlets, as demonstrated in studies with cats and monkeys

C. Patient selection

1. **Comprehensive intake evaluation,** which includes full radiographic or other tests as needed, history, and physical and psychological evaluation

2. **Pain syndrome is chronic** and is persistent for 6 months or more

3. **Patient has failed many previous treatments** such as epidural steroid injections, nerve root injections, and facet injections

D. Definitive contraindications

1. **Pathologic psychiatric disorders**
2. **Current street drug abuse**
3. **Medical problems that contraindicate the procedures**

E. Lumbosacral procedure. Lysis of adhesions in the epidural space can be undertaken in the cervical and thoracic regions, but is most commonly performed in the lumbar or sacral region.

1. **Equipment needed**

   a. R-K needle

   b. Epidural catheter
   c. R-K connector
   d. Syringes, 10 ml
   e. Glass syringe, 5 ml
   f. Bacteriostatic filter, 0.2 μm
   g. 0.25% bupivacaine (Marcaine MPF)
   h. Nonionic contrast material (Isovue 200)
   i. Betamethasone sodium phosphate and betamethasone acetate suspension (Celestone Soluspan) or triamcinolone
   j. Sterile drapes
   k. C-arm fluoroscopy
2. Technique
   a. Place the patient in a **prone position** on a fluoroscopy table. Prepare and drape the sacral area to ensure sterile conditions. Using sterile technique, place a 16-gauge modified Tuohy needle (available from Epimed Co., or a design manufactured by Medtronic that permits multiple passes) through the sacral hiatus and place the tip at S2–3. The needle should be directed toward the side of the painful area. This also provides protection from puncturing the dural sac.
   b. Fluoroscopy (with memory capacity) is used to confirm the position by anteroposterior and lateral views. All procedures should be carried out with protective measures for the physician (leaded gloves, apron, thyroid shield, and leaded glasses).
   c. Aspirate the needle. A patient with epidural scarring will have venous distention because scar formation interferes with venous runoff. If blood is aspirated, move the needle until no blood is aspirated.
   d. An **epidurogram** is obtained by injection of 10 ml of iohexol (Omnipaque) or metrizamide (Amipaque) or Isovue 200 under fluoroscopy. If venous runoff is noted while injecting, move the needle tip during injection until the contrast material is seen spreading within the epidural space. The spread of contrast medium shows up as a Christmas tree shape on fluoroscopy as the dye spreads into the perineural structures within the bony canal, or even follows the nerves to the outside of the vertebral column. Record the spread of the contrast material after the injection via a memory screen on the fluoroscope.
   e. Inject 10 to 15 ml of 0.25% **bupivacaine.** Note the displacement of previously injected contrast medium in the epidural space. This will outline the filling defect caused by epidural scarring.
   f. Under fluoroscopy, thread a stainless-steel, Teflon-coated, soft, spiral-tipped **epidural catheter** (RACZ Cauda-catheter) through the needle into the scar. Inject a mixture of 5 ml of 0.25% bupivacaine and 50% Isovue 200 contrast material into the scar area. Multiple passes may be required into the scar area. Finally after the lysis of adhesions, inject 6 mg of betamethasone into the scar area. A maximum volume of 40 to 50 ml can be injected in the lumbosacral area on the first day during lysis of adhesions. Be sure the patient is adequately sedated, as this procedure could be painful while dissection is underway.
   g. Note and record the scar dissection. At the termination of the procedure, obtain a hard copy of the radiographic image for the patient record. When the injections are completed, remove the needle and spray the area with tincture of benzoin. Cover the puncture site with an antibiotic ointment and secure the catheter with Tagaderm and sterile (Hypo-fix) tape. Place a bacteriostatic 0.2 μm filter on the end and cap the catheter. Remove the filter only for subsequent steroid injections.
   h. Approximately 30 minutes later, **inject** 10 to 15 ml of 10% sodium chloride **(hypertonic saline).** This provides further pain relief beyond the duration of the local anesthetic by its neurolytic effect on unmyelinated nerve fibers as well as by reduction of edema within previously scarred or inflamed nerves.
   i. Leave the catheter in place for 3 days. On the second and third days inject 15 ml of 0.25% bupivacaine and 30 minutes later inject 10 ml of 10% sodium chloride. There is no further benefit from injecting steroids again on days 2 and 3.
3. Undesirable effects. If hypertonic saline spreads farther than the local anesthetic, it can cause severe pain, never lasting more than 4 to 5 minutes, which

might require analgesia intravenously. Some of the undesirable effects that
have been reported from the intrathecal injection of hypertonic saline are

a. **Severe pain**
b. **Muscle cramps in affected segments**
c. **Hypertension**
d. **Cardiac arrhythmias**
e. **Pulmonary edema**
f. **Cerebral infarction**
g. **Localized paresthesia lasting many hours**
h. **Paresthesias sometimes persisting for weeks**
i. **Transient hemiplegia**
j. **Persistent loss of sphincter control with sacral anesthesia**
k. **Prolonged sensory deficit**
l. **Motor weakness up to 12 hours** (observed even though hypertonic saline
   was not injected; probably caused by high mechanical compression)

F. **Epiduroscopy.** Extensive work has been done to study the epidural space by
introducing a rigid scope into the area. More recently, however, flexible endoscopes
have become available that can be introduced into the caudal area to directly
visualize the epidural space. More work needs to be done, however, not only in
understanding the anatomy but also in differentiating normal from abnormal
tissue in the epidural space. Epiduroscopy is potentially an excellent diagnostic
and therapeutic tool to help solve some of the extremely difficult pain problems.

II. **Spinal cord stimulation**
   A. **Background.** Dorsal column stimulation is thought to provide analgesia by activation of the endogenous opiate pain suppression system and activation of synaptic
   gating mechanisms (Melzack and Wall, 1965, gate-control theory).

   Since the successful introduction of percutaneously placed electrodes for spinal
   cord stimulation by Shealy in 1967, significant advances have been made. These
   electrodes have increased the success rate for pain relief in previously nonre-
   sponding chronic pain sufferers from 25% to 30% to approximately 70%. New
   multiprogrammable systems, available from manufacturers such as Medtronic
   and Neuromed, increase the ability to deliver more satisfactory pain relief to
   patients. Other companies that manufacture spinal cord stimulators are Cordis
   and Avery.

   B. **Indications**
      1. **General indications.** The underlying pathology and topography of pain are
      amenable to **concordant paresthesias** (e.g., spinal stimulation for deafferen-
      tation, radicular, or ischemic pain rather than mechanical or nociceptive
      pain).
      2. **Specific indications**
         a. **Neuropathic**
         b. **Adhesive arachnoiditis, epidural fibrosis with radicular pain**
         c. **Peripheral causalgia**
         d. **Ischemic limb pain**
         e. **Phantom limb or stump pain**
         f. **Reflex sympathetic dystrophy**
         g. **Diabetic neuropathy**
         h. **Postherpetic neuralgia (intercostal)**
         i. **Thalamic pain**

   C. **Patient selection.** Adequate patient selection criteria are instrumental in improving the success of spinal cord stimulation.
      1. Norman Shealy and colleagues in 1970 developed **criteria for patient selection**
      that are still pertinent.
         a. No history of cingulotomy, cordotomy, or deep brain stimulation
         b. No history of dorsal root resection
         c. Able to tolerate a transcutaneous electrical nerve stimulation unit for 48
         hours and obtain partial relief
         d. Less than 5% of the patients a physician sees should receive an implant
         e. Willingness to undergo a pain rehabilitation program
         f. Has been on acceptable medications for at least 6 months without problems
         g. Minnesota Multiphasic Personality Inventory (MMPI) shows only depres-
         sion, not hypochondriasis or hysteria
         h. Emotional stability

2. Other recommendations
a. There is a demonstrated pathology, i.e., objective basis for pain complaints.
b. Further surgical intervention is not indicated.
c. Patient has primarily radiating extremity pain.
d. Trial stimulation has been successful.
e. No contraindications to implantation are present (sepsis, coagulopathy, etc.).

3. The most significant factor in patient selection is the **decision not to implant patients with abnormal psychosocial pathology.** In our experience, patients with high scores on the MMPI indicating problematic hysterical, neurotic, and hypochondriacal behavior should not be candidates. High anxiety or depression scores are not contraindications. Patients with severe drug addiction or pending litigation regarding their injury should undergo rigorous screening before implantation.

D. Procedure
1. Percutaneous screening trial. Prior to placing a permanent lead, a screening trial is usually performed (same-day procedure). This trial is very useful because it can help determine how much pain relief a given patient will achieve from a permanent device and whether the patient will be able to tolerate the device. It can also save a tremendous amount of time by clinically mapping the cord before the permanent implant, as this can be done with fluoroscopy. After a trial the patient is also better prepared to provide meaningful feedback to the physician implanting the permanent device.

2. Technique. Percutaneous electrode placement (same technique for screening and permanent lead placement)
   a. Positioning. Position the patient prone unless the electrode and pulse generator are implanted in the same sitting.
   b. Needle placement. Under fluoroscopy a modified Tuohy needle (see below) is introduced at a shallow angle (no more than 45 degrees so that the lead blank or electrode does not indent, encounter resistance from, or penetrate the dura) into the L1–2 or L2–3 interspace. The needle is placed paramedially using the loss-of-resistance technique. The side ipsilateral to the pain is usually chosen for needle placement. A guide wire can be passed through the needle, and easy passage will further ensure the epidural space.
   c. Passing the electrode. As correct placement of the stimulator electrode requires multiple passes through the needle, a regular Tuohy needle cannot be used because the catheter will be sheared if pulled back. To circumvent this, a modified Tuohy needle that has a much larger opening is used. Care must still be exercised, however, while passing electrodes back and forth.
   d. Electrode placement at T10–12 usually provides paresthesia in the lower extremities. Also, as the purpose of the procedure is to stimulate the dorsal column, electrode placement must be in the posterior epidural space. Stimulation can change with different body movements as the contact between the electrodes and dura changes. If the electrode is too lateral, it will stimulate the nerve roots, which will give radicular paresthesia of the chest wall or abdomen. This type of placement can be done intentionally to treat causalgic-type pain, but if that is not the goal, the electrode can be repositioned so that it is closer to the midline. Bed rest following the implant does not provide any additional benefit, especially because it takes up to 3 months for the electrodes to be fixed in the epidural tissue.
   e. Needle removal. One hand pulls the needle gently while the other hand "feeds" the electrodes under fluoroscopy. Immediately after removal of the needle, appropriateness of the stimulation is confirmed. The temporary screening lead is attached to a temporary battery source and is initially used to evaluate the feasibility of achieving worthwhile stimulation analgesia.
   The patient is discharged and monitored in office visits for 5 to 10 days. If adequate analgesia is obtained, the patient is scheduled for a procedure in which the permanent lead as well as the permanent battery source (pulse generator) are implanted (Medtronic) in the same setting.

E. Major problems with spinal cord stimulation
1. Lead movement (rarely needs to be repositioned)
2. Severe sensory dysesthesia
3. Lead fracture and current leakage

Selected Readings

Benzon HT. Review article: epidural steroid injections for low back pain and lumbosacral radiculopathy. *Pain* 24:277–295, 1986.

Jewett DL, King JS. Conduction block of monkey dorsal rootlets by water and hypertonic saline solutions. *Exp Neurol* 33:225–237, 1971.

King JS, Jewett DL, Sundberg HR. Differential blockade of cat dorsal root C-fibers by various chloride solutions. *J Neurosurg* 36:569–583, 1972.

Melzack R, Wall PD. Pain mechanisms: a new theory. *Science* 150:971, 1965.

North RB. Spinal cord stimulation for intractable pain: indications and technique. In *Current Therapy in Neurological Surgery,* Vol. 2. Philadelphia: Brian C. Decker, 1988.

Racz GB. Electrical stimulation analgesia. In Raj PP (ed.), *Practical Management of Pain* (2nd ed.). Chicago: Mosby–Year Book, 1992.

Racz GB, Sabonghy M, Gintautas J, Kline WM. Intractable pain therapy using a new epidural catheter. *JAMA* 148:579–581, 1982.

Shealy CN, Mortimer JT, Reswick J. Electrical inhibition of pain by stimulation of the dorsal column: preliminary clinical reports. *Anesth Analg* 46:489–491, 1967.

Shealy CN, Mortimer JT, Hagfors NR. Dorsal column electroanalgesia. *J Neurosurg* 32:560–564, 1970.

Squire QW, Calvillo O, Bromage PR. Painless intrathecal hypertonic saline. *Can Anaesth Soc J* 21:308–314, 1974.

Swerdlow M. Complication of neurolytic blockade. In Cousins MJ, Bridenbaugh PO (eds.), *Neural Blockade.* Philadelphia: J.B. Lippincott, 1980. Pp. 543–553.

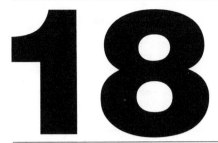

Hospitalization of the Chronic Pain Patient

Barry R. Snow
Paul Gusmorino
Isaac Pinter

I. **Background.** Treatment of the chronic pain patient is most effective when it is intensive, structured, wide-ranging, and rehabilitative. For this reason, and because the medical and behavioral history of the chronic pain patient is usually complex, successful treatment is often best conducted via inpatient hospitalization in a multidisciplinary program.

II. **Hospitalization**

    A. **Advantages of hospitalization.** Many chronic pain patients have extensive experience of unsuccessful treatment with a variety of outpatient therapies. These treatments are often organized in an uncoordinated manner because they are performed at different locations on a schedule that depends on both patient and therapist availability. Treatment in an inpatient unit offers several important benefits.

        1. **Intensive treatment in a coordinated manner on a regular basis**

        2. **The valuable experience of living with other patients also suffering with chronic pain conditions.** Patients with chronic pain often feel they are alone in their dilemma. Because they have a pain problem with no definitive etiology or treatment, these individuals believe that there is something fundamentally wrong with their body or character. Seeing that other people with varied backgrounds and life situations have experienced similar problems has a powerful role in improving the patient's psychological state. Furthermore, many patients trust their fellow pain sufferers (more than they trust their doctors). The inpatient setting provides them with a venue to learn new methods from fellow patients to alleviate or cope with their pain.

        3. **Treatment of patients with complex pain problems.** An intensive team approach and inpatient hospitalization can best address the problems of patients who

            a. Have severe deconditioning

            b. Live too far from treatment centers and would thus not benefit from outpatient treatment

            c. Have coexisting medical conditions

            d. Require detoxification from narcotic medication

    B. **Types of hospitalization care.** The physician can choose from two established methods of inpatient hospitalization care.

        1. The physician can maintain continuity of care throughout the treatment process when **admitting** the patient into a hospital with which the doctor is affiliated and calling on consultants from various disciplines as needed.

        2. **Referring** the patient to an existing comprehensive pain program has the advantage of providing the patient with an established group of professionals who have experience in pain management. Following treatment, the referring physician is sent a full report of the patient's progress in the program with recommendations for further treatment. A listing of these pain management centers can be obtained from the American Pain Society or from the Commission on Accreditation of Rehabilitation Facilities (CARF).

III. **Treatment plan**

    A. **Preadmission assessment.** For most patients, the assessment for inpatient hospitalization can be conducted on an outpatient basis and should include the following:

        1. **Comprehensive medical history and physical evaluation.** A complete medical, surgical, and medication history should be taken by the physician, and a comprehensive physical examination and appropriate laboratory and diagnostic studies should be conducted. In these steps, the clinician must exercise

care not to suggest (in the absence of physical findings) that the pain is not "real."

2. **Psychiatric or psychological examination.** It is imperative for the clinician to go beyond the traditional evaluation and obtain a basic understanding of the patients' lifestyle and the extent to which their chronic pain has affected their daily routine. An understanding of the patients' family setting and factors that contribute to "pain behavior" is also essential. Finally, asking for specific information on the nature of their pain experience is important because it helps to convince patients that the clinician is making a serious attempt to understand the nature and extent of their daily pain. Specific information on the "quality of pain" will be especially useful should the clinician choose to use pain-modifying imagery techniques.

3. **Setting behavioral goals.** Patients are urged to sign a preadmission goals contract. This contract specifies short-term goals during hospitalization and long-term goals for outpatient follow-up.

B. **In-depth psychological testing** can provide detailed information on important subjects, such as basic personality profile, general mood, typical coping strategies, and pain level. These instruments, described in Chapter 11, help the clinician go beyond clinical interview and examination procedures to make a more objective and accurate comparison of the individual's responses to those of appropriate reference groups.

IV. Treatment

A. **Chemical dependency**

1. **Narcotic abuse.** Chronic pain patients often abuse analgesic medications containing opioids such as oxycodone (Percocet, Percodan), codeine (Tylenol with codeine), and propoxyphene (Darvon). Some patients take these medications many times a day despite recognizing that the drugs provide little pain relief. Many patients spend a majority of their day in bed using the medication to help them sleep and avoid dealing with unhappy life circumstances. Some patients combine these medications with alcohol for the same purpose. Such prolonged use of opioid medications may, in addition to the obvious problem of drug dependency, produce such adverse reactions as constipation and lethargy.

One of the primary advantages of the inpatient treatment of those with chronic pain is the ability to detoxify patients who have become dependent on analgesics. It is critical that these patients understand that their medications are not improving their situation or their pain, because the drugs are interfering with their ability to learn more effective strategies for dealing with their pain.

2. **Detoxifying via a pain cocktail.** Patients are told on admission to the hospital the goals of the pain cocktail treatment, including a description of the taste, medication volume, and dosage frequency. Many patients will report being able to think more clearly and being happier than they were on narcotic analgesics. An important component of the cocktail treatment strategy is the maintenance of the same appearance of the medication and medication volume despite reducing its dosage so that patients do not expect their pain level to increase.

a. **On admission,** the patients are given the opioid analgesic they report to be taking at home. This dosage is observed over a period of 24 to 48 hours. The reason for this procedure is that sometimes the patients describe much larger quantities (or much smaller quantities) of home opioid medication use than what is actually seen to be taken once they are admitted to the hospital.

b. **After the evaluation period,** the 24-hour dose of opioid analgesic is given in an equivalent dose and is increased by approximately 20% (dose conversion tables may be found in the American Pain Society's guide for analgesic use).

c. **The patients then start on the pain cocktail,** which they receive every 6 hours. The drink is cherry flavored and a constant 10 ml in volume.

d. **The opioid analgesic content of the cocktail is reduced by approximately 20% a day** over the course of their hospital stay, but the total volume of the drink stays constant. When the total daily dose of opioid analgesic is less than 5 mg of methadone, the opioid analgesic is discontinued from the cocktail.

e. **Many patients continue on a pain cocktail** of acetaminophen or hydroxyzine for another few days.

B. Patient self-management and improvement. As medication usage is decreased, patients need to be encouraged to **increase their physical activity level, maintain responsibility for themselves, and regain their independence.**

    1. Physical well-being. The treatment plan should emphasize a wide range of physical therapies to increase **range of motion, muscle strength,** and **general mobility.** It is important to remind patients that these treatments are most effective as part of a complete rehabilitative program, and not as isolated pain relievers, and that they are **active partners in their own health care.** These therapies include

        a. Stretching and strengthening exercises

        b. Connective tissue massages

        c. Movement therapy

        d. Underwater range-of-motion exercises

        e. Other procedures such as **nerve blocks, transcutaneous electrical nerve stimulation (TENS),** or other **physical interventions**

        f. Instruction about the nature and source of pain as well as proper body mechanics. In an effort to increase patient strength and endurance, an **exercise program to wean patients from unnecessary assistive devices** should be executed. In addition to strengthening weakened muscles (which can complicate a patient's pain experience), these exercises help produce a general conditioning effect that has multiple benefits to the patient. Patients are expected to

          (1) Perform stretching and strengthening exercises on their own

          (2) Keep a record of the frequency and intensity of their exercise

          (3) Walk progressively longer distances and ride exercise bicycles for increasing periods of time

    2. Respect and responsibility. To enhance the impact of these therapies, the patient needs to be encouraged to conform to inpatient behavior that is consistent with the philosophy of self-care. Chronic pain patients must

        a. Spend the day out of their beds

        b. Be fully dressed in exercise clothes, not hospital pajamas

        c. Be responsible for making their beds and keeping their rooms in order

        d. Come to the desk to receive their prescribed medications

        e. Attend staff-patient-community meetings at which issues of mutual concern related to the functioning of the program are discussed. These meetings emphasize the important role the patient plays in the treatment of chronic pain. Patients are constantly reminded that they are not ill and will feel better if they perceive themselves as fully functioning individuals.

    3. Increased independence. At designated times during the program, patients are given a meal pass for use in the cafeteria. This arrangement stresses patients' independence and allows them to practice any dietary restrictions that were advised. The meal pass also affords the patients the opportunity to eat their meals in a more public and congenial setting. During the latter part of hospitalization, the patients are sent on a multichore time management mission. This project demands that patients manage their time effectively to achieve specified tasks.

    4. Vocational planning. If appropriate, patients are referred for vocational counseling to begin the process of return to work while they are still in the supportive hospital environment.

C. Emotional distress produced by chronic pain is also an important point of intervention. Many patients possess feelings of **helplessness, depression, anxiety, and agitation, as well as hostility** toward health care professionals.

    1. Psychological treatment

        a. Treatment plans that emphasize **supportive and cognitively oriented psychotherapy** can relieve the symptoms of depression and help patients understand their symptoms and change current behavior patterns.

        b. Patients should also be taught **assertiveness training** so that they can address their problems and concerns in a more direct and more effective way.

        c. Fundamentals of time management and leisure planning should be discussed. This will enable patients to identify pleasurable activities and incorporate them into their daily schedule. This activity is especially important, as many pain patients have stopped engaging in any pleasurable activities.

        d. The clinician may also want to **work with the patient's family members** who are also affected by the severe disability of the chronic pain patient. A better understanding of the patient's family dynamics will provide insight into determining the most effective treatment methods.

2. Psychotropic medications also have a significant role in treating depression. See Chapter 6 for a more complete discussion.

    a. Antidepressant medications have proved to be effective analgesics and partially effective hypnotics without some of the side effects associated with narcotic analgesics and sedative hypnotic medications. **Doxepin** has been found to be especially effective. **Doses** ranging from 25 to 75 mg given before sleep tend to be effective in improving patients' sleep and pain.

      (1) Complications

        (a) It is important that all patients be carefully screened for **cardiac conduction difficulty,** which is a relative contraindication to the use of doxepin.

        (b) In addition, some patients have problems with the **orthostatic hypotensive effect** of this medication. Patients should have their BP routinely checked in the supine and standing positions while they are on this drug.

        (c) When patients are unable to tolerate doxepin, a less sedating and less anticholinergic antidepressant, like **nortriptyline** 25–75 mg PO given at bedtime, has been effective in improving patients' sleep and pain.

      (2) Although the analgesic properties of the tricyclic antidepressants, independent of their antidepressant properties, have been recognized for some time, there have been no studies that suggest any one of the tricyclic antidepressants is a more effective analgesic than any other. Recently, there have been more studies reporting that the **serotonin-specific reuptake inhibitors (SSRIs)** such as fluoxetine (Prozac), sertraline (Zoloft), and paroxetine (Paxil) may be equally effective analgesics, independent of their antidepressant properties. Paroxetine 40 mg/day has been demonstrated to be as effective an analgesic as imipramine 100 mg/day in a population of patients with diabetic neuropathy. Although the advantages of the SSRIs are that there are no difficulties with cardiac conduction or orthostatic hypotensive effects, they lack some of the benefit in improving sleep difficulties often obtained with the more sedating tricyclic antidepressants.

    b. Antianxiety medications, primarily **benzodiazepines (Valium, Xanax, Ativan, and Tranxene),** should also be considered.

      (1) Drug selection and patient monitoring. An antianxiety medication with a relatively long duration of action may be a better choice. It is also essential to evaluate the patient's use of the medication to ensure that it is providing anxiety and pain relief and that it is being taken as prescribed.

      (2) Abuse and treatment. If abuse of these drugs is suspected, the antianxiety medications must be treated in the same manner as narcotic analgesics. The actual dosage taken by patients during the first few days of hospitalization must be evaluated, followed by a systematic reduction in dosage and detoxification with the use of a pain cocktail.

D. Stress and pain management. Many chronic pain patients show significant deficits in their ability to pace themselves during the day, are unable to maintain a low level of autonomic nervous system arousal in response to stress, and have difficulty returning to baseline levels of functioning after a period of increased activity. These patients can benefit from a stress management program that focuses on learning skills for self-regulation.

1. Advantages of hospitalization. Many patients have difficulty learning these skills at home, where they report significant distractions. By removing patients from their stressful home environment and daily routine, the hospital provides a secure environment for the learning and practice of behavioral self-regulation skills.

    a. Free of the necessity to cope with the multiple demands of daily living, patients can spend time focusing on improving their health.

    b. Patients can also support each other in learning these skills. These skills can then be carried into the difficult home environment following discharge.

2. Objective monitoring of self-regulation skills. To further define their pain problem, they initially undergo a sequence of biofeedback assessment sessions using techniques that provide specific information as to the **sites of muscular tension, patterns of protective guarding and bracing, shifts in postural adjustment,** and **specific patterns of physiologic arousal and recovery in response to pain.** In addition to their usefulness in providing targeted goals for relaxation, these assessment sessions often provide convincing information to the skeptical patient as to the direct relation between behavior and bodily response. They also often provide significant objective findings of pain-related functional deficits that do not appear in more structurally oriented medical procedures and scans. These sessions are followed by individual treatment sessions focusing on the responses that were found to be dysfunctional. These sessions employ the following procedures:

a. **Computer-driven diagnostic muscle scanning**
b. **Psychophysiologic stress profiling**
c. **Dynamic muscle evaluation**

3. **Group workshops and individualized training.** Stress management skills are best taught by a combined program of group stress management workshops and individualized behaviorally oriented training sessions. In these sessions, patients are given essential information on the **relation between stress and pain** and the nature of the **pain transmission system.** Specific strategies for altering their environment to reduce the frequency of stressful situations and increase personal resources are also discussed. Patients are next taught **self-control skills** such as

a. **Relaxation-oriented (diaphragmatic) breathing**
b. **Use of guided imagery and distraction**
c. **Strategies for cognitive restructuring of negative self-talk**
d. **Mental rehearsal techniques to help them practice imagining behaviors** that they had previously avoided
e. **sEMG (neuromuscular), temperature (thermal), and EEG (neurofeedback) biofeedback techniques**
f. **Hypnotic techniques** are taught to enable chronic pain patients to practice self-hypnosis on a regular basis. These techniques are useful for
   (1) **Relaxation and pain management**
   (2) **Reducing the psychological sequelae of trauma**
   (3) **Helping the patient become more self-sufficient**
   (4) In particular, patients with **posttraumatic stress disorders** resulting from traumatic injuries or driving-related phobias resulting from motor vehicle accidents benefit from these techniques.
   One should note that it is important to match the patient's personality and individual goals to the type of behavioral pain management strategy. This matching helps ensure the patient's continued interest and success in learning the skill.

4. **Therapeutic aids.** Patients in the hospital environment are also given therapeutic aids to help them practice the skills they are being taught.

a. **Relaxation tapes and tape players,** for example, may be used to provide patients with additional practice periods to build up their skills before discharge.
b. **Ambulatory biofeedback monitoring equipment** may also be provided to give patients specific feedback as they practice.
c. A variety of **educational and informational books** as well as **audio tapes** and **videotapes** are also made available. These materials provide information on anxiety and depression management, stress reduction, relaxation techniques, hypnosis, and other related topics. The availability of these alternative therapies while medications are being gradually reduced helps reinforce the use of behavioral self-regulation skills instead of opioid medications. To reinforce the self-regulation concept and practice, patients are given logs to record their sessions and monitor their progress.

V. **Follow-up.** Prior to discharge, the patient and physician need to review the progress the patient has made and design a personalized plan outlining the various possible outpatient therapies:

A. **A weekly regimen of physical and occupational therapy**
B. **More intensive training in hypnotherapy, biofeedback,** and **other self-regulation strategies**
C. **Family therapy and individual psychotherapy**

  D. A volunteer work program in the community. This work program is designed to provide patients with supervised, gradually increasing periods of work. Patients build up their tolerance for activity and are exposed to the social interaction that is an integral part of enhancing the pain patient's quality of life.

  E. Increased functioning. During follow-up in the office after the inpatient program, the physician's emphasis should not be on the patient's experience of pain, but on the patient's ability to

    1. Function in the home environment

    2. Maintain regular productive activity in and out of the home

    3. Pursue recreational or social activities

    4. Adhere to medication as prescribed

Selected Readings

American Pain Society. *Principles of Analgesic Use in the Treatment of Acute Pain and Chronic Cancer Pain: A Concise Guide to Medical Practice* (2nd ed.). Skokie, IL: American Pain Society, 1989.

American Pain Society/American Academy of Pain Medicine. *Directory of Pain Management Facilities.* Skokie, IL: American Pain Society, 1989.

Schwartz DP. Appropriate referral to inpatient vs. outpatient pain management programs. A clinician's guide. *Pain Digest* 1991. Pp. 1, 2–6.

Snow BR, Gusmorino P, Pinter I. Chronic pain and the geriatric patient: assessment and treatment. In Zuckerman JD (ed.), *Comprehensive Care of Orthopaedic Injuries in the Elderly.* Baltimore: Urban & Schwarzenberg, 1990.

Tollison CD, Satterthwaite JR, Tollison JW, Trent CG. *Handbook of Chronic Pain Management.* Baltimore: Williams & Wilkins, 1989.

Waldman SP. Providing pain management services: basic considerations. *Am J Pain Manage* 1994. Pp. 4, 86–88.

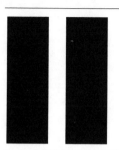

Pain Syndromes

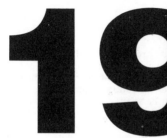

Cancer Pain

Russell K. Portenoy

I. **Background.** Pain is experienced by 30% to 50% of cancer patients in active treatment and more than 75% of those with advanced disease.[1,2] Unrelieved pain is common despite the availability of techniques that can provide adequate relief to most patients.[2] Unrelieved pain is profoundly debilitating to patients and their families, and all those involved in the care of cancer patients must acquire the skills necessary to manage this symptom.

II. **Approach to the patient**

    A. **Comprehensive assessment**

        1. Identify and characterize **underlying structural lesions** that may explain the pain. Such lesions are so common in the cancer population that all patients must be considered to have a structural cause for the pain unless another explanation is apparent.

        2. Clarify the **pathophysiology** of the pain, including nociception from injury to somatic or visceral structures, a neuropathic process, or psychological factors.

        3. Characterize the role of the pain in relation to the patient's **other symptoms.**

        4. Determine the contribution of the pain to the patient's **overall impairment** in quality of life.

    B. **Pain-oriented problem list.** This assessment can yield a problem list that guides the selection of treatments. Virtually all patients with cancer pain require multiple therapies, and such a problem list can help target these approaches.

    C. **Antineoplastic therapies.** As a first step in the management of cancer pain, the clinician should consider the potential analgesic consequences of primary antineoplastic therapies.

        1. **Radiotherapy** provides pain relief in approximately 50% of all patients and is commonly applied for the indication of pain.[3]

        2. **Chemotherapy** will alleviate some pain.[4]

        3. **Surgical intervention** performed for other indications, such as vertebral body resection for epidural cord compression or lysis of adhesions for bowel obstruction, may also produce analgesia as a benefit.[5]

    D. **Primary analgesic approaches** are the only options available to patients for whom antineoplastic therapy is inappropriate or ineffective. Pharmacotherapy is the most important of these approaches and typically involves the concurrent use of several drugs, supplemented in some cases by a coordinated application of other analgesic approaches. Pain and other symptoms continually change, and successful management also requires long-term follow-up and frequent monitoring.

III. **Pharmacologic approaches.** Three categories of analgesic medications are used in the treatment of cancer pain: **nonsteroidal anti-inflammatory drugs (NSAIDs); opioid analgesics;** and **adjuvant analgesics** (defined as drugs with other primary indications that are effective analgesics in specific settings).

    A. **Analgesic ladder.** The Cancer Pain Relief and Palliative Care program of the World Health Organization has advocated the analgesic ladder as a model approach to the selection of drugs for patients with cancer pain.[6] Early studies suggest that the optimal administration of drugs according to the analgesic ladder is capable of providing analgesia to at least 70% of patients with cancer pain.[7]

        1. **For mild to moderate pain,** acetaminophen or an NSAID should be used, combined with an adjuvant drug (an adjuvant analgesic or a drug to treat other symptoms) if needed.

        2. **For moderate to severe pain,** an opioid conventionally used for pain of this severity is used, combined with acetaminophen or NSAID and an adjuvant drug if needed.

3. For severe pain, an opioid conventionally used for pain of this severity is used with or without acetaminophen or an NSAID and with or without an adjuvant drug.

B. NSAIDs are believed to provide analgesia through a peripheral mechanism related to inhibition of the enzyme cyclo-oxygenase and consequent reduction of inflammatory mediators known to sensitize or activate peripheral nociceptors.[8] However, the marked disproportion between anti-inflammatory effect and analgesia observed with some of these drugs and the results of recent studies in animals and humans suggest that central mechanisms are also responsible for the analgesic effects. Central mechanisms are certainly involved in the analgesia produced by acetaminophen, a nonopioid analgesic often categorized with the NSAIDs.

A variety of subclasses comprise the NSAIDs (Table 19-1).[9] There is anecdotal evidence that efficacy and side effects vary not only in different subclasses but also within the subclass itself. This variability does not permit the clinician to reliably predict the analgesic response to any particular drug from the outcomes of previous trials.

1. Ceiling dose. NSAID analgesia is characterized by a ceiling dose, a dose above which additional increments in dose do not provide further analgesia. This characteristic restricts the utility of the NSAIDs to patients with relatively mild to moderate pain. It is important to recognize that the standard recommended dose of an NSAID may or may not reflect the minimum effective dose and the ceiling dose in any individual patient. Standard recommended doses are derived from studies conducted in patients who are not aged and who have a single inflammatory disease and no other significant medical problems. This population is very different from those with cancer pain, who are often elderly, have coexistent organ failure, or are receiving multiple other drugs.

2. Guidelines for the use of NSAIDs in patients with cancer pain are largely empirical, drawn from clinical experience, the pharmacology of these drugs, and the few studies available on the subject.

    a. Drug selection. NSAIDs are useful alone for mild to moderate pain and provide additive analgesia when combined with opioid drugs in the treatment of more severe pain.[10,11] They may be especially useful in patients with bone pain and pain related to inflammatory lesions; their efficacy in neuropathic pain appears to be limited.[10] Several factors are to be considered in the selection of an NSAID:

        (1) Favorable previous response to a particular drug

        (2) Concern about compliance with a prescribed regimen (may be lessened by the use of an NSAID with once-daily or twice-daily dosage)

        (3) The cost of the different NSAIDs (when this is an important issue, pharmacies can be screened for a schedule of charges)

    b. Side effects. The profile of adverse effects associated with NSAIDs (as a class, with each of the subclasses, and with specific agents) influences the process of drug selection.

    c. The pyrazole subclass, specifically phenylbutazone, carries a greater risk of adverse effects than the other NSAIDs and has been supplanted by newer drugs. All NSAIDs should be used cautiously in patients with renal insufficiency. Although lesser renal toxicity has been attributed to some drugs,[12] clinical experience has not sufficiently documented these differences. Unless anti-inflammatory effects are desired, acetaminophen is probably safer in the setting of renal insufficiency, notwithstanding one study that indicates a potential for renal toxicity from this drug as well.[13] Most agents are relatively contraindicated in patients with a diathesis for bleeding or peptic ulcer disease, common problems in cancer patients.

        Acetaminophen is again preferred in these settings. If anti-inflammatory effects are strongly desired, the use of a nonacetylated salicylate, choline magnesium trisalicylate or salsalate, is preferred. These salicylates have less ulcer potential than other NSAIDs and, at usual clinical doses, do not impair platelet aggregation.[14] NSAIDs may rarely cause or exacerbate encephalopathy and may be problematic in patients with preexisting organic brain syndrome. Finally, it should be noted that **significant hepatopathy mandates prudence in the administration of acetaminophen.**

    d. Dose-response relationship. Given the pharmacologic considerations discussed earlier, it is reasonable to begin administration of an NSAID for cancer pain at a relatively low dose, which is then increased gradually every

Table 19-1. Nonsteroidal anti-inflammatory drugs

Chemical class	Generic name	Approximate half-life (hr)	Dosage schedule	Recommended starting dose (mg/day)[a]	Maximum recommended dose (mg/day)	Comment
p-Aminophenol	Acetaminophen[b]	2–4	q4–6h	2600	6000	Overdosage produces hepatic toxicity. Not anti-inflammatory and therefore not preferred as first-line analgesic or co-analgesic in patients with bone pain. Lack of GI or platelet toxicity, however, may be important in some cancer patients. At high doses, platelet counts and liver function tests should be done periodically.
Salicylates	Aspirin[b]	3–12[c]	q4–6h	2600	6000	Standard for comparison. May not be tolerated as well as some of the newer NSAIDs.[d]
	Diflunisal[b]	8–12	q12h	1000 × 1, then 500 q12h	1500	Less GI toxicity than aspirin.[d]
	Choline magnesium trisalicylate[b]	8–12	q12h	1500 × 1, then 1000 q12h	4000	Unlike other NSAIDs, choline magnesium trisalicylate and salsalate have minimal GI toxicity and no effect on platelet aggregation, despite potent anti-inflammatory effects. May therefore be particularly useful in some cancer patients.[d]
	Salsalate	8–12	q12h	1500 × 1, then 1000 q12h	4000	
Propionic acids	Ibuprofen[b]	3–4	q4–8h	1600	4200	Available over-the-counter.[d]
	Naproxen[b]	13	q12h	500	1500	Available as a suspension and over-the-counter.[d]
	Naproxen sodium[b]	13	q12h	550	1375	—[d]
	Fenoprofen	2–3	q6h	800	3200	—[d]
	Ketoprofen	2–3	q6–8h	100	300	—[d]
	Flurbiprofen[b]	5–6	q8–12h	100	300	Experience is too limited to evaluate higher doses, though it is likely that some patients would benefit.[d]
	Oxaprozin	40	q24h	600	1800	

Table 19-1. Continued

Chemical class	Generic name	Approximate half-life (hr)	Dosage schedule	Recommended starting dose (mg/day)[a]	Maximum recommended dose (mg/day)	Comment
Acetic acids	Indomethacin	4–5	q8–12h	75	200	Available in sustained-release and rectal formulations. Higher incidence of side effects, particularly GI and CNS, than with propionic acids.[d]
	Tolmetin	1	q6–8h	600	2000	Short course recommended.[d]
	Sulindac	14	q12h	300	400	Less renal toxicity than other NSAIDs.[d]
	Diclofenac	2	q6h	75	200	—[d]
	Ketorolac (IM)	4–7	q4–6h	15–30 × 1	120	Parenteral formulation available. Experience is too limited to evaluate higher doses.[d]
	Etodolac	7	q8h	600	1200	
Oxicams	Piroxicam	45	q24h	20	40	Administration of 40 mg for over 3 weeks is associated with a high incidence of peptic ulcer, particularly in the elderly.[d]
Fenamates	Mefenamic acid[b]	2	q6h	500 × 1, then 250 q6h	1000	Not recommended for use longer than 1 week and therefore not indicated in cancer pain therapy.[d]
	Meclofenamic acid	2–4	q6–8h	150	400	—[d]
Pyrazoles	Phenylbutazone	50–100	q6–8h	300	400	Not a first-line drug owing to risk of serious bone marrow toxicity. Not preferred for cancer pain therapy.

[a]Starting dose should be one half to two thirds of the recommended dose in the elderly, those on multiple drugs, and those with renal insufficiency. Doses must be individualized. Low initial doses should be titrated upward if tolerated and clinical effect is inadequate. Doses can be incremented weekly. Studies of NSAIDs in the cancer population are meager; dosage guidelines are thus empiric.
[b]Pain is approved indication.
[c]Half-life of aspirin increases with dose.
[d]At high doses, stool guaiac and liver function tests, BUN, creatinine, and urinalysis should be checked periodically.

several days (or less often) to identify the minimal effective dose for the patient or, in the case of inefficacy, the ceiling dose or toxic dose. Should analgesia fail to accrue following an increase in dose, the ceiling has presumably been reached. When this occurs, the dose should be lowered to the previous level and continued, or the drug should be discontinued. If better analgesia occurs following an increase in dose, a trial at a higher dose should be considered, unless side effects are occurring or the dose has reached a level associated with an unacceptable risk of occult toxicity. Dose escalation cannot proceed indefinitely with the NSAIDs owing to their well-known dose-related toxicity. Unfortunately, there is little information available about the safety of long-term administration of NSAIDs at high doses for cancer patients. Based on clinical experience and customary use, maximal doses of 1.5 to 2 times the recommended starting dose are a prudent limit, below which the dose-response function can be explored to find the lowest dose that yields the greatest degree of analgesia. Patients who are maintained at doses above the standard level require relatively closer monitoring for occult fecal blood or changes in the urinalysis or renal function tests.

   e. Duration of trials. Several weeks are needed to judge the efficacy of a dose when NSAIDs are used in the treatment of grossly inflammatory lesions, such as arthritis. Clinical experience suggests that a briefer period, usually 1 week, is adequate for the same purpose in the cancer pain patient.

   f. Switching drugs. Given the variability in drug response, failure with one NSAID can be followed by success with another. There is no evidence that the failure of one drug renders success with any particular drug or class more likely. Hence, drug selection during these sequential trials is by trial and error.

C. Opioid analgesics. Expertise in the management of the opioid analgesics is the single most important factor in the successful treatment of the cancer pain patient. Guidelines, derived from pharmacologic principles and clinical experience, are summarized below.[15–17]

1. Selection. Similar to the NSAIDs, there is great variability in the response of a patient to different opioid drugs. Pharmacologic factors, however, strongly influence the initial selection of a drug, as well as the choice of subsequent drugs should a change become necessary.

   a. Opioid class. Opioid analgesics can be divided into agonist and agonist-antagonist classes based on specific patterns of drug-receptor interaction (Table 19-2).[18] The agonist-antagonist class can be further divided into the mixed agonist-antagonists (butorphanol, nalbuphine, and pentazocine) and the partial agonists (buprenorphine and probably dezocine). The agonist-antagonist drugs are seldom used in the management of cancer pain. These drugs all share the ability to reverse opioid effects and precipitate an abstinence syndrome in patients physically dependent on agonist drugs. All appear to have a ceiling dose for analgesia. These characteristics limit the potential of these agents to patients who are neither physically dependent nor tolerant to an agonist drug. In addition, some of these drugs, such as pentazocine and butorphanol, are associated with a relatively high incidence of psychotomimetic effects,[19] and most of them are not available in oral formulations, the preferred mode of delivery in the cancer pain population. These considerations explain the reliance on pure agonist drugs for the treatment of cancer pain.

   b. Weak versus strong opioids. Unlike the well-defined pharmacologic evidence that supports the division of opioids into different classes, the distinction between weak drugs advocated for the second rung of the analgesic ladder[6] and the strong opioids preferred for more severe pain is an operational one. Codeine is the prototype of the former group, but other drugs are also used in the United States, including oral propoxyphene, oxycodone (when combined with aspirin or acetaminophen), hydrocodone, and dihydrocodeine. Tramadol is a newly available opioid drug which has a unique mechanism of action and may also be appropriate for moderate cancer-related pain in the relatively nontolerant patient.

   There is no evidence from adequately controlled studies that codeine or the other drugs used for the second rung of the analgesic ladder have flatter dose-response curves or ceiling doses for analgesia. The designation as "weak" drugs, therefore, does not derive from an inherent inability to treat

Table 19-2. Opioid analgesics

	Equianalgesic doses[a]	Half-life (hr)	Peak effect (hr)	Duration (hr)	Toxicity	Comments
Morphine-like agonists						
Morphine	10 IM 20–60 PO[b]	2–3	0.5–1.0 1.5–2.0	3–6 4–7	Constipation, nausea, sedation most common; respiratory depression rare in cancer patients.	Standard comparison for opioids; multiple routes available (see Table 19-3).
Controlled-release morphine	20–60 PO[b]	—	3.0–4.0	8–12	Same as morphine.	Used for multiple routes (see Table 19-3).
Hydromorphone	1.5 IM 7.5 PO	2–3 —	0.5–1.0 1.0–2.0	3–4 3–4	Same as morphine.	Combined with aspirin or acetaminophen, for moderate pain; available orally without co-analgesic.
Oxycodone	20–30 PO	2–3	1.0	3–6	Same as morphine.	No oral formulation.
Oxymorphone	1 IM 10 PR	— —	0.5–1.0 1.5–3.0	3–6 4–6	Same as morphine.	Not preferred for cancer pain due to potential toxicity.
Meperidine	75 IM 300 PO	2–3 —	0.5–1.0 1.0–2.0	3–4 3–6	Same as morphine + CNS excitation; contraindicated in those on monoamine oxidase inhibitors.	Analgesic action due to metabolites, predominantly morphine; not available in U.S.
Heroin	5 IM	0.5	0.5–1.0	4–5	Same as morphine.	With long half-life, accumulation occurs after beginning or increasing dose.
Levorphanol	2 IM 4 PO	12–15	0.5–1.0	3–6	Same as morphine.	Risk of delayed toxicity due to accumulation; dosing should start on as-needed basis, with close monitoring.
Methadone	10 IM 20 PO	15–57	0.5–1.5	4–6	Same as morphine.	Anecdotally, 100 µg/hr is roughly equianalgesic to morphine 2 mg/hr.
Fentanyl transdermal system	—	—	—	48–72	Same as morphine.	Usually combined with an NSAID.
Codeine	130 IM 200 PO	2–3	1.5–2.0	3–6	Same as morphine.	

Drug	Dose				Effects	Comments
Propoxyphene	—	12	1.5–2.0	3–6	Same as morphine plus seizures with overdose.	Toxic metabolite accumulates but not significant at doses used clinically; often combined with an NSAID.
Propoxyphene napsylate	—	12	1.5–2.0	3–6	Same as hydrochloride.	Same as hydrochloride.
Hydrocodone	—	2–4	0.5–1.0	3–4	Same as morphine.	Only available combined with acetaminophen.
Partial agonists						
Buprenorphine	0.4 IM 0.8 SL	2–5	0.5–1.0 2.0–3.0	4–6 5–6	Same as morphine, except less risk of respiratory depression.	Can produce withdrawal in opioid-dependent patients; has ceiling for analgesia; sublingual tablet not yet available in U.S.; may be useful in cancer pain patients.
Mixed agonist-antagonist						
Pentazocine	60 IM 180 PO	2–3 —	0.5–1.0 1.0–2.0	3–6 3–6	Same profile of effects as buprenorphine, except for greater risk of psychotomimetic effects.	Produces withdrawal in opioid-dependent patients; oral preparation combined with naloxone in U.S.; ceiling doses and side-effect profile limits role in cancer pain.
Nalbuphine	10 IM	4–6	0.5–1.0	3–6	Same as buprenorphine except for greater risk of psychotomimetic effects, which is lower than pentazocine.	Produces withdrawal in opioid-dependent patients; no oral formulation; not preferred for cancer pain therapy.
Butorphanol	2 IM	2–3	0.5–1.0	3–4	Same profile of effects as nalbuphine.	Produces withdrawal in opioid-dependent patients; no oral formulation; not preferred for cancer pain therapy.

[a]Dose that provides analgesia equivalent to 10 mg IM morphine.
[b]Extensive survey data suggest that the relative potency ratio of 1:6 of IM to PO morphine changes to 1:2 to 1:3 with chronic use.

severe pain at higher doses, but rather is based on other factors such as a relatively high side-effect liability as doses are increased to levels adequate to treat severe pain (e.g., meperidine and propoxyphene), the unavailability until recently of a formulation that did not contain either acetaminophen or aspirin (hydrocodone), and conventional use.

In the United States, it has become common clinical practice to initiate opioid therapy with a drug containing codeine, propoxyphene, dihydrocodeine, oxycodone, or hydrocodone combined with aspirin or acetaminophen. Patients who fail to achieve adequate analgesia with doses of these drugs that yield maximally safe levels of the co-analgesic (e.g., 4–6 g acetaminophen, which is equivalent to 3 tablets of acetaminophen-containing combination product q4h) are then switched to a strong opioid, and the dose is titrated upward.

In the United States, the **strong opioids include morphine, methadone, hydromorphone, levorphanol,** and **oxycodone** (independent of a co-analgesic). **Fentanyl** is available in a transdermal formulation and **oxymorphone** is available in a formulation for rectal administration.

c. **Drug toxicities.** As noted previously, there is remarkable interindividual and intraindividual variability in the response to opioid drugs. This variability notwithstanding, there are several overriding drug-specific toxicities that influence opioid selection in the cancer pain patient:

(1) **The relatively high risk of psychotomimetic effects associated with the mixed agonist-antagonist subclass** was discussed above.

(2) **The use of meperidine is associated with the development of CNS hyperactivity,** including myoclonus, tremulousness, and seizures.[20] This is due to the accumulation of a toxic metabolite, normeperidine, and is most likely to become clinically evident in those patients with renal insufficiency and those who require high doses for prolonged periods. This effect contraindicates the use of this drug for the management of chronic cancer pain.

(3) **The metabolism of propoxyphene** also **yields** a toxic metabolite, **norpropoxyphene,** but the clinical relevance of this metabolite is limited at the doses used in common clinical practice.

d. **Pharmacokinetic differences.** Half-life is the most salient pharmacokinetic factor in the clinical management of the opioid drugs. Among those opioids currently in use, methadone (half-life variably reported from less than 12 hr to more than 100 hr) and levorphanol (half-life 12–16 hr) have relatively long terminal elimination half-lives. Since four to five half-lives are required to approach steady state plasma concentrations, regardless of drug, route of administration, or dosage interval, it is apparent that the accumulation of these drugs may occur for many days after dose adjustment has ceased. Furthermore, it must be emphasized that the **duration of analgesic effect is only loosely related to elimination half-life,** and dosing intervals of 4 hours for levorphanol and 4 to 6 hours for methadone are often needed clinically. The time required to approach steady state with these agents should thus be viewed as a period of increased risk, during which drug accumulation may result in delayed toxicity.[21] This phenomenon suggests that initiation of therapy with these drugs, methadone in particular, should be on an as-needed basis, with a switch to regularly scheduled doses after several days, during which the patient can establish an analgesic requirement.[22] Moreover, the drugs with a long half-life should be viewed as second-line agents in patients predisposed to adverse effects, including the elderly;[23] those with encephalopathy or other major organ failure; and those who will be difficult to follow or are suspected of noncompliance.

e. **Duration of effect.** Analgesic duration from each dose is another important factor in drug selection. As stated, most opioids require a dosing interval of 3 to 4 hours. Methadone, however, can be administered every 6 hours, or even less frequently in some patients. Controlled-release formulations of oral morphine (MS Contin and Oramorph SR) are effective at a dosing interval of 8 to 12 hours,[24] and the transdermal formulation of fentanyl can be administered every 48 to 72 hours.

f. **Previous favorable opioid exposure.** Given the great interindividual variability in opioid efficacy and occurrence of side effects, previous favorable experience with an opioid should be considered in selecting a drug. The exception to this is meperidine, with which the risk of toxic effects increases so dramatically with chronic oral administration at high doses that previous salutary postoperative experience cannot be used to predict future response in treating chronic cancer pain.

   g. In summary, opioid selection follows a logical process based on common clinical practice and pharmacologic principles.

     (1) Begin with a so-called weak opioid, typically a codeine or oxycodone combination product.

     (2) increase (in the absence of limiting side effects) until the maximum dose of the co-analgesic is attained.

     (3) Switch to a so-called strong opioid, which in the elderly or the medically frail is generally one of the short half-life drugs—morphine, hydromorphone, or oxycodone. In other patients, any of the pure agonists could be selected. A controlled-release oral formulation or the transdermal formulation should not be used for rapid dose titration in the patient with very severe pain owing to the relatively long period required to approach steady state plasma concentrations. In patients with very severe pain, dose titration with a short-acting drug can be followed by a switch to a long-acting formulation, if this is desired.

     (4) Finally, those patients who fail to benefit from a drug at maximally tolerated doses should be changed to an alternative approach, which may involve a switch to an alternative opioid, the use of an alternative route of opioid administration, the administration of an adjuvant analgesic, or the use of a nonpharmacologic analgesic approach (e.g., nerve blocks).

2. Dose-response relationship. A patient who is relatively nontolerant (for example, someone with limited exposure to a weak opioid) should generally begin one of the strong opioids at a dose equivalent to morphine 5–10 mg IM. If oral morphine is to be used, a ratio of intramuscular morphine to oral morphine of 3:1 should be used.[25] Patients on higher doses of opioids who are switched to another opioid should receive one half to two thirds the equianalgesic dose. Further reduction of the equianalgesic dose (to perhaps 25% to 33% of the equianalgesic dose) should be considered in the following:

   a. Aged patients

   b. Those with impaired hepatic or renal function

   c. Those undergoing a switch to methadone from another drug

3. Dose titration is essential at the start of therapy and is usually needed periodically throughout the patient's course. One reasonable approach to this process involves the concurrent use of a **regularly scheduled dose** and a **"rescue dose,"** which is usually offered every 2 hours on an as-needed basis.

4. Drug choice and dose size. The size of the rescue dose is based on empirical information; a quantity equivalent to approximately 5% to 15% of the total daily opioid intake is usually adequate. With the exception of methadone, controlled-release oral morphine, and transdermal fentanyl, the rescue dose can be of the same drug as that administered on a fixed-dose schedule. Given the pharmacokinetics of the latter drugs, it is appropriate to use an alternative opioid with a short half-life, such as morphine or hydromorphone, for the rescue dose. On a daily basis or less often, the quantity of supplemental analgesic can be summed to provide a guide for an appropriate increment in the regularly scheduled dose.

5. Dosage selection

   a. Fixed, around-the-clock dosing has achieved wide acceptance in the management of chronic cancer pain.

   b. As-needed dosing may also be beneficial in specific settings, such as the initiation of opioid therapy (particularly at the start of methadone therapy) and during periods of rapidly changing nociception (such as may follow radiotherapy to a bony lesion).

6. Route of administration

   a. The oral route is preferred in cancer pain management because of its relative safety, acceptability, economy, and duration of effect after each dose.

   b. Alternative routes are needed frequently, particularly in those with advanced cancer (Table 19-3).[26] Familiarity with these approaches, particularly those most commonly used, such as transdermal therapy, subcutaneous or

Table 19-3. Routes of administration

Route	Comment
Oral	Preferred in cancer pain management.
Buccal	Supporting data meager, and the method is generally unavailable and impracticable.
Sublingual	Buprenorphine is effective but not yet available in United States. Efficacy of morphine controversial. No clinical studies of other drugs.
Rectal	Available for morphine, oxymorphone, and hydromorphone. Although few studies are available, it is customarily used as if dose is equianalgesic to oral dose.
Transdermal	Available for fentanyl.
Intranasal	May be efficacious with some drugs; is available for butorphanol.

Subcutaneous
  Repetitive bolus
  Continuous infusion
  Continuous infusion with
    PCA
	Recent advent of ambulatory infusion pumps permits outpatient continuous infusion. Can be accomplished with any drug with a parenteral formulation.

Intravenous
  Repetitive bolus
  Continuous infusion PCA
    (with or without
    infusion)
	Intravenous route is indicated if other routes are unavailable or not tolerated. Infusion most useful in obviating bolus effect, i.e., peak concentration toxicity or pain infusion breakthrough at the trough. PCA is particularly useful for frequent breakthrough pain.

Epidural
  Repetitive bolus
  Continuous infusion
Intrathecal
  Repetitive bolus
  Continuous infusion
	Clearest indication is pain in lower body with poor relief and side effects from systemic opioids. Epidural catheter can be percutaneous (from lumbar region or tunneled to abdomen) or connected to subcutaneous portal, depending on patient's life expectancy. Intrathecal usually administered via subcutaneous pump. Morphine is the most common drug. Equianalgesic doses are not known. Usual starting doses are equivalent to morphine 5–10 mg IM for epidural and morphine 0.5–1.0 mg IM for intrathecal.

Intracerebroventricular	Rarely indicated.

PCA = patient-controlled analgesia

intravenous infusion therapy,[27] and spinal administration,[28] is requisite for the optimal management of cancer pain. Knowledge of relative potency is essential in switching opioid drugs or routes of administration.[29]

7. **Side effects.** The management of side effects is an essential component of the treatment of cancer pain, as symptomatic relief not only enhances patient comfort but also allows continued upward dose titration of the opioid to potentially analgesic levels. The most common side effects are constipation, nausea, and sedation.

a. **Constipation** is so common that a prophylactic regimen should be given to predisposed patients such as the elderly, patients with intrinsic bowel disease, the nonambulatory patient, and those concurrently taking other drugs with constipatory effects.[30]

b. Nausea should be aggressively managed with one of a variety of antiemetic drugs.[31]

c. Sedation that precludes the use of an otherwise effective analgesic can be managed by the addition of a psychostimulant, specifically dextroamphetamine, methylphenidate, or pemoline.[32]

d. Refractory side effects mandate a switch to an alternative drug, route of administration, or analgesic approach.

8. **Tolerance** is a poorly understood and complex phenomenon characterized by the need for higher opioid doses to maintain constant effects. Although tolerance is a potential reason for declining analgesic effects (or a need for higher doses to maintain effects), many surveys have demonstrated that patients with a stable disease state (whether malignant or nonmalignant in nature) can be maintained on the same analgesic dose for extremely long periods without loss of efficacy.[33,34] When the need for dose escalation arises in the cancer population, reevaluation usually demonstrates a progressive lesion. These observations suggest that concern about tolerance should not prevent the early use of opioids in patients with cancer pain. If a need for higher analgesic doses develops, alternative explanations, such as progression or recurrence of the neoplasm, must be considered.

9. **Physical and psychological dependence**

   a. **Physical dependence is** a pharmacologic property of opioid drugs **characterized by an abstinence syndrome** following administration of an antagonist or abrupt drug withdrawal. Although it is generally believed that physical dependence occurs during chronic opioid therapy, the dosage or duration of administration required to produce this outcome has not been established. Furthermore, the presumed relationship between tolerance and physical dependence is not well understood, and the degree of interindividual variability in both these phenomena is not known. In the management of cancer pain, the development of physical dependence does not pose a problem as long as

      (1) Opioid antagonists (including the agonist-antagonist opioids) **are avoided.**

      (2) Patients do not abruptly discontinue an opioid.

      (3) A tapering schedule is used when dose reduction is indicated.

   b. **Antagonists.** As patients receive higher doses of opioid drugs, and thereby develop both tolerance and physical dependence, the degree of sensitivity to the effects of antagonists increases.

      (1) Violent abstinence syndromes can be produced in the cancer patient on high doses of an opioid agonist after administration of very small doses of an antagonist drug. Given this risk, it is extremely important to **limit the use of naloxone** to those rare patients with symptomatic respiratory depression or the appearance of impending respiratory depression. Use of repetitive small doses of a dilute solution of naloxone (e.g., 0.4 mg/10 ml saline) further reduces the risk in this setting.

      (2) Adverse opioid effects that are not life-threatening can be more safely managed by withholding several doses, then reinstituting therapy at a lower level.

   c. **Addiction.** In contrast to the phenomena of physical dependence and tolerance, addiction is a psychological and behavioral syndrome with several fundamental characteristics.[35]

      (1) Loss of control over drug

      (2) Compulsive use

      (3) Continued use despite harm to the user or others

      (4) These characteristics, which reflect psychological dependence on the drug, are inferred on the basis of **observed aberrant drug-related behavior.** This behavior, when extreme, may include the theft, sale, and hoarding of drugs; acquisition of drugs from several physicians; and unsanctioned use. Concurrent abuse of alcohol or other nonopioid drugs may be an important indicator of prescription drug abuse.

      (5) Myth versus reality. Fear of addiction is a major reason for the undertreatment of cancer pain. The perception that addiction is a common outcome of opioid therapy persists despite abundant survey data demonstrating the contrary.[36-38] Extensive clinical experience in the cancer population,[33] as well as several surveys of patients with nonmalignant pain treated chronically with opioid drugs,[39] have also failed to support this concern. **Fear of addiction should not interfere with the appropriate administration of opioid drugs to patients with cancer pain.**

D. Adjuvant analgesics. There are many drugs with other indications that can be useful primary analgesics or co-analgesics in the management of cancer pain.

1. **Tricyclic antidepressants** have been demonstrated to be analgesic in many chronic, nonmalignant pain syndromes.[40] These drugs are preferred if an analgesic antidepressant is desired. The newer antidepressants, such as the serotonin-selective reuptake inhibitors, may be analgesic as well (demonstrated in a study of paroxetine), and such a drug should be considered if the patient is unable to tolerate a tricyclic drug. Of the tricyclic antidepressants, evidence of analgesic efficacy is best for the tricyclic compound **amitriptyline.** If the patient can tolerate this drug, it is preferred on this basis. If amitriptyline cannot be tolerated, desipramine can be recommended on the basis of strong evidence for analgesic efficacy. Initial doses of amitriptyline and desipramine should be very low (10–25 mg once daily), then titrated upward. Analgesic doses are usually in the range of 50 to 150 mg per day. All antidepressant drugs, like other adjuvants analgesics, are used after opioid dose escalation has failed to identify a dose associated with a favorable balance between analgesia and side effects. The most common situations are

   a. **Neuropathic pain syndromes** characterized by continuous dysesthesias, such as malignant plexopathy or chemotherapy-induced polyneuropathy

   b. **Cancer pain complicated by prominent depressive symptomatology or insomnia**

2. **Anticonvulsant drugs.** Extensive anecdotal reports (and reports of nonmalignant pain syndromes[41]) support the use of anticonvulsant drugs in the management of neuropathic pains that have a lancinating or paroxysmal character. For example, the shocklike head pains sometimes experienced by patients with recurrent head and neck cancer may respond dramatically to one of these drugs. **Carbamazepine, phenytoin, valproate** and **clonazepam** are the anticonvulsants currently used for pain management. **Baclofen,** a nonanticonvulsant with proven efficacy in trigeminal neuralgia,[42] may also be effective in this setting.

3. **Oral local anesthetics.** Recent studies have suggested that the oral local anesthetics **mexiletine** and **tocainide** can relieve neuropathic pains.[43,44] Mexiletine is the safer of the two, and is now used in patients with continuous or lancinating cancer-related pain. Because clinical experience with these drugs is limited, they should generally be used for

   a. Patients with continuous dysesthesias that have not responded to a tricyclic antidepressant

   b. Patients with lancinating dysesthesias who have not improved with anticonvulsant therapy

4. **Phenothiazines. Methotrimeprazine** is an analgesic[45] that has been used clinically in patients with advanced cancer for whom opioid drugs are problematic or pain is associated with nausea or anxiety. The sedative and hypotensive effects of this drug usually limit its use to bedridden patients with far-advanced cancer. There is very little evidence that other neuroleptics are analgesic, although some are commonly used in chronic nonmalignant pain syndromes.

5. **Corticosteroids** are important adjuvants in cancer pain management.[46] A controlled trial of **methylprednisolone** in patients with advanced cancer demonstrated that this drug **can improve analgesia, mood, and appetite,** at least for the short-term.[47] Although this study confirms clinical experience, there are no data from which to determine the best drug, dosage regimen, or duration of effects. Clinical experience suggests that short-term administration of high doses of a corticosteroid can provide dramatic pain relief in patients with severe pain due to bone metastases or tumor infiltration of neural structures. Doses can usually be tapered rapidly as alternative approaches are implemented. In those with advanced disease, more long-term, open-ended treatment is often undertaken in an effort to ameliorate pain and a variety of other symptoms such as anorexia, lassitude, and dysphoria.[46]

6. Other adjuvant analgesics
  a. Methylphenidate and dextroamphetamine are co-analgesic in low doses and, along with pemoline, are effective remedies for opioid-induced sedation.[32]
  b. Hydroxyzine is analgesic at relatively high parenteral doses,[48] and although the drug has been disappointing as an analgesic at the relatively low doses usually employed orally, it may be considered for cancer pain patients who have a primary indication for an anxiolytic or antiemetic.
  c. Bisphosphonates, calcitonin, or strontium-89 may benefit patients with refractory bone pain.[49]
  d. Anticholinergic drugs (e.g., scopolamine) and octreotide have been used to treat refractory pain from bowel obstruction.
IV. Alternative approaches. Surveys suggest that the need for invasive analgesic approaches (Table 19-4) is present in less than 20% of cancer pain patients.[50] Some type of alternative analgesic therapy should be considered **in all patients who fail to achieve a favorable balance between analgesia and side effects during opioid dose titration.**
 A. Anesthetic approaches
   1. Trigger point injections are the simplest anesthetic approach that is within the purview of most clinicians and may be useful in treating cancer-related myofascial pains.[51]
   2. Nitrous oxide inhalation has been used for those with advanced cancer, particularly for those patients with severe pain precipitated by predictable activities such as dressing changes.[52]
   3. Regional anesthetic techniques comprise a large group of procedures potentially useful in the management of localized pains.[53,54]
    a. Nerve blocks may be temporary or permanent and may be targeted at somatic or sympathetic nerves.
    b. Neurolytic blocks may be appropriate after nondestructive techniques have been exhausted. The possible exception to this is celiac plexus blockade, which appears to have a therapeutic index sufficient to warrant earlier use in patients with epigastric pain due to neoplasms in the region of the celiac axis.[55]
 B. Neurostimulatory approaches
   1. Stimulation of afferent neural pathways may produce analgesia. Published experience in the cancer pain population with these procedures is anecdotal. It is commonly observed that early results are favorable, but are not long-lasting.[56] Results also appear to be relatively better in pains of neuropathic origin. The techniques founded on this principle include
    a. Counterirritation (systematic rubbing of the painful part)
    b. Transcutaneous electrical nerve stimulation
    c. Percutaneous electrical nerve stimulation
    d. Dorsal column stimulation
    e. Deep brain stimulation
    f. Acupuncture
   2. Given the possibility of short-lived effects and the limited supporting data, the **techniques that have gained clinical acceptance are the noninvasive ones, particularly transcutaneous electrical nerve stimulation.** This approach should be considered most strongly in patients with severe neuropathic pains, in whom some degree of immediate relief may provide the time needed for an adequate trial of opioids or adjuvant analgesics, and in those with transitory pains (such as postoperative pain) in whom opioid use is relatively contraindicated.
 C. Physiatric approaches. The analgesic potential of physiatric techniques, including the use of physical and occupational therapies, orthoses, and prostheses, is underrecognized. Bracing can benefit movement-related pain unresponsive to opioid drugs. For example, refractory arm pain from malignant brachial plexopathy may be improved by a splint that supports the shoulder and limits abduction, while persistent back pain from vertebral metastases may be reduced with a surgical corset. In some patients, prosthetic devices may similarly help relieve stump and phantom pain. Physical therapy can limit the development of the myofascial pains, joint ankyloses, and contractures that may complicate immobility and abnormal motor function. Finally, both physical and occupational therapy emphasize rehabilitation and offer the patient some degree of personal control,

Table 19-4. Invasive procedures used in the management of cancer pain

Site	Anesthetic approach	Neurosurgical approach[a]	Neuroaugmentative approach
Pelvis, perineum[b]	Chemical rhizotomy	Bilateral cordotomy; midline myelotomy	Dorsal column stimulation
Epigastrium[c]	Celiac plexus block	—	—
Abdomen, chest	Chemical neurectomy; chemical rhizotomy	Neurectomy; rhizotomy; cordotomy	Percutaneous electrical stimulation
Arms, legs[b]	Chemical rhizotomy	Neurectomy; rhizotomy; cordotomy	Percutaneous electrical stimulation
Head, neck	Chemical rhizotomy; chemical gangliolysis	Rhizotomy	—
Generalized pain	Chemical hypophysectomy	Bilateral cordotomy	Deep brain stimulation

[a]Unilateral pain can also be treated by surgical procedures directed at the brain stem, specifically tractotomies and thalamotomy; other procedures, lobotomy and cingulumotomy, were designed to reduce suffering by producing an asymbolia for pain, if not pain relief, and are rarely done.
[b]Spinal administration of opioids is commonly used in this setting.
[c]Celiac plexus blockade is often utilized early in the management of patients with malignant epigastric visceral pain.

elements that may be particularly salutary as the patient increasingly perceives an inability to control either the cancer itself or the treatments undertaken to combat it.

D. Neurosurgical approaches. Localized pains may be amenable to procedures that denervate the painful part. Accordingly, neuroablative techniques have been devised for every level of the nervous system from peripheral nerve to cerebral cortex (see Table 19-4).[57] These procedures are fundamentally antinociceptive, and should not be considered for pains in which the presumed pathophysiologic substrate is central, including neuropathic pains believed to be due to deafferentation and pains of psychological origin. In support of this view, there is ample evidence that the efficacy of ablative procedures declines in the treatment of deafferentation pain.[58] These approaches should be considered after adequate trials of pharmacologic therapies have failed. Lobotomy and cingulumotomy are now rarely considered. Hypophysectomy is an ablative procedure performed surgically or via injection of a neurolytic solution. Usually advocated for patients with generalized pains, this procedure is capable of providing relief, at least transiently, to some patients, without regard for the hormonal sensitivity of the neoplasm.[59,60]

E. Psychological approaches. All cancer patients need psychological support. Disease-related issues should be addressed openly and efforts made to buttress and coordinate the resources of the patient and family. The acute and compelling need for support of this kind provided the impetus for the development of continuing care programs, the most comprehensive of which utilize a multidisciplinary team approach.[61] The spectrum of psychological approaches to pain management (discussed in more detail in Chap. 12) is extremely broad.[62,63] Formal psychotherapy, supportive in some instances and usually cognitive or behaviorally oriented in others, is necessary with some patients.

  1. Consultation with a specialist should be considered early in patients with
    a. A past history of a psychiatric disorder
    b. Current evidence of marked psychological distress
    c. Maladaptive patterns of behavior, such as social withdrawal, insistence on unnecessary help in activities of daily living, or substance abuse
    d. Distress in family members

  2. A variety of **specific cognitive approaches** have been advocated in the management of cancer pain.[62–67] These approaches, which include hypnosis, relaxation training, distraction techniques, and others, may be particularly useful in patients with prominent anxiety and those with a pattern of predictable pain. Although these techniques are time-consuming, presume a cognitively intact patient, and often require trained personnel, the simpler types, such as relaxation training, are within the purview of most clinicians to teach and most patients to learn. These approaches **are underutilized and deserve greater emphasis** in the clinical management of pain.

References

1. Portenoy RK. Cancer pain: epidemiology and syndromes. *Cancer* 63:2298–2307, 1989.
2. Bonica JJ. Treatment of cancer pain: current status and future needs. In Fields HL, Dubner R, Cervero F (eds.), *Advances in Pain Research and Therapy*, vol. 9. New York: Raven, 1985. Pp. 589–616.
3. Salazar OM, Rubin P, Hendrickson FR, et al. Single-dose half-body irradiation for palliation of multiple bone metastases from solid tumors. *Cancer* 58:29–36, 1986.
4. Bonadonna G, Molinari R. Role and limits of anticancer drugs in the treatment of advanced pain. In Bonica JJ, Ventafridda V (eds.), *Advances in Pain Research and Therapy*, vol. 2. New York: Raven, 1979. Pp. 131–138.
5. Sundaresan N, DiGiacinto GV. Antitumor and antinociceptive approaches to control cancer pain. *Med Clin North Am* 71:329–348, 1987.
6. World Health Organization. *Cancer Pain Relief and Palliative Care*. Geneva: World Health Organization, 1990.
7. Ventafridda V, Tamburini M, Caraceni A, et al. A validation study of the WHO method for cancer pain relief. *Cancer* 59:850–856, 1987.
8. Vane JR. Inhibition of prostaglandin synthesis as a mechanism of action for aspirin-like drugs. *Nature New Biol* 234:231–238, 1971.

9. Sunshine A, Olson NZ. Non-narcotic analgesics. In Wall PD, Melzack R (eds.), *Textbook of Pain* (2nd ed). New York: Churchill-Livingstone, 1989. Pp. 670–685.
10. Ventafridda V, Fochi C, DeConno F, Sganzerla E. Use of nonsteroidal anti-inflammatory drugs in the treatment of pain in cancer. *Br J Clin Pharmacol* 10:343–346, 1980.
11. Ferrer-Brechner T, Ganz P. Combination therapy with ibuprofen and methadone for chronic cancer pain. *Am J Med* 77:78–83, 1984.
12. Swainson CP, Griffiths P. Acute and chronic effects of sulindac on renal function in chronic renal disease. *Clin Pharmacol Ther* 37:298–300, 1985.
13. Sandler DP, Smith JC, Weinberg CR, et al. Analgesic use and chronic renal disease. *N Engl J Med* 320:1238–1243, 1989.
14. Cohen A, Thomas GB, Coen EE. Serum concentration, safety and tolerance of oral doses of choline magnesium trisalicylate. *Curr Ther Res* 23:358–364, 1978.
15. Agency for Health Care Policy and Research, Cancer Pain Management Panel. *Clinical Practice Guideline Number 9. Management of Cancer Pain.* Washington, DC: US Department of Health and Human Services, 1994.
16. Foley KM. The treatment of cancer pain. *N Engl J Med* 313:84–95, 1985.
17. Cherny NI, Portenoy RK. Practical issues in the management of cancer pain. In Wall PD, Melzack R (eds.), *Textbook of Pain* (3rd ed.). Edinburgh: Churchill-Livingstone, 1994. Pp. 1437–1467.
18. Houde RW. Analgesic effectiveness of the narcotic agonist-antagonists. *Br J Clin Pharmacol* 7:297S–308S, 1979.
19. Kantor TG, Hopper M, Laska E. Adverse effects of commonly ordered oral narcotics. *J Clin Pharmacol* 21:1–8, 1981.
20. Kaiko RF, Foley KM, Grabinski PY, et al. Central nervous system excitatory effects of meperidine in cancer patients. *Ann Neurol* 13:180–185, 1983.
21. Ettinger DS, Vitale PJ, Trump DL. Important clinical pharmacologic considerations in the use of methadone in cancer patients. *Cancer Treat Rep* 63:457–459, 1979.
22. Sawe J, Hansen J, Ginman C, et al. Patient-controlled dose regimen for methadone for chronic cancer pain. *Br Med J* 282:771–773, 1981.
23. Portenoy RK. Optimal pain control in elderly cancer patients. *Geriatrics* 42:33–44, 1987.
24. Portenoy RK, Maldonado M, Fitzmartin R, et al. Controlled-release morphine sulfate: analgesic efficacy and side effects of a 100 mg tablet in cancer pain patients. *Cancer* 63:2284–2288, 1989.
25. Kaiko RF. Commentary: equianalgesic dose ratio of intramuscular/oral morphine, 1:6 versus 1:3. In Foley KM, Inturrisi CE (eds.), *Advances in Pain Research and Therapy,* vol. 8. New York: Raven, 1986. Pp. 87–94.
26. Coyle N, Adelhardt J, Foley KM, Portenoy R. Character of terminal illness in the advanced cancer patient: pain and other symptoms in the last 4 weeks of life. *J Pain Symptom Manage* 5:83–93, 1990.
27. Portenoy RK, Moulin DE, Rogers A, et al. Intravenous infusion of opioids in cancer pain: clinical review and guidelines for use. *Cancer Treat Rep* 70:575–581, 1986.
28. Payne R. Role of epidural and intrathecal narcotics and peptides in the management of cancer pain. *Med Clin North Am* 71:413–428, 1987.
29. Houde RW. Misinformation: side effects and drug interactions. In Hill CS, Fields WS (eds.), *Advances in Pain Research and Therapy,* vol. 11. New York: Raven, 1989. Pp. 145–161.
30. Portenoy RK. Constipation in the cancer patient: causes and management. *Med Clin North Am* 71:303–312, 1987.
31. Baines M. Nausea and vomiting in the patient with advanced cancer. *J Pain Symptom Manage* 3:81–85, 1988.
32. Pruera E, Chadwick S, Brenneis C, et al. Methylphenidate associated with narcotics for the treatment of cancer pain. *Cancer Treat Rep* 71:67–70, 1987.
33. Kanner RM, Foley KM. Patterns of narcotic drug use in a cancer pain clinic. *Ann NY Acad Sci* 362:161–172, 1981.
34. Twycross RG. Clinical experience with diamorphine in advanced malignant disease. *Int J Clin Pharmacol Ther Toxicol* 9:184–198, 1974.
35. Jaffe JH. Drug addiction and drug abuse. In Gilman AG, Goodman LS, Rall TW, Murad F (eds.), *The Pharmacological Basis of Therapeutics* (7th ed.). New York: Macmillan, 1985. Pp. 532–581.
36. Porter J, Jick H. Addiction rare in patients treated with narcotics. *N Engl J Med* 302:123, 1980.

37. Perry S, Heidrich G. Management of pain during debridement: a survey of U.S. burn units. *Pain* 13:267–280, 1982.
38. Medina JL, Diamond S. Drug dependency in patients with chronic headache. *Headache* 17:12–14, 1977.
39. Portenoy RK. Chronic opioid therapy in non-malignant pain. *J Pain Symptom Manage* 5:S46–S62, 1990.
40. Portenoy RK. Adjuvant analgesics in pain management. In Doyle D, Hanks GW, MacDonald N (eds.), *Oxford Textbook of Palliative Medicine*. Oxford, UK: Oxford University Press, 1993. Pp. 187–203.
41. Swerdlow M. Anticonvulsant drugs and chronic pain. *Clin Neuropharmacol* 7:51–82, 1984.
42. Fromm GH, Terence CF, Chatta AS. Baclofen in the treatment of trigeminal neuralgia. *Ann Neurol* 15:240–247, 1984.
43. Dejgard A, Petersen P, Kastrup J. Mexiletine for treatment of chronic painful diabetic neuropathy. *Lancet* 1:9, 1988.
44. Lindstrom P, Lindblom U. The analgesic effect of tocainide in trigeminal neuralgia. *Pain* 28:45, 1987.
45. Beaver WT, Wallenstein SM, Houde RW, Rogers A. A comparison of the analgesic effects of methotrimeprazine and morphine in patients with cancer. *Clin Pharmacol Ther* 7:436–446, 1966.
46. Ettinger AB, Portenoy RK. The use of corticosteroids in the treatment of symptoms associated with cancer. *J Pain Symptom Manage* 3:99–104, 1988.
47. Bruera E, Roca E, Cedaro L, et al. Action of oral methylprednisolone in terminal cancer patients: a prospective randomized double-blind study. *Cancer Treat Rep* 69:751–754, 1985.
48. Stambaugh JE, Lane C. Analgesic efficacy and pharmacokinetic evaluation of meperidine and hydroxyzine, alone and in combination. *Cancer Invest* 1:111–117, 1983.
49. Payne R. Pharmacologic management of bone pain in the cancer patient. *Clin J Pain* 5 (Suppl 2):S35–S42, 1989.
50. Ventafridda V, Tamburini M, DeConno F. Comprehensive treatment in cancer pain. In Fields HL, Dubner R, Cervero F (eds.), *Advances in Pain Research and Therapy*, Vol. 9. New York: Raven, 1985. Pp. 617–628.
51. Twycross RG, Fairfield S. Pain in far-advanced cancer. *Pain* 14:303–310, 1982.
52. Fosburg MT, Crone RK. Nitrous oxide analgesia for refractory pain in the terminally ill. *JAMA* 250:511–513, 1983.
53. Raj PP. Prognostic and therapeutic local anesthetic blockade. In Cousins MJ, Bridenbaugh PO (eds.), *Neural Blockade in Clinical Anesthesia and Management of Pain* (2nd ed.). Philadelphia: J.B. Lippincott, 1988. Pp. 899–933.
54. Cousins MJ, Dwyer B, Gibb D. Chronic pain and neurolytic neural blockade. In Cousins MJ, Bridenbaugh PO (eds.), *Neural Blockade in Clinical Anesthesia and Management of Pain* (2nd ed.). Philadelphia: J.B. Lippincott, 1988. Pp. 1053–1084.
55. Bridenbough LD, Moore DC, Campbell DD. Management of upper abdominal cancer pain: treatment with celiac plexus block with alcohol. *JAMA* 190:877–880, 1964.
56. Ventafridda V, Sganzerla EP, Fochi C. Transcutaneous nerve stimulation in cancer pain. In Bonica JJ, Ventafridda V (eds.), *Advances in Pain Research and Therapy*, vol. 2. New York: Raven, 1979. Pp. 509–515.
57. Pagni CA. Role of neurosurgery in cancer pain: re-evaluation of old methods and new trends. In Beneditti C, Chapman CR, Morrica G (eds.), *Advances in Pain Research and Therapy*, vol. 7. New York: Raven, 1984. Pp. 603–629.
58. Tasker RR. Deafferentation. In Wall PD, Melzack R (eds.), *Textbook of Pain*. New York: Churchill-Livingstone, 1984. Pp. 119–132.
59. Gianasi G. Neuroadenolysis of the pituitary: an overview of development, mechanisms, techniques, and results. In Beneditti C, Chapman CR, Morica G (eds.), *Advances in Pain Research and Therapy*, vol. 7. New York: Raven, 1984. Pp. 647–678.
60. Lipton S, Miles JB, Williams N, Bark-Jones N. Pituitary injection of alcohol for widespread cancer pain. *Pain* 5:78–82, 1978.
61. Coyle N. A model of continuity of care for cancer patients with chronic pain. *Med Clin North Am* 71:259–270, 1987.
62. Cleeland CS, Tearnan BH. Behavioral control of cancer pain. In Holzman AD, Turk DC (eds.), *Pain Management*. New York: Pergamon, 1986.

63. Fishman B, Loscalzo M. Cognitive-behavioral interventions in management of cancer pain: principles and applications. *Med Clin North Am* 71:271–289, 1987.
64. Cagnello VW. The use of hypnotic suggestion for relief of malignant disease. *Int J Clin Exp Hypn* 9:17–22, 1961.
65. Fotopoulos SS, Graham C, Cook MR. Psychophysiologic control of cancer pain. In Bonica JJ, Ventafridda V (eds.), *Advances in Pain Research and Therapy,* vol. 2. New York: Raven, 1979. Pp. 231–243.
66. Simonton O, Matthews-Simonton S, Sparks T. Psychological intervention in the treatment of cancer. *Psychosomatics* 21:226–233, 1980.
67. Fleming U. Relaxation therapy for far-advanced cancer. *Practitioner* 229:471–475, 1985.

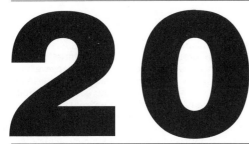

Pain in Children
Barbara S. Shapiro

I. Background
A. Perception of pain.
Parents know by observation and intuition that their children feel pain. Observation has now been validated by research. It is clear that babies and children, when exposed to painful stimuli, hurt. The responsibility of physicians and nurses to relieve pain and suffering applies to patients of all ages.

Many principles of pain assessment and treatment are the same for all age groups. Pain, as a multifaceted experience, must be approached in a multimodal manner, with the therapy adjusted to the type of pain and the context in which it occurs.
B. Undertreatment of pain.
Until recently, pain in children has been viewed as a symptom of disease or trauma, and not as a problem that deserves assessment and treatment. There are many reasons for the undertreatment of pain in children:
1. A lack of knowledge of age-specific assessment and treatment technique has been a major barrier. The experience and communication of pain is shaped by age and cognitive development. Anatomic and physiologic variables affect types of pain problems and use of medication.
2. Although family issues must be considered for patients of all ages, inclusion of the family is vital for the adequate treatment of pain in children. Health care professionals may not realize this.
3. Children are essentially powerless in the medical system, and cannot act as their own advocates to demand treatment. This places greater responsibility squarely on the shoulders of physicians and nurses.

II. Types of pain
A. Etiology.
Stimulation of nociceptors, changes in the central and peripheral nervous system, and emotional factors can all produce pain and are all involved in the experience of pain. The classification of pain according to etiology can be helpful in determining therapy. However, rigid classification schemes ignore the complexity of the pain experience. For example, postoperative pain may be viewed as a somatic nociceptive pain syndrome. However, neuropathic pain can sometimes occur in the postoperative period, and emotional factors always influence the perception of pain. Successful treatment of pain rests on understanding and assessing the several possible determinants.
B. Duration.
The classification of pain as acute or chronic defines the approach to treatment, with immediate and aggressive treatment (usually pharmacologic) for acute pain, and a carefully planned multimodal approach for chronic pain.
1. **Acute pain.** The causes of acute pain are similar in children and adults:
   a. **Postoperative** pain
   b. Pain from **trauma**
   c. Pain from **infectious and inflammatory processes**
   d. **Procedural pain.** Children have special problems with pain and anxiety from procedures such as **venipunctures, lumbar punctures, bone marrow aspirations and biopsies, and burn dressing changes.** Although these procedures are also distressing to adults, children may not understand the reasons for such procedures and that the duration of the pain is limited. Often procedures are performed without the consent of the patient. The resultant anxiety and loss of control can be overwhelming, and coping skills are eroded. Procedures are particularly difficult for babies and young children and for children with chronic illnesses, such as cancer, in which repeated and frequent procedures are necessary.

   e. Pain related to **acute illness**
   2. Chronic pain
      a. Chronic pain in adults is commonly defined as pain that lasts for more than 3 months. However, **young children often exhibit characteristics associated with chronic pain after just a few days of continuing severe pain.** The interaction of time with pain is very complex, and the rigid classification of pain as acute or chronic, based solely on duration, ignores the underlying forces. When pain starts, the patient reacts with a variety of emotions and behaviors, including anxiety and anger, and attempts to escape from or reduce the unpleasant feeling. These reactions are predicated on the belief that the pain will stop. If the pain continues, the expectation of relief gradually fades. Eventually, the individual has no perception of the temporal limitation of the pain. Anxiety fades into apathy and depression, avoidance into passivity, and the emotions and behaviors associated with the pain become increasingly pervasive and fixed. The perception of duration is influenced by age, cognition, reactions of others, context, and intensity of the pain. **The young child or baby with pain cannot understand that some situations are temporary, and a tolerable length of a time for an adult can be unbearably long for a child.**
      b. Chronic pain may be steady or recurrent. Although steady pain is common in adults, **recurrent pain problems,** such as headaches and abdominal pain, **are more often seen in children.** The frequency and intensity of the recurrences, as well as individual, familial, and social factors, influence the extent to which the pain becomes a part of daily life.
III. The experience of pain is shaped by the meaning, context, memory, and understanding of pain, all of which vary with age. Neonates and babies respond to nociceptive stimuli and may develop conditioned responses to nonpainful stimuli that have been paired with painful stimuli. However, the experience differs from that in older persons. A baby suffers as we suffer, but the pain is interpreted differently than it is by older individuals.
   A. Babies. During the first 2 years of life, babies develop a repertoire of responses to painful events that vary with the severity of the pain, the reactions of adults, and the memory of past events. For example, the 1-year-old baby who falls when walking may not cry unless an alarm is cued by the caregiver. The 15-month-old baby about to receive an immunization reacts with anticipatory fear and anger. Separating babies from parents provokes intense anxiety; soothing physical contact with them can help ease pain and distress.
   B. Children. As the child develops verbal and cognitive abilities, the meaning of the pain becomes important. Preschool children do not usually worry about pain being a harbinger of serious illness, but they are sensitive to the worries of their parents about the meaning of the pain. Children up to the age of 11 or 12 years commonly believe that pain is a punishment for misbehavior.
   C. Adolescents. As children approach adolescence, they begin to view pain as a symptom, and worries about the significance of the symptom influence the perception of the pain. The experience begins to approach that of an adult, but the reaction is shaped by the issues of adolescence.
IV. Assessment. The care provider must be cognizant of the presence and intensity of pain in order to determine appropriate treatment. Pain can be communicated by words, expressions, and behavior (crying, guarding a body part, grimacing). In children, it is necessary to adjust the pain assessment to age, developmental level, and context.
   Pain assessment should be adapted to the pain problem and the patient. Acute pain can be assessed quickly, with attention to specific factors such as intensity, region, radiation, quality, and provocative and palliative factors. However, more complex or chronic pain problems warrant a detailed assessment of the psychosocial status of the family and patient, as well as of the pain. An initial focus on the pain validates to the child and the family that the care provider believes the patient and takes the problem seriously. Once the pain has been described, other issues that may be related to the pain, such as family functioning, school performance, mood, stresses, and social relationships, can be explored.
   A. Neonates and babies. Adequate assessment of pain in this age group requires an awareness of painful stimuli; situations that are painful for older children and adults can be expected to be painful for babies. Examples are surgery, bone marrow aspirations and biopsies, chest intubations, osteomyelitis, fractures, and

burns. In a situation in which pain is expected or suspected, the baby should be given analgesia. Subsequent behavior suggesting increased comfort is an indication for continued pain management.

  1. Signs of acute pain in babies include
  a. Crying or moaning
  b. Muscle rigidity
  c. Flexion or flailing of the extremities
  d. Diaphoresis
  e. Irritability
  f. Guarding
  g. Changes in vital signs
  h. Pupillary dilation

  2. Signs of chronic pain. Chronic pain in babies is more difficult to assess. Signs of pain overlap with signs of illness; therefore, a careful history, physical examination, and laboratory evaluation are essential. After a short period of persistent pain, babies sometimes exhibit
  a. Apathy
  b. Irritability
  c. Changes in sleeping and eating
  d. A lack of interest in their surroundings

  3. Factors influencing signs of pain
  a. Babies who are ill may not have the vigor to cry.
  b. The baby who is intubated and receiving paralyzing agents cannot exhibit signs of pain; in this situation, anticipatory analgesia is indicated.

  4. Continued assessment. Once analgesia has been implemented, behavior must be assessed at regular intervals to determine the adequacy of analgesia. A particular behavior may be targeted for ongoing assessment. For example, a baby with bone pain from leukemia may cry when held and when the diaper is changed. Adequate analgesia would allow the baby to be content during these maneuvers. Nurses and parents can rate the apparent comfort, and record this on a log to facilitate adjustment of the dose of analgesic.

B. Older children

  1. Pain severity scale. The child over the age of about 6 years who understands the concepts of rank and order can use numerical or visual analogue scales to rate the pain severity. Numerical scales are easy to use and can be recorded on the bedside chart. Visual analogue scales may be more sensitive to small changes and can sometimes be used by children who do not understand numbers. Categorical scales can be utilized if the vocabulary is adjusted to the age of the child (e.g., none, a little, some, or a lot of pain).

  2. Verbal descriptors. Children over the age of 5 years can describe the characteristics of their pain, although it may be necessary to suggest choices of descriptive words. Children understand the qualities implied by "burning," "stinging," and "pins and needles." The distinction between throbbing and steady pain can be made by grasping the forearm of the child and replicating the sensation. Some children may understand a graphic representation of temporal qualities (spikes, straight).

  3. Faces scales. Children over the age of 4 years who do not yet understand order and number can be shown a series of faces ranging from smiling to neutral to frowning to crying and asked to point to the face corresponding to the pain. Several series of faces, cartoon and photographed, have been developed for pain assessment. A faces scale with established reliability and validity should be used for research; however, the clinician at the bedside with no tools but a piece of paper and pencil can draw a series of cartoon faces.

  4. Body map. Children over the age of 3 years can use an outline of the body to indicate the location and the severity of the pain. The child is asked to pick four crayon colors representing pain intensities from none to the worst and to color an anterior and a posterior body outline. Children vary in their choices of colors, so colors should not be preassigned. This method can be used to follow conditions of migrating and radiating pain, such as in polyarticular juvenile rheumatoid arthritis. Also, children who are very anxious and reluctant to talk about their pain may relax with the activity of filling out the body map.

C. Factors influencing pain ratings

  1. Cognitive ability affects the understanding of age-appropriate assessment scales. When understanding of the scale is in doubt, the child can be asked to score very recent events and to rate the pain several times during the interview. Children who are very ill or very apprehensive may regress, and a faces scale may become necessary for a child who usually would be able to use a numerical or visual analogue scale.

2. **Context** influences pain ratings. If children fear possible consequences of admitting to pain, such as further procedures, they may deny or minimize their pain. Other environmental factors may augment the pain report. If the child feels that the pain is not believed by parents or medical care providers, pain may be overrated or underrated.

3. **Timing** of pain assessments is important. Children in pain may find repeated questions about pain intrusive or nonsensical; they may refuse to answer or give meaningless answers. Many children are naturally able to use coping techniques such as diversion and spontaneous imagery, and frequent assessments may subvert this activity. Children under the age of 9 or 10 may be unable to see the relationship between answering questions about pain and relief of the pain.

4. **Interviewer.** The relationship with the interviewer may shape the response. Children are quick to sense a desired answer from nuances of language and expression, and may answer to please (or displease) the care provider or parent. Establishment of rapport, honesty, flexibility, and validation of the child's experience are crucial in obtaining a meaningful assessment.

5. **Behavioral observation versus verbal reports.** Observation of behavior complements the verbal report in the evaluation of pain, and is the only way for the clinician to assess pain in a nonverbal child. Behavior and verbal pain reports are influenced by the patient's as well as the care provider's personality style, ethnocultural factors, and social expectations. For verbal children, reliance on observations of behavior to guide intervention can result in overtreatment or undertreatment. Obtaining a verbal report validates the care provider's concern to the child, enlists the child as a therapeutic ally, and encourages verbal communication rather than "acting out" behavior. Behavioral observation then aids in evaluating coping skills and style and the effects of context.

6. **Fear** and pain exacerbate one another. Ordered scales can be used to assess fear as well as pain in the child over the age of 7 or 8 and can be useful in planning therapy. For example, the child with burns who is having difficulty with dressing changes may be asked to differentiate fear and pain. If the pain is severe, even if accompanied by fear, it can be considered primary, and therapy should be directed at pain control. Conversely, if fear is predominant, pharmacologic, psychological, and behavioral management can include anxiolysis.

7. **The extent to which pain is bothersome** to the child is more important than the reported pain intensity in determining treatment. Sometimes children report pain of a high intensity that bothers them relatively little, and vice versa. This reflects individual differences in pain rating, coping skills, meaning of the pain, and tolerance. Many older children understand the difference between intensity and bother, and the ranked scales can be used to rate both.

V. **Treatment.** The clinician chooses from a variety of pharmacologic, cognitive-behavioral, psychological, and physical approaches. If more than one method is used, they are introduced within an integrated and cohesive framework for the family and the patient. The primary physician maintains contact with all professionals involved in the treatment, so that treatment goals are complementary and changes in the regimen can be made when necessary.

A. **Pharmacologic management.** A stepwise approach is useful for both children and adults. **Mild pain** is managed with acetaminophen or an anti-inflammatory drug. A mild opioid is added for **moderate pain,** and a strong opioid is added for **severe pain.** Medications such as tricyclic antidepressants, stimulants, or centrally acting agents may be used as adjuvants or as primary therapy.

1. **Nonopioid analgesics.** Acetaminophen is well tolerated and can be administered orally or rectally. Because there is some evidence that chronic daily use of acetaminophen in adults may be correlated with renal insufficiency, children with chronic pain problems should be advised not to use acetaminophen daily for long periods of time. If acetaminophen does not provide adequate analgesia, or if inflammation contributes to pain, the nonsteroidal anti-inflammatory agents are indicated. Because Reye's syndrome is correlated with the adminis-

tration of salicylates to children with varicella or influenza, **aspirin should not be used for children with a fever or other evidence of viral infection.** The side effects of **aspirin or ibuprofen are often intolerable,** and the frequency of administration can pose a problem for children with chronic daily pain. In these situations, other anti-inflammatory agents such as **naproxen, choline magnesium trisalicylate,** or **indomethacin** can be employed.

2. **Opioid analgesics.** Opioid doses must be adjusted to size. When oral administration is possible, **codeine,** in conjunction with acetaminophen or an anti-inflammatory agent, is effective for moderate pain. Some children may experience an upset stomach or agitation when taking codeine; if so, or if analgesia is inadequate, alternative agents can be use. **Oxycodone, morphine,** and **hydromorphone** can be used in lower doses for moderate pain, and in higher doses for severe pain. If a child cannot swallow tablets, morphine is available in a liquid preparation, and hydromorphone can easily be crushed and suspended in liquid by the pharmacist or nurse. Suspensions can be diluted so that small amounts can be administered accurately to the baby or young child. **Meperidine** is poorly absorbed from the GI tract, and **methadone** is difficult to titrate because of the very long half-life; these drugs **should be used only when other agents are not tolerated.**

   Morphine and hydromorphone are recommended when parenteral administration is needed. Intravenous meperidine has a short duration of action, and use for more than 24 hours in adults has been associated with dysphoria. Thus, although useful in a single dose given before a painful procedure, it should be used for ongoing analgesia only when other agents are not tolerated. The safe and effective use of intravenous methadone requires experience with titration. It may be useful in the recovery room after surgery, or when many intravenous medications are being administered and intravenous access is available only intermittently. The mixed agonist-antagonist agents cause less spasm of the sphincter of Oddi than opioid agonists and may cause less of a decrease in intestinal motility. Agents such as **nalbuphine** can be used **for children with pancreatitis, cholecystitis, or inflammatory bowel disease.**

3. **Routes of administration.** Analgesia should be administered in a manner that is not feared by the child. If the oral route is not possible, the intravenous route should be used, as most children would rather have pain than an intramuscular injection. Continuous subcutaneous infusion can be used if the child cannot take oral medication and there is no intravenous access. It should be used cautiously in an acute situation, especially when the patient is dehydrated. Rectal administration is useful for babies and toddlers; however, older children and adolescents usually despise this route.

4. **Patient-controlled analgesia** has become an accepted method for administering analgesics. Commercial devices are available for intravenous analgesia that provide a patient-controlled dose, usually in response to the patient's pressing a button. There is a refractory time, called the "lockout interval" during which another dose cannot be administered, and a maximal dose limit is prescribed.

   Patient-controlled analgesia can be used as successfully with children as it has been used with adults. The patient needs to be able to understand the relation between a stimulus (pain), a behavior (pushing the button), and a slightly delayed effect (pain relief). Children over the age of 8 or 9 years can use patient-controlled analgesia for acute pain if their cognitive and emotional development is appropriate to their chronologic age. In chronic situations, such as pain associated with cancer, bone marrow transplantation, or burns, children as young as 6 years can use patient-controlled analgesia. There are some potential difficulties with patient-controlled analgesia:

   a. When first starting to use patient-controlled analgesia, young children may need reminders to press the button if the pain is bothersome.

   b. If the dose is too small, adults often stop using the button; this reaction is intensified in children.

   c. Children already disoriented by the experience of being in the hospital who wake up from sleep in pain may have a very difficult time remembering to utilize the device.

   d. The button must always be accessible. Although an adult may be able to search for a button that has fallen by the side of the bed, children are rarely able to do this.

   e. Children who are depressed or who have learning disabilities may not be able to use patient-controlled analgesia. Patients and their families should be interviewed to determine appropriateness.

5. **Oral administration of patient-controlled analgesia.** Patient-controlled analgesia is a concept, and not just a machine. Patients with chronic or cancer-related pain usually prefer to take medication by mouth when possible. Oral bedside patient-controlled analgesia can be used to bolster the perception of control. A small number of tablets, such as a 4-hour supply, can be kept at the bedside; tablets are then replaced by the nurse at regular intervals. The number of tablets at the bedside and the frequency of replacement are determined by calculating the maximal safe dose for the patient. The patient may keep a diary of medication use. To use oral bedside patient-controlled analgesia, the patient should be at least 12 or 13 years of age, and the family and patient should be well known to the staff. This approach relies on and enhances responsibility and independence and cannot be used for all patients. In the hospital, the nurse also must determine whether it is safe for the roommates to have analgesics at the bedside.

6. **Parent-controlled analgesia** utilizing the commercial devices can be used when children are unable to control the analgesia and are expected to have continuing severe pain, for example, when the child is at home dying of cancer. When analgesia is controlled by a person other than the patient, the approach is different from that in patient-controlled analgesia:

   a. The dose should supplement the basal infusion rather than being the mainstay of therapy. The sum of the doses required over 8 to 12 hours is added to the basal infusion.

   b. The dose should be large, as parents cannot be expected to use the button frequently.

   c. The lockout interval should be long, as the dose is based on observed rather than subjective experience. Parents should be instructed never to press the button when the patient is asleep.

   d. This method should be discussed with the family before implementation. Many families welcome participation in increasing the comfort of their child, but for some the responsibility may be onerous, and may detract from the parent's ability to participate in other interactions with the child and the medical staff. For example, when the diagnosis of cancer is made, most parents are overwhelmed, and have not yet learned about the disease, medications, and hospital operating procedures. However, a few months later, most parents become familiar with the hospital and medications and, if present at the child's bedside, may welcome the opportunity to ensure comfort.

7. **Side effects.** Most people do not like the alteration of sensorium associated with opioids. Children, however, may not be able to articulate a dysphoric reaction, and behavior resulting from dysphoria may be ascribed to regression, anxiety, or impulsivity. Parents can usually judge whether behavior is consistent with the usual personality of the child. Unusual agitation, impulsivity, or anxiety, without obvious precipitants, may warrant a change to an alternative opioid.

   Side effects such as **pruritus, nausea,** and **vomiting** can be troublesome in children. Younger children often do not communicate the experiences of pruritus and nausea, whereas vomiting can be seen by the observer and is usually treated. Side effects should be monitored with a high index of suspicion in young children and babies; a trial of antiemetics or antihistamines may be necessary. For older children and adolescents, ordering antiemetics or antihistamines on an as-needed schedule can be problematic. A schedule is preferable in which the child is asked at regular intervals whether or not there are problems and whether or not medication is desired.

8. **Opioids in neonates and babies.** The use of opioids in neonates and babies under about 6 months of age must be approached with caution. The elimination half-life for opioids in babies, although highly variable, is far longer than that in adults.

   a. Babies under the age of 3 months who are not intubated are susceptible to dose-related respiratory depression and apnea, especially if they are premature. Initial doses should be one quarter to one third of the usual starting dose.

   b. A 1-month-old baby with severe burns who is not intubated should be given morphine at 0.02–0.03 mg/kg of body weight as a starting dose. The effect and duration of action of the initial dose should be observed to determine subsequent intervals and doses. If an infusion is used, it should be at an initial dose of about 0.01 mg/kg/hr, with additional small "rescue doses" given hourly if needed. The infusion is then titrated to the needs of the infant.

c. Close cardiorespiratory monitoring, including the use of pulse oximetry, is necessary. The monitoring should be continued for at least 24 hours after the opioids are discontinued. Much higher starting doses of opioids can be used for the baby who is intubated. Rapid development of tolerance in babies may necessitate a rapid increase in the dose.

d. Babies requiring parenteral opioids are most commonly treated with fentanyl or morphine. Fentanyl causes less histamine release than morphine, and thus may be preferable when bronchospasm is a concern. Codeine, hydromorphone, and morphine solutions can be used for enteral analgesia. It is best to use small doses administered at frequent intervals to avoid wide swings in pain control.

e. Babies may experience dysphoria, nausea, or pruritus as side effects from opioids, although this cannot be assessed directly. Unusual agitation may signal an opioid side effect; a trial of adjuvants or a change to an alternative opioid may be warranted.

9. **Adjuvants**

a. **Tricyclic antidepressants** are effective in a variety of pain syndromes. Except for the use of imipramine for enuresis, these medications, however, **have not been approved for routine use in children,** and published clinical experience with these drugs for pain in children is limited. **Tricyclics** such as amitriptyline can be used as adjuvants or as primary pain therapy for children with problems such as cancer pain, headaches, or neuropathic pain. However, until more data are available they **should be used only for a significant pain problem,** and when there is reason to believe that alternative methods, both pharmacologic and nonpharmacologic, will not be effective or will have unacceptable side effects. Usually starting doses for amitriptyline are 0.1–0.3 mg/kg, administered in a single dose at night. The dose can then be increased in increments to a total dose of 1 or 2 mg/kg per day. If the dose is to be administered on a chronic basis, and if the dose is greater than 2 mg/kg, levels can be obtained to guide use.

b. **Stimulants,** such as methylphenidate, dextroamphetamine, and caffeine, can be useful for patients with cancer pain. The starting dose can be extrapolated from the usual starting dose for an adult with cancer pain and adjusted to the size of the child. For example, one could initiate methylphenidate at 0.1 mg/kg, given in the morning and the afternoon.

c. **Centrally acting agents,** such as **carbamazepine, dilantin,** and **clonazepam** can be used for neuropathic pain syndromes, such as spinal cord trauma or trigeminal neuralgia. Other agents, such as intravenous **lidocaine,** which have been used in adults, can be used **for children with very severe pain that has not responded to other modalities.**

B. **Cognitive-behavioral and psychological approaches** are as useful for children as they are for adults. Because pain is a multifaceted experience, it is crucial that therapy not rely on pharmacologic intervention alone. For some pain problems, cognitive-behavioral approaches will be the mainstay of therapy; for others, these techniques will complement other methods.

Additionally, the child is part of a family. Pain and its treatment can raise powerful issues for the patient, the family, and the medical care providers. Treatment of the patient in isolation from the larger social context may doom intervention to failure.

Some families have a difficult time accepting the psychological components of pain and may regard the recommendation for such treatment as a dismissal of the reality or intensity of the pain. During the assessment, the clinician sets the stage for acceptance of psychological factors by interweaving questions about psychosocial issues throughout the pain assessment, with an explanation of the interrelationships. Validation of the clinician's belief in the reality and importance of the pain is essential for future acceptance of recommendations for psychological approaches. The primary physician must explain the power and usefulness of cognitive-behavioral approaches at the time of recommendation or referral, and should maintain communication with the family and with the mental health provider so that treatment is seen as collaboration rather than as abandonment by the primary care physician.

1. **Hypnosis and relaxation.** Children over the age of 3 or 4 years can learn techniques of self-hypnosis for pain control. As in adults, hypnotic abilities vary greatly among individuals, but in general, children have greater hypnotic ability than adults. A patient can learn self-hypnosis more easily when the pain is mild. Patients with acute severe pain usually need pharmacologic analgesia before they can effectively learn and practice self-hypnosis.

   Children with intermittent pain may not practice the techniques during pain-free times, and without practice, use of self-hypnosis for severe pain may not be effective. Inclusion of the family may help provide an atmosphere in which the child will practice at regular intervals. However, this must be approached with care to avoid a power struggle between the child and the parents. Similarly, when a hospitalized child or adolescent is using self-hypnosis, the technique must be perceived by medical and nursing care providers as belonging to the child. If the child is frequently reminded by several care providers to use self-hypnosis, this undermines the perception of autonomy and control.

2. **Distraction.** Children with good coping skills use distraction to alter the experience of pain. This may be misunderstood by care providers, who believe that if a child is able to play or watch television, the pain cannot be very severe. It is important to praise a child's ability to cope with pain in a constructive manner, rather than using the ability as a reason to withdraw other treatments. In chronic and recurrent pain problems, it is important to distinguish distraction from secondary gain. The concept of distraction can be used to encourage responsibility and functional activity.

3. **Education.** Pain is regarded by most adolescents and adults as a sign of pathology. Children quickly sense their parents' anxiety about disease and become anxious themselves. The pain of some problems, such as reflex sympathetic dystrophy and tension headaches, does not indicate immediate harm. Demystification of the pain, by discussing the difference between hurt and harm, can help restore a patient's ability to function despite the pain. Education about pain, its treatment, and the disease (if present) is necessary.

4. **Psychotherapy** is useful when there is significant family or individual psychopathology that may be contributing to the pain or impairing function. The presence of chronic pain in a child or adolescent can place considerable stress on the family. However, for the majority of patients and families, treating the pain and teaching cognitive-behavioral approaches reduces the stress. Psychotherapy may be oriented to the family or to the individual depending on the problems and the context.

5. **Contracts** are written or unwritten agreements between the health care team and the patient (and family).
   a. For adolescents with chronic, complex, and severe pain syndromes, contracts help to
      (1) Facilitate discussion
      (2) Underscore the patient's role as a therapeutic ally
      (3) Establish clear expectations of behavior and responsibility for all concerned
      (4) Defuse mistrust
   b. An adolescent with sickle cell disease and frequent admissions for crisis pain, for example, might with his or her family and physician formalize the following into a written document:
      (1) Criteria for admission
      (2) Pharmacologic treatment (perhaps including drug, dose, route, and schedule)
      (3) Weaning from medication
      (4) Patient responsibilities while hospitalized
      (5) Staff responsibilities during hospitalization
   c. Copies of the document should be kept by all participants, and other copies could be made available to the emergency room and hospital staff. The contract can be very flexible or very specific, and the issues in the contract should reflect the pertinent problems for that patient. The terms of the contract should not be changed without the agreement of all those involved in formulating the contract.

6. Operant conditioning. Patterns of behavior that reflect the presence of pain may help or hinder the child's participation in activities necessary for normal development. The reactions of others in the environment may reinforce maladaptive behavioral patterns that are deleterious to the child's well-being. Family and health care providers can be taught to change their reactions so that more healthy functioning is encouraged.

C. Physical approaches can be useful for children and adolescents with chronic pain. Physical methods reinforce the physician's concern about the pain to the patient and encourage patient participation in reducing the pain.

1. Physical therapy and aerobic conditioning may help to restore a sense of well-being.

2. Transcutaneous electrical nerve stimulation and other physical modalities are usually well accepted by children and adolescents.

VI. Pain syndromes

A. Acute pain

1. Postoperative pain is the most common cause of severe acute pain in children. Management depends on age and type of surgery. Although recovery after surgery varies from patient to patient, the physician can usually assess the expected duration and intensity of pain.

a. When postoperative pain is mild and short, regional nerve blockade can be employed. If this is not feasible, one or two doses of intravenous medication can be given before changing to oral management. Medication should be administered at scheduled intervals during the period when pain is expected to be a problem.

b. For major surgery, parenteral or peridural analgesics are necessary. As the child improves, it is best to decrease the dose rather than increase the interval. The use of oral medication facilitates ambulation.

c. Constipation often develops after surgery. The pain of constipation should be distinguished from incision pain, and appropriate therapy should be instituted, because opioids will worsen the problem. Likewise, the child using a patient-controlled analgesia device who is experiencing gas pains as bowel motility returns can be taught to use the device for incisional pain only.

d. For patients who are very anxious about surgery, the hospital, and the pain, stress management techniques can be helpful. Transcutaneous electrical nerve stimulation also works well for some patients.

e. Adolescent substance abusers with postoperative pain often need special treatment. These patients may be tolerant of opioids and require large doses of analgesics for adequate pain control. They often have poor coping skills for anxiety and pain. Poor pain control, which should be avoided, results in a craving for medication. Clear expectations and structure should be provided, and patients should be told how and when the medication will be decreased. Teaching cognitive-behavioral techniques of pain and anxiety control can be helpful.

2. Burns. The management of pain in children with severe burns is a challenging problem. The child with burns who can be managed at home usually needs analgesia for only 1 or 2 days. However, the hospitalized child may require dressing changes over many weeks.

a. In the acute phase of burn management, the child has ongoing pain of varying degrees of severity, punctuated by the often excruciating pain of debridement and dressing changes. Sometimes there is little pain for the first few days, followed by severe pain. As healing takes place, the ongoing pain lessens, although dressing changes may continue to be a problem.

b. Initial management of severe burns requires parenteral analgesia. When the child is stable and intravenous access is no longer required for the administration of fluids and other medications, a change to oral management can facilitate ambulation. Analgesia should be provided around the clock; very high doses may be necessary.

c. Dressing changes are usually accompanied by both pain and anxiety, and the concurrent administration of an analgesic and an anxiolytic can be helpful. For some children, only an analgesic is required, as adequate pain relief assuages the anxiety. Analgesic doses before dressing changes may need to be two or three times higher than the usual scheduled dose.

d. The use of tricyclic antidepressants for burns has not been investigated.

Nighttime administration of a small dose may aid in sleep. If long-term administration of opioids is expected, the addition of a tricyclic antidepressant may be synergistic.

e. The management of a child with severe burns must be multidisciplinary, because providing adequate analgesia is often not sufficient to prevent the emergence of anxiety and behavior problems. Prolonged hospitalization, daily painful procedures, and loss of body integrity are difficult for the child. In addition, burns are often sustained in situations in which the child misbehaved or was inadequately supervised. Issues of family dysfunction, dissension, and guilt influence the child's reaction to the injury.

Multidisciplinary management includes the teaching of stress management techniques, the institution of a behavioral reinforcement program, and providing children with the means to express their anxieties and fears. Expectations of the care providers should be consistent and reasonable, and the child should have a daily schedule so that difficult procedures are predictable and interspersed with more normal activity. As much as possible, the child should perceive some control over the environment, including the dressing changes. This includes the use of patient "time out" and having the child participate in the changes by removing the dressing. Painful procedures should not be performed by nurses whom the child trusts. Rather, a different person should perform the procedure, in a place other than the child's bed.

B. Chronic pain without illness

1. Recurrent headaches are a common cause of pain in childhood. Some headaches are symptoms of a serious condition, such as meningitis, sinusitis, or tumor. However, the majority of head pain is similar in etiology to head pain experienced by adults. Children may have vascular (migraine) headaches, tension headaches, and headaches of both vascular and myofascial etiology (mixed headache syndrome). The diagnosis is made after a careful history and physical examination. The child who has an occasional headache can easily be treated with a single dose of acetaminophen or a nonsteroidal anti-inflammatory agent. Some patients with infrequent but severe headaches respond well to the addition of a single dose of codeine or oxycodone to these medications. Ergotamines are rarely necessary for children.

The child with daily headaches, like the adult with this problem, usually has a mixed headache syndrome or headaches from muscle spasm. In the mixed headache syndrome, the muscle spasm and pain perpetuate the vascular component. Bruxism may be present with resultant spasm and pain in the temporomandibular joint and muscles of mastication. Careful examination of children with daily or frequent headaches may reveal trigger points in the head and neck. Like the adult, the child with frequent or daily headaches benefits from a multidisciplinary program.

a. Pharmacologic management for the child with frequent headaches includes

(1) A nonsteroidal anti-inflammatory drug for abortive treatment

(2) Prophylaxis with **propranolol** or a **tricyclic antidepressant** can be instituted at the same time. The athletic child may not tolerate the side effects of propranolol. Because tricyclic antidepressants are effective in myofascial pain syndromes and for prophylaxis of migraines, they are the medication of choice for a mixed headache syndrome.

(3) Periactin has been reported to be **efficacious,** but sedation can be a problem.

(4) Calcium channel blockers or **centrally acting agents** are **rarely needed** for headache prophylaxis in children, especially if a multidisciplinary program is instituted.

b. Cognitive-behavioral approaches, including **self-hypnosis** and **biofeedback,** work well for children with frequent headaches. Pharmacologic treatment reduces pain while the child is learning other techniques. The onset of frequent headaches may be associated with stresses in the family or at school, and psychotherapy may be indicated.

c. Physical approaches decrease spasm and tenderness of the muscles of the head and neck. Often postural habits aggravate muscle spasm; the child may be watching television while lying down with the neck flexed to a 90-degree angle. Physical measures include

(1) Regular application of heat or cold, as well as massage

(2) Transcutaneous electrical nerve stimulation

(3) Stretching and strengthening exercises

(4) Trigger point injections

d. **The multidisciplinary program** includes the institution of appropriate pharmacologic, psychological, and physical methods, along with education and reassurance about the benign nature of the headaches. The child over the age of 6 or 7 years should be an active participant in treating the problem, with the support and understanding of the family.

2. **Myofascial pain syndromes**

a. Children often have myofascial pain resulting from trauma and overuse. This pain usually can be resolved with the use of

(1) Rest

(2) Ice

(3) Compression

(4) Elevation

(5) Followed by **gradual mobilization**

b. Prolonged pain with trigger points is seen far less frequently in children than in adults. Treatment of prolonged myofascial pain syndromes involves

(1) **Physical therapy**

(2) **Postural remediation**

(3) **Application of heat and cold**

(4) **Relaxation techniques**

(5) **Teaching of coping skills**

(6) **Psychotherapy when indicated**

(7) **Trigger point injections** may be helpful but should be approached with an awareness of the fear that children have for needles. Children respond better to massage and heat or ice.

(8) **A short course of tricyclic antidepressants** can be used if the pain interferes with mobilization.

3. **Reflex sympathetic dystrophy** is easier to treat in children than in adults, and is less likely to be associated with irreversible trophic changes. It usually responds readily to physical therapy. Transcutaneous electrical nerve stimulation, self-hypnosis, and tricyclic antidepressants decrease the pain while the child is mobilizing the affected body part. The role of regional sympathetic blockade in childhood reflex sympathetic dystrophy is not clear. If the patient does not respond to physical therapy after a reasonable length of time, such as 2 weeks, or if trophic changes are developing, a block may be indicated.

4. **Recurrent abdominal pain** is a common problem for children. In the absence of localized pain or symptoms and signs of a systemic disorder, a disease-related etiology is unlikely. Individual variation in intestinal motility patterns or constipation may be responsible for the pain. Although stress and emotional problems can cause or aggravate abdominal pain, most children with recurrent abdominal pain probably have functional physiologic variations. Treatment is multimodal, with cognitive-behavioral and psychological interventions as the mainstay of therapy. A high-fiber diet is also helpful.

5. **Chest pain,** in the absence of signs and symptoms of serious cardiac or pulmonary problems, is usually self-limited in children. An anti-inflammatory agent is helpful for costochondritis or myofascial tenderness. Esophagitis may cause chest pain; if the pain is burning in character, the empiric use of an antacid may be warranted. Esophageal spasm is usually paroxysmal, short-lived, and intense.

6. **Limb pain.** History, physical examination, and simple laboratory testing usually indicate the presence of pathophysiologic entities that need specific treatment. Otherwise, physical methods and cognitive-behavioral coping techniques are the mainstay of therapy.

C. **Pain within the context of nonmalignant chronic illness.** The care provider, in consultation with the patient and the family, must consider the disease, individual and contextual factors, the severity of the pain, and the patient's ability to cope with the pain. Pain that is severe erodes the child's psychological reserves.

Children with diseases such as sickle cell disease, hemophilia, juvenile rheumatoid arthritis, and inflammatory bowel disease commonly experience pain as a result of the illness. The treatment of this pain depends on the intensity and context of the pain.

1. Pain in **sickle cell disease** often requires repeated and liberal use of opioids for management.
2. The child with **hemophilia** has pain as a symptom of a bleeding episode; the pain usually resolves rapidly on receiving factor correction. Therefore, patients with hemophilia rarely become opioid tolerant.
3. Children with **juvenile rheumatoid arthritis** usually respond well to nonsteroidal anti-inflammatory agents, physical therapy, transcutaneous electrical nerve stimulation, and cognitive-behavioral techniques. For some children who are severely affected, the tricyclic antidepressants can provide some analgesia, so that the child can more readily participate in physical therapy and activities of daily living. Opioids are not usually necessary; during a flare of disease activity, mild opioids usually provide adequate pain control.
4. The pain of **inflammatory bowel disease** responds to therapy for the disease. However, at times the pain can be severe and recalcitrant. The use of opioid agonists is problematic because of the effect on intestinal motility. Although opioids are necessary for severe pain episodes, the pain is generally managed with disease-directed therapy and cognitive-behavioral techniques with the occasional use of tricyclic antidepressants. When opioids are necessary, the use of an agonist-antagonist preparation should be considered.

D. Cancer pain. Childhood cancer differs from cancer in adults in type and natural history. Whereas adults may experience disease-related pain for months or years, cancer in children tends to be either rapidly progressive or rapidly responsive to treatment. Disease-related pain occurs at diagnosis and relapse; persistent and intense pain is most often seen in the palliative and terminal phases of the disease. Treatment-related pain, as with mucositis and painful neuropathies, occurs throughout the course of the illness.

1. One of the major causes of pain and anxiety in children with cancer is **repeated procedures**, such as bone marrow aspiration and lumbar puncture. Leukemia and lymphoma are the most common malignancies in childhood, and often require frequent procedures. Children cite these procedures as being the worst part of having cancer.
2. **Management of treatment and disease-related pain is similar in children and adults.** However, because most children with cancer are thrombocytopenic from chemotherapy at the time they experience pain, most nonsteroidal anti-inflammatory drugs are contraindicated, and acetaminophen is the only agent that can be used. Opioid therapy is similar in adults and children. Tricyclic antidepressants and stimulants can be used as adjunctive therapy, even in babies and very young children with cancer.
3. **Procedural pain** and anxiety **should be aggressively managed** in children and adolescents with cancer. If pharmacologic and cognitive-behavioral interventions are not provided, the resulting pain and stress can profoundly erode the child's already limited emotional resources, and impair quality of life. Mild anxiety during the first procedure may subsequently become a phobia. **Children do not become desensitized as a result of multiple procedures.**
4. **The extent of pain and anxiety associated with procedures should be evaluated.** Procedures mostly associated with anxiety, such as venipunctures, are best treated with cognitive-behavioral techniques. Pharmacologic anxiolysis may be helpful in a cycle of escalating anxiety. Procedures that can be very painful, such as bone marrow aspiration and biopsy, require a combination of analgesia and anxiolysis. Some institutions routinely use general anesthesia for children having bone marrow examinations. If this option is not available, the combination of an opioid analgesic (such as morphine or fentanyl) and an anxiolytic (such as midazolam) can be employed. These medications should be titrated to the desired effect. For example, a child could receive midazolam in small incremental doses of about 0.03 mg/kg of body weight, followed by morphine in small incremental doses of 0.03 mg/kg. For many children, cognitive-behavioral skills decrease the pain and anxiety associated with procedures. However, it takes time to learn these techniques, and pharmacologic intervention is necessary in the meantime.

Selected Readings

Anand KJS, McGrath PJ (eds). *Pain in Neonates.* New York: Elsevier Science, 1993.

Carr DB, Jacox AK (eds). *Acute Pain Management: Operative or Medical Procedures and Trauma.* Washington, DC: Agency for Health Care Policy and Research, Public Health Service, U.S. Department of Health and Human Services, 1992.

Gardner GG, Olness K. *Hypnosis and Hypnotherapy with Children.* New York: Grune & Stratton, 1981.

Pjetterbaum B, Hagberg CA. Pharmacologic management of pain in children. *J Am Acad Child Adolesc Psychiatry* 32:235–242, 1993.

Ross DM, Ross SA. *Childhood Pain: Current Issues, Research and Management.* Baltimore: Urban & Schwarzenberg, 1988.

Schechter NL, Berde CB, Yaster M (eds). *Pain in Infants, Children, and Adolescents.* Baltimore: Williams & Wilkins, 1993.

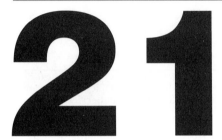

Low Back Pain
Joseph G. Sankoorikal
Sridhar V. Vasudevan

I. Background. Despite significant improvements in the understanding of pain, low back pain continues to be a major problem throughout the world and a great challenge to medical professionals. It is estimated that 80% of Americans will experience pain in their lower back severe enough to disrupt their job or normal daily activities at some time during their lives.[1-3] Currently, more than 14 million Americans experience low back pain.[4] The annual cost of this problem is estimated to be about 20 billion dollars. It is the leading cause of disability in patients under 45 years of age and is the third most prevalent disability in people over 45 years of age. Several problems affect its management:[5]
  A. The lack of a uniform definition
  B. Difficulty identifying a specific diagnosis
  C. The lack of objective pain measurement techniques
  D. A host of psychological and environmental factors that relate to low back pain
  E. Cognitive and individual variability of pain perception based on ethnic background and social structure[6]
II. Nociceptive anatomy. Several parts of the lumbosacral spinal column are pain sensitive. These are the anterior and posterior **longitudinal ligaments, vertebral body, synovia of articulating facets, nerve roots, muscle, and related connective tissues.** The intervertebral disk itself is pain insensitive, but the most peripheral annular fibers may have some innervation. Acute trauma, inflammation, or other injuries to any of the above structures can cause acute low back pain with or without radiation.[7]
III. Biomechanics. The low back (i.e., the lumbosacral spine) should be considered as a mobile structure and not a static column. The activity of the lumbar spine exerts compression and shearing stress on the bony components of the back and tensile stress on the ligamentous and muscular components.[8] Restriction of the motion of the spine is provided by connective tissue and muscular elements. These muscles provide intermittent forces to balance the vertebral column at rest or support it during activity. When the body is in a particular posture for a long time, the muscles relax and the vertebrae sag against the ligaments further restricting motion.

Extension of the spine is provided mainly by various muscles and fascia, including lumbosacral fascia, superficial multisegmental muscles, collectively named the erector spinae muscle, and deeper muscles, namely the multifidus and rotators. The multifidus extends the spine and rotates it toward the opposite side.[9]

The forward and lateral flexor muscles of the lumbar spine are located anterior and lateral to vertebral bodies and the transverse process. The iliopsoas muscle flexes the lumbar spine and bends it toward the same side. Anterior abdominal muscles also have a role in lumbar spine flexion.[9]

Lateral motion is restricted by the fibers of the anulus fibrosus and the lateral vertebral ligament.[7,8]
IV. Causes of low back pain
  A. Stress. Injury to the low back may be caused by **compressive** or **tensile** stresses.
    1. Compression. Compressive stresses are exerted on the vertebral bodies, the intervertebral disks, the apophyseal joints, and the pedicles. In normal conditions, only extremely severe trauma will exceed the strength of the vertebral body, causing collapse. When chronic inflammation, malnutrition, endocrine imbalance, and osteoporosis weaken the vertebrae, however, even relatively mild stress can damage the vertebrae, resulting in pain. The compressive stresses on the apophyseal joints (facets) can lead to osteoarthritic changes and pain.

    2. Tension. Compressive stress **within the disk** increases hydraulic pressure causing tensile stress.[8]
- **B. Poor posture.** The majority of posture-related low back pain is attributed to deviations from normal posture in the static spine. These include an increase in pelvic tilt and an increase in the lumbosacral angle with a concomitant increase in lumbar lordosis. In the latter condition, pain can originate from irritation of the facet joint synovial tissue.[7]
- **C. Kinetic dysfunction.** Deviations of normal function in the kinetic spine also lead to irritation of pain-sensitive tissues. Disruption of the normal lumbar-pelvic rhythm causes pain and is caused by abnormal strain on a normal back, normal strain on an abnormal back, or normal stress on an unprepared normal back. Tight hamstrings can also alter the lumbar-pelvic rhythm.[7,8]
- **D. Inflammation** decreases the tensile strength of the ligaments and periarticular connective tissue.[8] The disk may be the source of pain when there are degenerative changes in the anulus. Although the disk itself may rarely be the source of pain, disk degeneration more commonly produces symptoms by virtue of its secondary effects on surrounding spinal structures—the paraspinal muscles, spinal ligaments, posterior joints, and nerve roots.
- **E. Facet joint subluxation** is concomitant with disk degeneration. Instability of the spine can predispose a person to fracture of articular facets. A sudden twist or strain gives rise to effusion and locking of a loose body in the arthritic facet joint, causing the clinical picture of sudden severe pain with lock of the back. The facet joints resist most of the intervertebral shear force and in lordotic postures share in resisting intervertebral compressions. They also prevent excessive motions from damaging the disks.[9]

V. Clinical manifestations
- **A. Acute lumbosacral strain.** Pain is often limited to the low back or buttocks.
- **B. Intervertebral disk protrusions.** Approximately 50% of patients with intervertebral disk protrusion first come to medical attention with low backache, which is followed by radicular sciatic pain. Nearly one third of these patients will have a history of sciatica and backache having begun simultaneously.[7] The onset of symptoms may be acute or gradual. In acute onset, patients describe an accident as a causative factor, such as lifting a heavy object in the stooping position, or a twisting of the spine. In gradual onset, there may not be a precipitating factor while the patient feels increasing pain.
- **C. Herniated disk syndrome** is secondary to an increase in intradiskal pressure, which causes rupture of the anulus fibrosus with a resultant extrusion of the nucleus pulposus. The herniated nucleus compresses nerve roots and produces sciatic pain, which radiates into either extremity, mostly on the posterior aspect of the thigh and leg. Occasionally, pain may be described as cramping or tightness. Other symptoms include tingling, numbness, and weakness as well as possible problems with bowel and bladder control. Pain may be aggravated by prolonged sitting or standing, walking, or climbing up and down stairs.
- **D. Myofascial trigger points** in the paraspinal muscles may, at times, mimic radicular symptoms and should also be considered in patients with sciatica.[7]

VI. Diagnosis
- **A. History.** Obtain a detailed history that includes the mechanism of injury, onset of pain, duration and frequency, location and radiation, aggravating and relieving factors, and bowel and bladder changes. Other factors including past medical history, family history, social and occupational history, and review of systems should be part of the history taking. Have the patient fill out a pain diagram and pain scale.
- **B. Physical examination**
  - **1. Inspection.** Undress the patient sufficiently to provide full inspection and palpation of the spine. This is important because pelvic tilt and listing of the trunk due to muscle guarding (spasm) cannot be observed unless the entire contours of the body are exposed. Inspect the spine anteriorly and posteriorly. Note any increase or decrease of lumbar lordosis and the presence of any kyphosis or scoliosis. Note any antalgic behavior in walking and any guarding of either extremity.
  - **2. Range of motion.** Assess the spinal range of motion in all directions: i.e., flexion-extension, lateral flexion, and rotation. The modified Schober's test is a valuable test for spinal mobility because it provides an objective assessment. Patients with spondyloarthropathies have decreased lumbar flexion and an

abnormal test result. A point between the sacroiliac dimple is marked along with another mark 10 cm above the lower one. The patient is asked to bend forward, and the increased distance is measured. In patients with normal lumbar flexion the distance increases 4 to 5 cm. Patients with limited flexion will have a distance less than 4 cm.

3. **Palpation** of the back muscles for any **voluntary** or **involuntary guarding** (spasm), **focal tenderness**, or **trigger points.** Involuntary guarding is objective and characterized by sustained muscular contraction rather than by repeated and voluntary brief contraction. It can be induced by palpating the paraspinal muscles while the patient alternately bears weight on the lower extremities. The paraspinal muscles on the side of the weight-bearing limb should relax while the opposite side contracts. Lack of relaxation in a specific area of the lumbosacral paraspinal muscles is indicative of involuntary guarding.

4. **Specific tests**
   a. Place the patient supine and perform the straight leg raising (SLR) test. The purpose of this test is to stretch the dura. Raise the leg with the knee extended. When the sciatic nerve is stretched and its nerve roots and corresponding dural attachments are inflamed, the patient will experience pain along its anatomic course to the lower extremity. Between 30 and 70 degrees of tension is applied to the dura and nerve roots. A positive test may also be related to mechanical low back pain. It is important to note that for the SLR test to be positive, the pain should be reproduced in the nerve root distribution, with pain and neurologic symptoms below the knee level. Pain produced only in the lumbar or gluteal region can occur with a muscular strain or spasm. Leg length should be measured to determine whether one leg is significantly longer than the other.
   b. In **Lasègue's test,** the patient is supine with hip flexed to 90 degrees and the knee is slowly extended until sciatic pain is elicited. A positive test is suggestive of nerve root irritation.
   c. Another test that stresses both the hip and sacroiliac joints is **Patrick's test,** also called the **fabere sign** (flexion, abduction, external rotation, extension). The test is done by positioning the lateral malleolus of the tested leg on the patella of the opposite leg. Downward pressure is then placed on the medial aspect of the knee. Pain originates in the sacroiliac joint.
   d. **Naffziger's test** is done by compressing the jugular veins in the neck for approximately 10 seconds until the patient's face begins to flush. The patient is then asked to cough to increase the intrathecal pressure. Sciatic pain will be aggravated if there is dural sensitivity.

5. **Special maneuvers.** The lateral flexion and torsion maneuver and backward extension are performed with hands clasped behind the neck. This motion can aggravate the pain symptoms in the affected side in patients with nerve root compression. Jarring percussion over the lumbar paravertebral area may reproduce sciatic pain from disk herniation and may aid in diagnosis.

6. **Neurologic evaluation.** A full evaluation is mandatory. Note any muscle, atrophy, weakness, change in deep tendon reflexes, or sensory changes in the nerve root distribution.

VII. **Other diagnostic tests**
   A. **Plain x-ray films** of the lumbar spine assist in ruling out fracture, tumor, and major structural defects. Anteroposterior and lateral views show the bony configuration and intervertebral spaces. Spot views best evaluate the L5–S1 disk space. Oblique views best evaluate spondylolysis, as they show the intervertebral foramina, lesions of the neural arches, and facets. Flexion-extension views should be included whenever spinal instability is suspected.
   B. **A CT scan** is used to rule out significant disk bulge and protrusions causing nerve root compression.
   C. **Myelography,** a sensitive test to determine the presence of disk herniation, can also differentiate lesions, such as tumors, and detect partial or complete blocks secondary to the degeneration of intervertebral joint complexes when such degeneration is complicated by spondylolisthesis or osteophyte formation.
   D. **MRI** provides further sophistication in anatomic diagnosis. Conjoined nerve roots, neurofibromas, internal disk disruption, epidural fibrosis, and a variety of other findings can be apparent with MRI.
   E. **Diskography,** a visualization technique of specific lumbar disks, is infrequently

performed now, as it fails to differentiate consistently between symptomatic and asymptomatic disk disease.

F. Electromyography (EMG) is useful in localizing the presence of nerve root compression due to a herniated disk. EMG can demonstrate ongoing nerve injury as well as signs of nerve recovery.[10-12]

VIII. Differential diagnosis includes a large array of regional and referred causes.

  A. Osseous
  1. Congenital
  2. Traumatic
  3. Infectious
  4. Neoplastic
  5. Arthritic

  B. Soft tissue
  1. Postural
  2. Myofascial pain and strain
  3. Fibrositis, fibromyalgia
  4. Tendinitis

  C. Diskogenic
  1. Acute herniated nucleus pulposus
  2. Disk degeneration

  D. Viscerogenic
  E. Vascular
  F. Neurogenic
  G. Metabolic
  H. Psychosomatic

IX. Treatment. The importance of tensile forces that strain or tear connective tissue has been stressed above. In cases of fracture, there is additional bony trauma to treat, and in cases of definite radicular compression, decompression may be needed. Treatment, in any case, can be divided into the acute and chronic phases.

  A. Acute phase
  1. **Rest.** Restriction of physical activity eliminates the stress of gravity and relieves muscular spasm. The patient should rest on a firm mattress with hips and knees in a flexed (semi-Fowler) position. Traditional recommended treatment is 1 to 2 weeks of rest. Recent evidence, however, indicates that a maximum of 3 to 4 days of complete rest, followed by early remobilization, provides better results and is therefore the treatment of choice.
  2. **Pharmacotherapy.** Nonnarcotic analgesics are used first. Narcotics should be used only in the presence of severe pain. Their use should be limited for the first 2 to 4 weeks owing to the potential of abuse and dependence. Anti-inflammatory agents are extremely helpful in relieving inflammatory edema and the associated pain.[13] Tranquilizers and muscle relaxants are also commonly used to ease the tension and apprehension during the first few weeks after the acute onset. Oral steroids or injections with anesthetics are also considered, depending on the etiology and severity of the problem.
  3. **Physical modalities**
      a. **Heat.** The application of heat, especially moist heat, is very helpful in relieving spasm. Superficial heat modalities such as hydrocollator packs and hydrotherapy are beneficial, as are deep heat modalities such as diathermy and ultrasound, which are used less often.[14,15] The physiologic effects of heat include
          (1) Increasing the pain threshold of skin and peripheral nerves
          (2) Raising the distensibility of fibrous collagen tissues
          (3) Decreasing the sensitivity of muscle spindles to stretch, which relaxes striated muscles
          (4) Increasing the viscoelastic properties of joints, producing a relaxing sedative effect
      b. **Cold** has therapeutic effects that include decreasing
          (1) Inflammation
          (2) Nerve conduction velocity and thus pain
          (3) Muscle spindle activity and its resultant muscle spasm[14,15]
      c. **Massage,** although usually not tolerated by patients in an early acute phase, can be added as an adjunct to therapy. It is especially valuable in muscular

strains and in the treatment of chronic myofascial pain syndromes with active trigger points.

   d. Traction (4–10 lb) is used to assist in keeping the patient at "rest." Traction in a semi-Fowler position, by tilting the pelvis anteriorly and flattening the lumbar curvature, opens the posterior aspects of the vertebrae.[16] In the lumbar area, 200 to 300 lb of traction force is needed to widen the space between disks and therefore is impractical.[14,15]

   e. Transcutaneous electrical nerve stimulation (TENS). Conventional TENS uses high-frequency, low-intensity stimulation, while "acupuncture-like TENS" uses low-frequency, high-intensity stimulation. Although the former one is based on the gate-control mechanism, the latter seems to be mediated through an endorphinergic system. TENS has the major advantage of being an excellent nonpharmacologic method of pain control while increasing self-reliance.[14,15,17–20]

4. Exercise

   a. Six specific **flexion exercises** (devised by Williams in 1953) are commonly used.[21]

   (1) Abdominal strengthening (sit-ups)

   (2) Gluteus maximus strengthening (pelvic tilt)

   (3) Erector spinae and low back stretching (pelvic roll)

   (4) Hamstring stretching

   (5) Hip flexor stretching

   (6) Gluteus maximus strengthening

   b. Spinal extension exercises have not been recommended as part of an exercise regimen until recently. Studies now suggest that, in addition to Williams' exercises, **strengthening of spinal extensors** and the **promotion of extension positioning** can be beneficial.[14,15]

5. Orthotics such as corsets and braces permit an earlier mobilization and resumption of normal activities. Some rigid braces may also restrict motion in those derangements in which instability of vertebral segments is the predominant factor in producing pain. Corsets do not eliminate the stress of gravity, although they do minimally restrict spinal mobility. They act as an "external conscience" by decreasing excessive mobility and thereby reminding patients to avoid troublesome positions.[7] A therapeutic exercise program should be prescribed, along with supportive devices to prevent any deconditioning of muscular support from disuse.[22]

6. Patient education regarding proper body mechanics during activities of daily living, home exercise programs to maintain strength, flexibility, mobility, and proper posture, weight reduction, and proper nutrition should be emphasized.

B. Chronic phase. Chronic pain is characterized by symptoms that persist beyond the expected healing time of an injury or illness, or beyond 6 months. There are few objective clinical and laboratory findings or residual structural defects that could reasonably cause or explain the reported symptoms. It is often associated with significant lifestyle changes that include deconditioning, drug misuse, depression, sleep disorders, dramatic pain behavior, and disabilities that far exceed any underlying pathology. It is considered to be a biologic and psychosocial process as well, and often does not benefit from medical or surgical treatment alone.[23]

1. Rehabilitation. The rehabilitation model of treatment attempts to maximize the patient's function and restore his or her usual role. It addresses the medical, physical, emotional, psychosocial, and vocational aspects of the individual. In addition to physicians, the treatment team should include occupational therapists, physical therapists, social workers, psychologists, and other medical consultants. Treatment goals include

   a. Elimination or decrease of nonessential medication use

   b. Elimination or decrease of pain behavior by behavior modification

   c. Increase of physical conditioning by structured and graded physical activities

   d. Increase of coping skills and proper education regarding correct body mechanics

   e. Return to usual roles such as gainful employment or homemaking

   f. Improved sleeping pattern

2. Medications

   a. Medication originally given on an as-needed basis must be given at regular intervals and in decreasing strength.

b. Sedative, anxiolytic, and analgesic drugs should be avoided.

c. Narcotics should be limited to hospitalized patients with clear pathology.

d. Tricyclic antidepressants are beneficial, not only for pain management but also for improving sleep patterns.[24]

3. Other modalities such as TENS units and nerve blocks have achieved good results. Relaxation techniques accomplished through biofeedback[6] or audiotapes have also been helpful in reducing pain behavior. Behavior modification is a well-established program that rewards constructive behavior and deemphasizes or ignores pain behavior.[23,25,26]

References

1. Horal J. The clinical appearance of low back pain disorders in the city of Gothenburg, Sweden. *Acta Orthop Scand Suppl* 118, 1969.
2. Hult L. Cervical, dorsal and lumbar spine syndrome. *Acta Orthop Scand Suppl* 17, 1954.
3. Nachemson, AL. Work for all—for those with low back pain as well. *Clin Orthop* 170:77, 1983.
4. Chaffin, DB, Herrin, GD, Keyserling WM. Pre-employment strength testing: an updated position. *J Occup Med* 20:403, 1978.
5. Vasudevan SV. Clinical perspectives on the relationship between pain and disability. *Neurol Clin* 7:429, 1989.
6. Lee PWH, Chow FL, Cham KC, Wong S. Psychosocial factors influencing outcome in patients with low back pain. *Spine* 14:838–843, 1989.
7. Cailliet R. *Low Back Pain Syndrome* (3rd ed.). Philadelphia: F.A. Davis, 1981.
8. Kottke PJ. Evaluation and treatment of low back pain due to mechanical causes. *Arch Phys Med Rehabil* 42:426, 1961.
9. Borenstein DG, Wiesel SW. *Low Back Pain: Medical Diagnosis and Comprehensive Management.* Philadelphia: W.B. Saunders, 1989.
10. Kimura J. *Electrodiagnosis in Diseases of Nerve and Muscle: Principles and Practice* (2nd ed.). Philadelphia: F.A. Davis, 1989.
11. Johnson EW. *Electrodiagnosis of Radiculopathy.* In Johnson EW (ed.), *Practical Electromyography.* Baltimore: Williams & Wilkins, 1980. Pp. 229–245.
12. Johnson EW, Melvin JL. Value of electromyography in lumbar radiculopathy. *Arch Phys Med Rehabil* 52:239–243, 1971.
13. Saal JA. The role of inflammation in lumbar pain. In Physical Medicine and Rehabilitation. *State of the Art Reviews* 4:191–199, 1990.
14. Kottke FJ, Stillwell GK, Lehmann JF. *Krusen's Handbook of Physical Medicine and Rehabilitation* (3rd ed.). Philadelphia: W.B. Saunders, 1982.
15. Vasudevan SV, Hegmann K, Moore A, Cerletty S. Physical methods of pain management. In Raj RP (ed.), *Practical Management of Pain* (2nd ed.). Chicago: Year Book Medical Publishers, 1990.
16. Kester NC. Low back pain—pathomechanics and a regime of treatment. *Arch Phys Med Rehabil* 49:98, 1968.
17. Melzack R, Wall PD. Pain mechanisms: a new theory. *Science* 150:971–979, 1965.
18. Lehmann TR, Russell DW. Efficacy of electroacupuncture and TENS in the rehabilitation of chronic low back patients. *Pain* 26:277–290, 1986.
19. Johansson F, Almay BG. Predictors for the outcome of treatment with high frequency TENS in patients with chronic pain. *Pain* 9:55–61, 1980.
20. Fried T, Johnson R. TENS: its role in the control of chronic pain. *Arch Phys Med Rehabil* 65:228–231, 1984.
21. Williams PC. The conservative management of lesions of the lumbosacral spine. *Instr Course Lect* 10, 1953.
22. Kester NC. Evaluation and medical management of low back pain. *Med Clin North Am* 53:525, 1969.
23. Vasudevan SV, Lynch NT. Pain centers—organization and outcome. *West J Med* 154:532–535, 1991.
24. Krishnan K, Rama R, France RD. Antidepressants in chronic pain syndromes. *Am Fam Physician* 39:233–237, 1989.
25. Vasudevan SV. Rehabilitation of the patient with chronic pain—is it cost effective? *Pain Digest* 2:99–101, 1992.
26. Charmaz K. Loss of self: a fundamental form of suffering in the chronically ill. *Sociol Health Illness* 5:168–195, 1983.

Selected Readings

Acute Low Back Problems in Adults—Clinical Practice Guideline No. 14. Washington, DC: U.S. Department of Health and Human Services, 1994.

Bonica JJ (ed.). *General Considerations of Chronic Pain. The Management of Pain.* Philadelphia: Lea & Febiger, 1990. Pp. 180–196.

Hansen TJ, Merritt JL. *Rehabilitation of the Patient with Lower Back Pain—Rehabilitation Medicine Principles and Practice.* Philadelphia: Lippincott, 1988. Pp. 728–749.

Prithvi Raj P. *Practical Management of Pain.* St. Louis: Mosby–Year Book, 1992.

Schwab CD (ed.). *Physical Medicine and Rehabilitation. Musculoskeletal Pain.* Hanley & Belfus, 5(3), 1991.

Travell J, Simons D. *Myofascial Pain and Dysfunction. The Trigger Point Manual,* vols. I and II. Baltimore: Williams & Wilkins, 1991.

Walsh NE (ed.). *Physical Medicine and Rehabilitation. Rehabilitation of Chronic Pain.* Hanley & Belfus, 5(1), 1991.

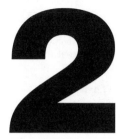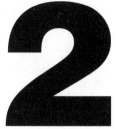

Failed Back Surgery Syndrome

Thomas R. Haher
Joseph Dryer
Robert C. Nucci
Mark A. Liker

I. Background

A. Of the 250,000 spinal operations that are performed annually in the United States, 10% to 15% will fail to relieve initial presenting symptoms or enable the patient to return to work,[1] leaving patients and their physicians with the problem of chronic pain. **Failed back surgery syndrome (FBSS)**[2,3] can be due to
   1. Recurrent disk herniation
   2. Infection
   3. Epidural fibrosis
   4. Lateral canal stenosis and instability
   5. Psychological factors, particularly depression
B. The indication for initial surgery is usually nerve root or cord compression from adjacent soft tissue or bony elements. The most common cause of nerve compression for individuals 25 to 55 years old is a herniated nucleus pulposus. For older patients or those on steroid therapy, the most common cause is spinal stenosis.
C. The **presenting symptoms** consistent with a herniated disk are
   1. Radicular pain
   2. Weakness
   3. Paresthesias
   4. Numbness in the distribution of the affected nerve root
D. Objective findings often consist of
   1. Loss of the associated reflex
   2. Loss of motor strength
   3. Reproduction of the radicular pain with stretching of the root
   4. Decreased sensation to touch
   5. In spinal stenosis the symptoms include neurologic claudication with relief of pain with sitting or flexing the lumbar spine.
E. Diagnostic tests to demonstrate nerve root compression include
   1. **Myelography**
   2. **CT scan**
   3. **MRI**
   4. **Electromyography (EMG)**
F. The physician must anatomically correlate the objective findings on physical examination with the location of the lesion on the diagnostic tests. It is the responsibility of the patient to assess the pain, after appropriate conservative therapy, with respect to its **effect on quality of life** and the ability to perform activities of daily living.
G. If pain persists despite appropriate conservative therapy and physical and diagnostic tests coincide with respect to the anatomic level of the lesion, then **surgery** is offered **to decrease nerve compression.** The onus of success therefore rests on the patient as well as the physician.
H. A less frequent indication for surgery is **spinal instability,** a condition in which abnormal spinal motion exists between or among intervertebral bodies. A diskogram is indicated by some clinicians to document this lesion. Spinal fusion eliminates the abnormal motion that produces low back pain.

II. Definition: the persistence or recurrence of the initial subjective or objective physical findings in the immediate, midterm, or chronic postoperative period.

III. Etiology. The causes of FBSS are multifactorial.[4–8]

A. Herniated nucleus pulposus and low back pain. Disk excision gives relief of radicular pain more often than low back pain. Careful diagnosis is paramount because disk excision does not relieve back pain. If back pain exists, then causes other than a herniated disk must be investigated.

B. Lateral stenosis is a bony compression of the exiting nerve root caused by hypertrophied degenerative facet joints. Lateral stenosis may be present with a herniated disk. The diagnosis of lateral stenosis must be made preoperatively and is amenable to surgical intervention. Failure to identify and treat lateral stenosis will result in FBSS. Up to 60% of patients diagnosed as having a herniated disk may have associated or isolated lateral stenosis.[9,10]

C. Central stenosis is diffuse narrowing of the spinal canal. Up to 15% of FBSS patients have unrecognized central stenosis. The lesion is treated surgically by a wide decompressive laminectomy. Failure to recognize this entity while performing a disk excision will result in FBSS.[9]

D. Recurrent herniated disk

1. **Retained disk material** within the anulus may exit the posterior lateral region of the anulus and cause nerve root compression. A sequestered disk fragment in the lateral recess may be difficult to find and remove during surgery.

2. The existence of **an inferior or superior disk herniation** is also possible with resulting radiculopathy and other similar symptomatology. The diagnosis may be aided by an MRI with contrast material (galadinium) that differentiates scar tissue from sequestered or new disk material. The time period from the date of surgery to the onset of symptoms may also aid in the diagnosis. The treatment consists of reexploration of the canal and nerve root, followed by adequate decompression and removal of the offending disk material.

E. Infection

1. Approximately 5% of surgical wounds become infected. The presentation of a wound infection is usually 5 to 7 days after the procedure. **Signs of an acute infection** are
   a. Persistent fever
   b. Increasing paraincisional pain
   c. Flucetulence

2. **Treatment** consists of
   a. Rapid evacuation of the purulent fluid
   b. Copious irrigation followed by antibiotic treatment

3. **Chronic infection** with or without osteomyelitis is a difficult problem to diagnose and treat. It may mimic low back pain secondary to any of the preceding causes. A tissue diagnosis is mandatory in conjunction with proper antibiotic coverage.[11,12] The presence of chronic infection is indicated by
   a. Persistently elevated erythrocyte sedimentation rate
   b. Bony destruction as evidenced by serial x-rays
   c. An enlarging paraspinal mass imaged on CT or MRI

F. Epidural fibrosis is often an unavoidable sequela of spinal surgery reflecting the formation of scar tissue adjacent to the dura. Because it is to some extent always present after surgery, its role as a causative factor in FBSS is uncertain and episodic at best. The diagnosis is entertained when abnormal EMG findings are present with usually no other positive diagnostic tests for root compression. CT scans may show fibrosis around the affected nerve root.[13]

G. Arachnoiditis. Scar tissue leading to arachnoiditis may form within the dura, causing clumping, ischemia, and atrophy of nerve roots. It may be caused by an inflammatory stimulus resulting from a herniated disk, blood, or a chemical irritant in the subarachnoid space, such as contrast medium used in myelography. The pia-arachnoid membrane may react to minor trauma with an inflammatory response producing adhesions. The traumatic event may occur outside the dura compressing the roots and pia-arachnoid.[14-16]

H. Missed lesions. Postoperative persistent symptoms may reflect missed pathology at the time of surgery[17,18]:

1. **Far out syndrome** is impingement of the sacral alar and the L5 transverse process upon the L5 nerve root as seen with spondylolisthesis.[19]

2. Negative disk exploration at the time of surgery may reflect one of the following:[20]
   a. Disk fragment in the intervertebral foramen
   b. Nerve root kinking by the pedicle
   c. Articular process compressing on the nerve root
   d. Lateral disk herniation
   e. Spinal stenosis
   f. Surgery performed at the wrong level

I. Mechanical pain (instability). Removal of bone and soft tissue during surgery may result in the inability of the spine to support physiologic loads. This removal of load-supporting structures causes load sharing or alternative loading paths to be established, with transference to adjacent structures that cannot tolerate the increased stresses. This painful condition is difficult to confirm unless abnormal motion can be documented on flexion and extension of the spine.[21,22]

J. Pseudarthrosis. The goal of a spinal fusion is to eliminate motion between the vertebral bodies. Failure to eliminate this motion would result in the persistence of pain. The same problems and techniques in defining instability apply to the diagnosis of pseudarthrosis.

K. Chronic intrinsic radiculopathy. When the nerve root is subjected to prolonged compression-induced ischemia, nutritional insufficiency, and edema, the condition may no longer be amenable to surgical intervention because the pain may originate from the nerve root itself. This condition may exist in up to 30% of patients with FBSS.

L. Psychological factors in FBSS must always be considered for proper management and treatment. Psychological factors and secondary gain can influence the patients' desire for surgical intervention as well as their perception of a good result. Depression, anxiety, maladaptive behavior, and an obsession with personal well-being can prolong or indefinitely extend the recuperative period. As a result of this, poor results are often encountered in cases covered by workmen's compensation insurance.

IV. Onset of symptoms with respect to diagnosis. The onset of the patient's symptomatology after surgery may guide the clinician to the cause of FBSS.
  A. Immediate onset of symptoms[2,8,17,18]
   1. Wrong diagnosis
     a. Occult infection
     b. Spinal infection
     c. Disk space infection
     d. Retroperitoneal tumors
     e. Viral plexopathics
     f. Peripheral neuropathies (diabetes)
     g. Vascular disease
   2. Discogenic pain. Internal disk derangement produced by compressive loading of the disk exceeding structural tolerance.
   3. Delayed surgery. Irreversible damage to the nerve roots due to chronic changes.
   4. Wrong level
   5. Inadequate decompression of the affected nerve root
  B. Delayed onset (6 months to 1 year)[2,14,16]
   1. Recurrent disk herniation
   2. Ischemic root
   3. Epidural fibrosis
   4. Arachnoiditis
  C. Prolonged delay (>1 year)
   1. Disk space collapse causing root compression
   2. Instability
V. Nonoperative treatment of FBSS
  A. Bed rest is indicated for postoperative radicular pain secondary to irritation of the nerve roots. It decreases irritation by decreasing the motion of the surrounding structures.[23]
  B. Physical therapy. If the etiology of the pain is muscle spasm or muscle weakness, a period of inactivity followed by muscle-strengthening exercises will provide relief.
  C. Acupuncture relieves pain by increasing tactile stimulation thereby interfering with the sensory transmission of painful stimuli.
  D. Medications. Narcotics and muscle relaxants should be avoided in all but acute episodes of pain. Nonsteroidal anti-inflammatory drugs should be the mainstay of therapy if contraindications do not exist.
  E. Injections may be used to decrease pain locally or to destroy the neurologic tissue that transmits painful stimuli to the CNS. In order to use injections effectively, the location of the region causing or transmitting the pain must be known. The injection may be given in the region of
   1. Localized soft tissue pain called **trigger points**
   2. The **facet joints** for localization and ablation of the pain
   3. The **nerve root** for therapeutic and diagnostic reasons

4. Injections into the **intervertebral disk** have been reported to be beneficial not only in localizing the disk in question but also to decrease the pressure on an affected nerve root secondary to a bulging disk.

5. **Epidural** injections in the failed back have been shown to decrease inflammation in nerve entrapment and dural compression from scar tissue.

F. **Dorsal column stimulator.** This is another modality of competitive stimulation to decrease the effect of painful stimuli. It is not a destructive procedure such as ablative injections and has proved to be effective especially when a transcutaneous electrical nerve stimulation (TENS) unit has been successfully used locally. The advantage of a dorsal column stimulator is in its ability to affect a larger region than a TENS unit.

G. **Psychological intervention**[24]

References

1. Kelsey JL, White WW. Epidemiology and impact of low back pain. *Spine* 5:133–142, 1980.
2. LaRocca H. Failed lumbar surgery syndromes: causes and correctives. In Bridwell K, DeWald R (eds.), *Textbook of Spinal Surgery.* Philadelphia: J.B. Lippincott, 1991. Pp. 719–737.
3. Zucherman J, Schofferman J. Pathology of failed back surgery syndrome. *Spine: State of the Art Reviews* 1:1–3, 1986.
4. Mixter W, Barr J. Rupture of the intervertebral disc with involvement of the spinal cord. *N Engl J Med* 211:210–215, 1934.
5. Jackson R. The long term effects of wide laminectomy for lumbar disc excision. *J Bone Joint Surg Br* 53:609, 1971.
6. Weber H. Lumbar disc herniation. A prospective study of prognostic factors including a controlled trial. *J Oslo City Hosp* 28:33, 1978.
7. Dvorak J, Gauchat MH, Valach L. The outcome for surgery for lumbar disc herniation. 1. A 4–17 years follow-up with emphasis on somatic aspects. *Spine* 13:1418, 1984.
8. Burton C, Kirkaldy-Willis H, Yong-Hing K, Heithoff K. Causes of failure of surgery on the lumbar spine. *Clin Orthop* 157:191–199, 1981.
9. Frymoyer J. The role of spine fusion. *Spine* 6:284, 1981.
10. Epstein J, Lavine B, Epstein B. Recurrent herniation of the lumbar intervertebral disc. *Clin Orthop* 52:169, 1967.
11. Kostuik P, Frymoyer J. Failure after spinal fusion. In Frymoyer J (ed.), *The Adult Spine: Principles and Practice.* New York: Raven 1991. P. 650.
12. Wiffen J, Neuwirth M. Spinal stenosis. In Bridwell K, DeWald R (eds.), *Textbook of Spinal Surgery.* Philadelphia: J.B. Lippincott, 1991. Pp. 637–656.
13. Zucherman J, Schofferman J. Pathology of failed back surgery syndrome. Lesions that cause pain. *Spine: State of the Art Reviews* 1:9, 1986.
14. Burton C. Lumbosacral arachnoiditis. *Spine* 3:24–30, 1977.
15. Wilkinson H. The role of improper surgery in the etiology of the failed back syndrome. In Wilkinson H (ed.), *The Failed Back Syndrome.* Philadelphia: J.B. Lippincott, 1993. Pp. 5–16.
16. Pheasant H. Sources of failure in laminectomies. *Clin Orthop* 6:319–329, 1975.
17. Crock H. Observations on the management of failed spinal operations. *J Bone Joint Surg Br* 58:193, 1976.
18. Crock H. Isolated lumbar disc resorption as a cause of nerve root canal stenosis. *Clin Orthop* 115:109, 1976.
19. Wiltse L, Guyer R, Spencer C, et al. Alar transverse process impingement of the L_5 spinal nerve: the far out syndrome. *Spine* 9:31–41, 1984.
20. MacNab I. Negative disc exploration. *J Bone Joint Surg* 53A:891, 1971.
21. Haher T, Tozzi J, Lospinuso M. The contribution of the three columns of the spine to spinal stability: a biomechanical model. *Paraplegia* 27:432, 1989.
22. Haher T, Dryer J, Slhoub J, O'Brien M. The role of the lumbar facet joints in spinal stability: identification of alternative paths of loading. *Spine* 19:2667–2671, 1994.
23. Wilkinson H. Alternative therapies for the failed back syndrome. In Frymoyer J (ed.), *The Adult Spine: Principles and Practices.* New York: Raven, 1991. Pp. 2069–2091.
24. Goldstein R. Psychological evaluation of low back pain. *Spine: State of the Art Reviews* 1:103–114, 1986.

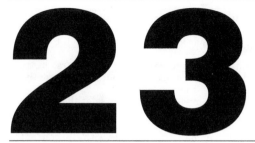

Nonarticular and Myofascial Pain Syndromes

Mark G. Greenbaum
Stuart A. Rubin

I. **Background.** Nonarticular and myofascial pain syndromes can have a significant effect on a patient's comfort and function. These syndromes include bursitis, tendinitis, regional myofascial pain syndromes, and fibromyalgia. Although differentiating these conditions from one another may be difficult, proper diagnosis is essential for proper treatment and preventing the development of chronicity.

Although nonarticular and myofascial tissue constitute the largest percentage of body tissue, they receive relatively little attention in contemporary medical education. In assessing pain and dysfunction, clinicians often focus on the bones, joints, and nerves and do not consider the overlying nonarticular and myofascial tissues as a possible nociceptive source. Unfortunately, this has led to frequent misdiagnoses and inadequate treatment of many of these syndromes.

II. **General principles**
- A. **Functional anatomic context.** The pain must be understood in the correct anatomic context. Knowledge of the relationship of position and movement to functional anatomy can help clarify the cause of pain that is produced by a certain position or movement.
- B. **Closed kinetic chain.** The body has been described as a closed kinetic chain when the foot is weight-bearing and an open kinetic chain when it is in space. Any biomechanical or external force that produces pain or pressure anywhere along the closed kinetic chain can transmit abnormal biomechanical forces proximally or distally, ipsilaterally or contralaterally, and produce secondary pain. These secondary pains (e.g., low back pain) are often the presenting symptoms. If the primary pain is not treated (e.g., metatarsalgia, which causes an antalgic gait placing abnormal forces on the low back), treatment for secondary pain will not be as effective.
- C. **Multiple causation.** A patient's pain can have more than one component. For example, a painful subacromial bursitis could cause painful spasm of the surrounding musculature. Both of these aspects should be addressed for optimal treatment.
- D. **Psychosocial and functional aspects.** Understanding the psychosocial and functional life of a patient is essential in evaluating the patient's pain. A stressed patient will often assume certain postures and maintain a heightened muscle tone, which could increase the biomechanical forces exerted on the tissues.
- E. **Muscle physiology.** Muscle is a dynamic tissue that can exert high forces on neighboring muscles, nonarticular tissues, and nerves. All muscles have reflexes that must be respected and modulated to successfully treat a myofascial process.
- F. **Concurrent medical conditions** might cause underlying pain or increase the susceptibility of nonarticular and myofascial tissues to damage.
- G. **Nerve entrapments.** Entrapments of peripheral nerves and radiculopathies can cause pain in the respectively innervated and neighboring muscles.

III. **Bursitis.** Bursae are closed filled sacs lined by synovial cells, which facilitate the motion of tendons, muscles, and skin over bones. There are more than 80 bursae on each side of the body. Inflammation of the bursal wall (bursitis) may be caused by excessive friction, trauma, or infection. The most commonly inflamed bursae include
- A. **Subacromial bursitis,** which is the most common, with its extension onto the subdeltoid bursae often associated with a rotator cuff tendinitis. It can calcify and usually responds to physical modalities with aggressive stretching and therapeutic exercise. It may require injection of corticosteroids.
- B. **Pes anserine bursitis,** which is inflammation of the bursa under the tendons of

the semitendinosus, sartorius, and gracilis muscles as they insert onto the medial aspect of the upper tibia. It is most common in overweight women. Often there is pain on stair climbing. This superficial bursa responds well to corticosteroid injection.

C. Greater trochanteric bursitis, which is inflammation of the bursa at the gluteal insertion onto the femoral trochanter. A deep-lying bursa, it frequently requires injection of corticosteroids.

D. Prepatellar bursitis, which is inflammation of the bursa at the lower patella or under the patellar tendon. It usually results from frequent kneeling (housemaid's knee).

E. Olecranon bursitis, which is inflammation (sometimes with effusion) at the point of the elbow. It commonly occurs with gout, rheumatoid arthritis, or trauma and is occasionally septic. Additional pressure or trauma should be avoided.

F. Achilles bursitis, which is inflammation of the bursa just above the insertion of the Achilles tendon to the calcaneus. It can present as "pump bumps" caused by closely contoured heel counters. Neither the deep bursa nor the Achilles tendon sheath should be routinely injected because of the possibility of rupture of this heavily stressed tendon. Treatment in general is conservative with avoidance of irritation and trauma by modifying the patient's activities or posture. Appropriate padding and splinting may be useful. Physical modalities such as heat, ultrasound, and phonophoresis with therapeutic exercises are beneficial. Anti-inflammatory medication and antibiotics should be used when indicated.

IV. Tendinitis

A. Inflammation of tendon, tendon sheath, or its attachment to bone caused by excessive repetitive trauma muscular or systemic disorders. Nodular hypertrophy of the tendon and stenosis of its sheath can result. Simultaneous deposition of calcium, usually at the shoulder, wrist, and ankle, can result in calcific tendinitis. A few of the more common examples include

  1. Lateral epicondylitis (tennis elbow)—inflammation of the tendinous origin of the wrist and finger extensors at the lateral epicondyle. There is pain on resisted wrist extension and supination. If it is refractory to massage, ultrasound, or anti-inflammatory drugs, local corticosteroid injection is usually curative.

  2. Bicipital tendinitis—inflammation of the tendon of the long head of the biceps brachii with possible dislocation, subluxation, or rupture. There is pain on resisted supination of the forearm (Yergason's sign). Treatment initially is with physical modalities and exercise. In resistant cases local injection of corticosteroids into the tendon sheath is indicated.

  3. De Quervain's disease—stenosing tenosynovitis of the abductor pollicis longus and extensor pollicis brevis at the radial styloid. It is common with repetitive grasping with movement of the hand in a ulnar direction. When the thumb is placed in the palm and grasped by the fingers, ulnar deviation of the wrist causes sharp pain (Finkelstein's sign). Avoiding the provoking activity and splinting is sometimes curative. Local corticosteroid injection into the tendon sheath often results in improvement.

B. General treatment guidelines

  1. Injection of corticosteroid directly into the tendon should be avoided, especially in athletes who will be doing severe loading of the tendon, which may result in a tear.

  2. Injection should be around, rather than directly into, the tendon. Overexertion after injection should be avoided for at least 1 week.

  3. Repeated administration of local steroids (more than three per year) should be performed with caution.

  4. Insoluble steroid preparations should be mixed with lidocaine to prevent calcium deposits.

V. Myofascial pain syndrome

is pain or autonomic phenomena referred from active myofascial **trigger points,** which are hyperirritable loci within a taut band of skeletal muscle or its fascia. They are painful on compression and can evoke specific patterns of referred pain and autonomic phenomena. Active trigger points cause pain; latent trigger points cause painless restriction of motion and muscle weakness.

A. General Overview

  1. Etiology. An initiating stimulus (i.e., trauma, fatigue, stress) causes a physiologic response, which generates a hyperirritable locus (trigger point). The CNS is excited, and often pain and autonomic phenomena are referred. Muscles associated with the trigger point become tense, which leads to fatigue. Local ischemia occurs, leading to release of nociceptive agents. A vicious circle of increasing motor and sympathetic activity then ensues, which leads to increased pain.

2. **History.** Onset may be sudden or gradual. Specific movement or activity associated with the onset of pain should be inquired about. Patients should try to pinpoint which muscles may have been overloaded and strained thereby developing the active trigger points.

3. **Physical examination**
   a. **Functional examination**—look for deviations in posture, body asymmetry, restricted range of motion of muscles. There should be no neurologic deficits.
   b. **Examination of a muscle for trigger points**
      (1) Stretch the muscle (just short of pain).
      (2) Palpate for a taut band.
   c. **Palpate along the taut band** to its maximum point of tenderness, the trigger point.
   d. **Local twitch response** is a major diagnostic criteria for trigger points, which consists of a transient contraction of the muscle fibers in the taut band with muscle in a neutral position. Quick palpation or needle contact with the trigger point causes a vigorous local twitch response.
   e. **Jump sign**—strong digital pressure on an active trigger point can cause severe pain with an involuntary reflexlike flinching and jerking of the body.

4. **Laboratory findings.** Radiologic, electrodiagnostic, and laboratory studies are useless in the diagnosis of myofascial trigger points. Some laboratory studies may be helpful in identifying perpetuating or predisposing factors.

B. **Perpetuating factors**
   1. **Mechanical stress** is caused by structural inadequacies:
      a. Leg length discrepancy, pelvic and head tilt
      b. Scoliosis
   2. **Postural stress**
      a. Misfitting chair
      b. Poor posture, round shoulders, kyphosis, and head tilt
      c. Abuse of muscles
         (1) Sustained isometric contraction or immobility of muscle
         (2) Excessive repetitions of same movement; excessively quick and jerky movements
   3. **Constriction of muscles—prolonged pressure**
   4. **Nerve entrapments**
   5. **Psychological factors**
      a. Misunderstanding of condition
      b. Depression
      c. Anxiety, tension
      d. Secondary gain
   6. **Nutritional, metabolic, and endocrinologic imbalances**
   7. **Chronic infection**
   8. **Impaired sleep**

C. **Treatment is to inactivate the trigger points by restoring the muscle to its full stretch range of motion.**
   1. **Stretch and spray**
      a. **Material**—chlorofluoromethane vapocoolant with jet-stream nozzle. Clinically this is preferred to ethylchloride spray (which is flammable, explosive, and colder than desirable) despite its minimal contribution to ozone layer depletion. One can also use stroking with an edge of plastic-covered ice. Cooling helps to block reflex spasm and pain during passive stretching of the involved muscle.
      b. **Technique**
         (1) Position the patient in a comfortable manner with the affected muscle at maximal stretch.
         (2) Apply parallel sweeps of vapocoolant to the skin at a distance of 18 inches at a speed of about 4 inches/sec. The sweeps should be unidirectional and cover the muscle containing the trigger point. The direction of spray should progress in the same direction as the muscle fibers proceed toward the referred pain pattern. The spray stream should be diverted at an acute angle to the skin of approximately 30 degrees, and

frosting of the skin should be avoided. The involved muscle should be sprayed first, then the referred area, and the application repeated with two or three superimposed sweeps.

(3) During each sweep, maintain gentle, smooth, steady tension on the muscle.

(4) Warm the skin with a hot pack.

(5) The muscle should be moved through the full active range of motion.

(6) The entire procedure can be repeated if needed.

(7) Instruct the patient on specific stretching exercises to be done at home.

2. Trigger point injection

    a. Materials—1% lidocaine, 0.5% procaine or 0.25% bupivacaine, dry needling or isotonic saline (no epinephrine), 21- to 25-gauge needle.

    b. Technique

        (1) Prepare the skin.

        (2) Localize the trigger point.

        (3) Stretch the muscle sufficiently to tighten the muscle fibers containing the trigger point.

        (4) Fix the trigger point in position by holding it between the fingers or with a pincer grip between the thumb and fingertips.

        (5) Inject 0.5–1.0 ml when the trigger point is contracted by the needle. The local twitch response and referred pain should be elicited when the needle tip penetrates the point (that is, if they were elicited by palpation prior to the injection).

        (6) Progressively stretch the muscle to its full length. This maneuver may require a few sweeps of vapocoolant spray beforehand to relax any remaining tense fibers.

        (7) Apply hot pack over all trigger points that have been injected.

        (8) Have the patient actively move the muscle through its full range of motion.

        (9) Instruct the patient in specific stretching exercises to be done at home.

        (10) The procedure can be repeated 3 to 4 days later.

3. Alternative treatments to inactivate myofascial trigger points

    a. Ischemic compression

        (1) Stretch the relaxed muscle to the verge of discomfort.

        (2) Apply sustained, tolerably painful pressure with a thumb (or strong finger) directly over the trigger point. As the discomfort tends to decrease, gradually increase the pressure by adding pressure from another finger. Continue this maneuver up to 1 minute with as much as 20 or 30 lb of pressure. Follow with stretching of the muscle.

    b. Postisometric relaxation

        (1) Have the patient isometrically contract the tense muscle against resistance. Hold it for 3 to 10 seconds.

        (2) The patient then relaxes, and the clinician gently stretches the muscle.

4. Corrective actions

    a. Avoid strenuous activity for 1 week after stretch and spray. However, gentle full range of motion of the muscle is encouraged.

    b. The patient should learn which activities aggravate the pain and avoid them. Bad habits should be unlearned. Nonpainful muscles should be substituted when possible.

    c. Avoid sustained muscle contraction. Avoid maximum effort or overload of muscles.

    d. Maintain mobility and full range of motion of muscles.

    e. Relaxation, biofeedback

    f. Correct standing, sitting, and sleeping posture

    g. Conditioning and strengthening exercise for latent, not active, trigger points

D. Specific example—upper trapezius. Of all the muscles in the body, the trapezius is considered to have the most potential myofascial trigger points. Trigger points in the upper trapezius refer pain unilaterally upward along the posterolateral aspect of the neck to the mastoid process and are a major source of neck pain secondary to sustained muscular contractions. Pain can also be referred to the temple, back of the orbit, and jaw. The whole muscle can contract and cause pain or activate trigger points within it. Trigger points can also be activated by external mechanisms such as chronically poor neck and head posture. Vague

Table 23-1. Comparison of fibromyalgia and myofascial pain syndrome

	Myofascial pain syndrome	Fibromyalgia
Sex	M ≈ F	F > M (73–88%)
Onset	Sudden, related to specific muscle movement, overload	Insidious, no specific precipitatory factors
Physical examination	Dysfunctional postures, asymmetries, decreased range of motion	(−)
	Trigger point taut band → referred pain, twitch response	Tender points Diffusely tender muscles, soft and doughy, widespread distribution
Laboratory findings	(−)	(−)
Chronicity	Caused by perpetuating, usually correctable factors	Inherent to the disease
Sleep disturbance, fatigue, depression	Unusual	Usual
Overlap of trigger points vs. tender myofascial trigger points	More than half of the designated tender points are also common trigger points.	Many patients with fibromyalgia also have active or latent myofascial trigger points.

chronic overloads such as tight bra straps, heavy pocket books, as well as anxiety and depression have been implicated as well.

VI. Fibromyalgia. Also known as fibrositis, fibromyalgia is a generalized soft tissue rheumatic disorder with widespread aching, stiffness, and tender points with associated symptoms including fatigue, depression, and sleeplessness. There are usually no precipitatory trauma, provocative repetitive motion, or physical stress and no known cause. Although they are superficially similar, fibromyalgia is distinct from the myofascial pain syndrome (Table 23-1).

A. Treatment (total cures are rare)
1. Reassurance and education by the physician
2. General mobilization and stretching exercise program
3. Sports, cardiovascular fitness training
4. Tricyclic antidepressants or muscle relaxants for pain relief or sleep disturbances
5. Biofeedback, relaxation, cognitive-behavioral therapy

Selected Readings

Bennet RM. Confounding features of the fibromyalgia syndrome: a current perspective of differential diagnosis. *J Rheumatol Suppl* 19:58–61, 1989.

Cailliet R. *Soft Tissue Pain and Disability* (2nd ed.). Philadelphia: F.A. Davis, 1988.

Friction J, Awad E (eds.). *Myofascial Pain and Fibromyalgia.* New York: Raven, 1990.

Sheon RP, Moskowitz RW, Goldberg VM. *Soft Tissue Rheumatic Pain* (2nd ed.). Philadelphia: Lea & Febiger, 1987.

Simons DG. Myofascial trigger points: a need for understanding. *Arch Phys Med Rehabil* 62:97–99, 1981.

Smyth HA. Non-articular rheumatic and psychogenic musculoskeletal syndromes. In McCarty DJ (ed.), *Arthritis and Allied Conditions* (10th ed.). Philadelphia: Lea & Febiger, 1989. Pp. 1241–1254.

Travell JG, Simons DG. Myofascial pain and dysfunction. *The Trigger Point Manual.* Baltimore: Williams & Wilkins, 1983.

Travell JG, Simons DG. Myofascial pain and dysfunction. *The Trigger Point Manual,* Vol. 2. *The Lower Extremities.* Baltimore: Williams & Wilkins, 1992.

Wolf F, Smyth HA, Yunus MB, et al. The American College of Rheumatology 1990 criteria for the classification of fibromyalgia. *Arthritis Rheum* 33:160–172, 1990.

Yanus MB, Masi AT, Aldaj TC. Criteria studies of primary fibromyalgia syndrome (PFS). *Arthritis Rheum* 30(Suppl):550, 1987.

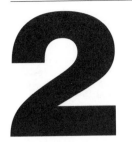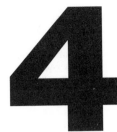

Reflex Sympathetic Dystrophy

Robert J. Schwartzman

I. Background

A. Reflex sympathetic dystrophy (RSD) is a syndrome of **pain, hyperesthesia, vaso-motor disturbance,** and **dystrophic changes** that usually follows peripheral nerve or soft tissue injury. The symptoms are complex and involve the sensory, motor, and autonomic systems.[1–4] Although there is no specific test that will unequivocally diagnose it, the diagnostic tests are helpful in confirming a clinical impression. The illness evolves over time, the early stages are sympathetically maintained, and the later stages are sympathetically independent. The evolution through the stages has general time boundaries, but there are marked variations among patients.[5]

B. Perhaps the most disturbing part of the illness is that it is **frequently initiated by trivial trauma** such as brachial plexus traction injury, carpal tunnel surgical procedure, sprain, or fracture.[5] At least 50% of patients who get RSD have suffered a soft tissue injury. Casting and immobilization of the injured part may be seen in at least half of the patients who develop RSD.[5]

C. Another aspect of the illness that is hard to comprehend and becomes devastating to patients is that it **spreads proximally from a distal injury but may spread to the contralateral extremity.**[6–8] A patient frequently develops RSD symptomatology in the upper extremity following the use of crutches for lower extremity disease. It appears as if nerves are sensitized to the process once it begins in areas distant from the site of injury. Major nerves in areas compromised by RSD may become symptomatic if they traverse the involved area. A patient suffering RSD in the lower extremity may develop sciatic nerve somatic lancinating pain in addition to the burning pain from the RSD. The process may generalize to involve the entire body surface.[6] Patients may have both dissociation of RSD by stage as well as predominant symptoms in different parts of their body simultaneously.

D. RSD has **six major components** (in general, the first three are seen early in the illness, while the next three dominate its later stages):[6]

    1. Pain
    2. Edema
    3. Autonomic abnormality
    4. Movement disorder
    5. Trophic changes
    6. Autoimmune phenomena

E. The key to successful treatment of this illness is **diagnosis and treatment within 3 to 6 months.**[9] The disease must be treated while the pain is sympathetically maintained. The underlying cause must be identified and treated. If the problem progresses to sympathetically independent status, the patient can be helped but not cured.[10,11]

F. The pain of RSD is **frequently associated with**

    1. Hyperalgesia—lowered pain threshold and enhanced pain perception
    2. Allodynia—pain from innocuous mechanical or thermal stimuli
    3. Hyperpathia—higher pain threshold that once exceeded causes severe pain that reaches maximum intensity rapidly and is not stimulus-bound
    4. Some patients have limbs that are **almost anesthetic to somatic stimuli** but may suffer a **concomitant deep ache.**

II. Stages of RSD.
The clinical signs and symptoms of each stage of RSD insidiously merge one into another, but in general stage I lasts for 6 months, stage II for 2 years, and stage III supervenes after this. Some patients may remain in a specific stage for months and years and then rapidly progress to end-stage disease. From

our experience of approximately 2000 patients, approximately 2% to 5% of patients will get generalized disease, and approximately 25% of patients will have their disease spread to either the contralateral or ipsilateral extremity.

In any stage of RSD, the symptom complex may be dissociated in affected extremities. One extremity may be extremely painful while the contralateral extremity demonstrates autonomic dysfunction. Conversely, patients may have severe livedo reticularis, dusky cyanosis, and circulatory abnormalities but have skin with little pain and no movement abnormality.

A. **In stage I disease,** the pain following peripheral injury is more severe than would be expected for the degree of tissue damage and progressively worsens.[5] It is usually described as burning, intense, diffuse, deep, and distal to the site of injury. The pain quickly spreads out of a nerve or dermatomal distribution and is exacerbated by movement, emotional upset, and dependent posture. Allodynia, hyperalgesia, and hyperpathia are objective concomitants of the pain. Patients suffer spontaneous exacerbations of their pain and frequently complain of an unremitting deep ache. Both a painful warm extremity (angry backfiring C-fiber nociceptors [ABC] syndrome) and a cold extremity that is hypoanesthetic to cold, but if stimulated with a cold stimulus is reported as burning pain (triple cold syndrome), have been described.[12,13] A subset of patients obtain pain relief by packing the extremity in ice or wrapping it tightly with elastic bandages or cloth. Sympathetic blocks may increase the pain of some patients, who have higher-temperature-sensitized C-fiber polymodal receptors (increasing the temperature of the vasodilated extremity) and may suffer further pain as C-fiber polymodal cold afferents fire as the leg cools. Many patients adapt a protective posture to shield the affected part from all stimuli. In this stage of RSD, the nails become ridged, thick, and brittle while the hair darkens and grows quickly. Edema, temperature change (hypothermia or hyperthermia), hyperhidrosis, livedo reticularis, dusky cyanosis, and diffuse mottling are present distally, although the inciting injury may be proximal. Thermography, which evaluates the effects of small fiber activity that cannot be shown by ordinary electromyography (EMG) recordings, will show temperature changes in many dermatomal distributions that would be unexpected from the location of the injury.[14]

B. **In stage II disease** (dystrophic), the constant burning pain, hyperalgesia, and allodynia intensify and are accompanied by sleep disruption, anxiety, and severe depression.[5] The skin demonstrates brawny edema and is usually hyperhidrotic, cool, cyanotic, and mottled. Hair loss occurs in the areas where it was previously stimulated, and the nails continue to thicken and become more ridged and brittle. The bones frequently reveal cystic and subchondral erosion as well as diffuse osteoporosis (Sudek's atrophy). Frequently, a triple-phase bone scan will demonstrate abnormal pooling at this stage.[5]

C. **Stage III disease** is dominated by ever-increasing pain that has spread to areas remote from the injury. The skin becomes shiny, the integument atrophies, the joints become tender and contract, and there is diffuse muscle atrophy. The movement disorder is seen as frequently as is pain, but is not generally appreciated.[4] Most clinicians misdiagnose the **movement disorder** as secondary to pain or hysteria. It consists of five components:

1. **Difficulty in initiating movement**
2. **Weakness**
3. **Spasms**
4. **Tremor**
5. **Increased reflexes**

D. Patients with **longstanding RSD** suffer skin ulcerations, infections in edematous areas, and autoerythrocytic phagocytosis.[15]

III. **Pathogenesis**

A. A great deal of experimental work in animal models of RSD and clinical studies of patients have given new insight into pathogenetic mechanisms that may cause the disease.[16,17] Peripheral nerve injury or **damage to deep C-fiber afferents** is the overwhelming cause of RSD. Damage to these afferents causes the expression of early response genes (c-*fos* proto-oncogene), which leads to the production of excitatory neuropeptides (dymorphan) that may change the excitability of central-pain-projecting (CPP) neurons (origin of the spinothalamic tract) in the dorsal horn.[18] The peripheral afferent C-fiber projection to the spinal cord excites the sympathetic outflow through the intermediolateral column, several segments above and below the afferent segment that subserves the affected dermatome.[19]

Pain projections may activate central sympathetic nuclei (nucleus magnus raphus), which may activate sympathetic efferents bilaterally.[20] Thus, a painful afferent impulse may activate multisegmental spinal sympathetic efferent activity (somatic-sympathetic reflexes) that can be reinforced from central sympathetic nuclear discharge. Damaged nerves fire ectopically and repetitively, which may also drive spinal sympathetic activity.[21] Repetitive nociceptor firing may cause up-regulation of alpha receptors on these same C-fiber nociceptors.[22]

B. Allodynia and hyperalgesia, so characteristic of RSD patients, may result both from peripheral C-fiber nociceptor sensitization to thermal and mechanical stimuli and from central sensitization of dorsal horn CPP neurons.[23,24] **Cross-modality threshold sensitization at the receptor level** has been demonstrated in the ABC syndrome.[1,12] These patients pack the affected extremity in ice so that their polymodal C-fiber nociceptors cannot discharge to touch when the extremity is cold. The quantity and degree of spontaneous pain perceived in patients with RSD is related to the frequency of discharge in specific groups of nociceptors, which in turn is related to their resting thresholds. Algogenic agents or inflammatory mediators released at the site of injury may profoundly influence peripheral C-fiber nociceptor discharge.[25] Nerve block studies in patients with RSD reveal that allodynia to touch and cold is maintained by alpha$_1$-responsive receptors, myelinated fibers, and sensitized C fibers.[23,26,27]

C. The strongest evidence for sympathetic involvement, at least in patients with stage I RSD, is **pain relief by sympathetic block**.[28,29] Stimulation of the sympathetic efferents in awake patients with causalgia increases their pain.[30] Subcutaneous injection of noradrenaline into an asymptomatic extremity of a patient with RSD cured by prior sympathectomy reproduced burning pain after a delay of 10 minutes.[28]

D. Studies of **experimental models** of causalgia and neuropathic pain have shown that sprouts of regenerating afferent axons fire spontaneously and that these ectopic discharges can be driven by systemic noradrenaline and blocked by phentolamine.[31] Recent studies in a model of mixed peripheral nerve injury demonstrated that a subset of C-fiber nociceptor units increase their discharge rate with sympathetic stimulation that is mediated by alpha$_1$-adrenergic receptors and occurs days after injury in those C-fiber nociceptors that retain their connectivity to the periphery.[32] Sympathetic stimulation may also activate A delta nociceptors.[33]

E. The importance of **central mechanisms** in the pain of RSD is most apparent in its **later stages.**
   1. Recent studies have demonstrated that nociceptive afferent projections induce central sensitization in pain-projecting neurons of Rexed layers I and II.[34] This is manifested by
      a. A lowered threshold to fire
      b. A greater number of discharges per stimulus
      c. Enlarged cutaneous receptive fields
   2. Conditioning stimuli from C-fiber nociceptors produce incremental action potential discharges from CPP neurons to successive stimuli, the wind-up phenomenon.[35] The afferent C-fiber input releases excitatory amino acids and neuropeptides that produce long-lasting excitatory postsynaptic potentials. These potentials summate and depolarize a population of dorsal horn (DH) interneurons whose projections decrease the voltage-dependent Mg^{2+} block of the N-methyl-D-aspartate ion channel complex of the CPP neuron.[35] Central sensitization of the CPP of the DH may be the spinal mechanism underlying the hyperalgesia and persistent pain seen after C-fiber injury in these patients.

F. The pathologic pain of RSD is maintained by **both peripheral sensitization of receptors and central sensitization of CPP neurons** of the DH. Clinical studies in patients with RSD demonstrate that the low-threshold mechanoreceptors and myelinated A beta fibers are involved in hyperalgesia and touch-evoked pain.[26] The sympathetic nervous system modulation of C-fiber afferents in a partially damaged nerve and the suprasegmental spread and amplification of this interaction by spinal cord somatosympathetic reflexes supports the importance of sympathetic activity in stage I disease. The appearance of small dark neurons in the DH of the experimental rat painful peripheral nerve model, as well as the transsynaptic degeneration of putative inhibitory interneurons, could be anatomic markers of the centralization of this evolving process that is characteristic of stage II and III disease.[36,37] A great deal of both clinical and animal experimentation suggests mechanisms that underlie the edema, autonomic dysfunction, and motor abnormalities commonly encountered in patients with RSD.[38]

IV. **Treatment.** The successful treatment of RSD rests with early diagnosis while the patient has sympathetically maintained pain. This is a clinical diagnosis that is supported by a clinical response to sympathetic block (bupivacaine, sufentanil, phentolamine), triple-phase bone scan, detailed bone x-ray, and infrared thermography.[14,39–41] Patients must be able to utilize the extremity or the process cannot be aborted.

A. **Major treatment principles**
  1. Early diagnosis within 3 to 6 months
  2. Eliminate the underlying cause (disk, carpal tunnel syndrome, brachial plexus traction injury)
  3. Sympathetic block to eliminate pain
  4. Aggressive physical therapy

B. **Stage I disease**
  1. **Pharmacologic management.** In stage I disease, steroids, calcium channel blockers, phenoxybenzamine, prazocin (alpha$_1$) antagonist, and clonidine (alpha$_2$) antagonist may offer relief.[5] If these agents do not offer enough relief to allow for aggressive physical therapy, sympathetic blockade of the affected region is the most effective treatment.
  2. **Sympathetic blockade.** If the RSD is localized to one upper extremity, we proceed with 0.25% bupivacaine blocks in a series of five, administered every other day. If the first set of five blocks is effective but short-lived, fentanyl (Sufenta 5 μg) is used in the second series of blocks. In general, we will employ up to 15 to 20 blocks over 3 to 4 months with intensive physical therapy. Subsequent to each block patients go to physical therapy. Stress loading and intensive functional-hand physical therapy are imperative. In the lower extremity, we utilize a Hubbard tank to help patients bear weight on the lower extremity. If two series of five paravertebral blocks are not effective in producing pain relief, a 5-day epidural block is employed.[8]
  3. **Sympathectomy.** If blocks are effective but do not last, we consider sympathectomy. Although sympathectomy should be avoided, if possible, once the process escapes from sympathetic maintenance it will not be curable. In males, we are particularly concerned about lower extremity sympathectomy due to possible sexual dysfunction, although we have not encountered this complication. In the upper extremity, the T2 ganglion must be denervated as this primarily innervates the hand. In the lower extremity there is frequent crossover innervation at the L1–2 level. Unfortunately, aberrant sympathetic tissue has been encountered, and this usually lies in the nerve exit foramina. Sympathetic tissue may regenerate, and we have seen this more frequently in the upper extremity. Following sympathectomy, the patient may experience sympathalgia or increased burning pain in the denervated area. In the lower extremity this usually occurs on the inner thigh in the ilioinguinal nerve distribution. It may be delayed up to 10 days following surgery, and is usually self-limited in 6 weeks but does respond to carbamazepine (Tegretol).[9]
  4. **After sympathectomy.** In those patients who have undergone sympathectomy and are relieved of pain for 2 to 3 months but note its gradual return, we proceed in the following manner:
     a. A trial of paravertebral blocks of the ipsilateral side to determine the status of the sympathetic chain. If this relieves the pain, we will proceed with a series of three blocks and physical therapy.
     b. If this proves to be unsuccessful after initially interrupting the pain, we will block the contralateral side and continue with intensive physical therapy.
     c. If we have determined that there is residual sympathetic activity in the ipsilateral extremity that is responsible for pain, we will proceed with a chemical sympathectomy under fluoroscopic guidance. Occasionally guanethidine or bretylium Bier blocks will be effective after sympathectomy when they had failed before surgery.[9]

C. **Stage II or III disease.** In those patients who have failed sympathectomy and progressed to stage II or III RSD, we employ dorsal column stimulation, particularly in the lower extremity.[11] The parameters of stimulation and electrode placement must be adjusted and monitored so that the area of pain is covered by the stimulation. In our experience, this will diminish the pain approximately 50%. At this level of pain reduction concomitant oral pain medication (nonsteroidal anti-inflammatory medications) and amitriptyline may be effective in maintaining adequate comfort and function for the patient.

D. **Beyond stage III disease** the treatment for RSD, particularly in late sympathetic independent pain stages, is unsatisfactory. Immediate diagnosis, alleviation of the underlying cause, sympathetic blocks while the process is still in stage I, and intensive physical therapy are the best chance for cure.

1. **Morphine pump.** Those patients who suffer intractable overwhelming pain or whose RSD has spread to their entire body, we treat with a morphine pump.[10] All of these patients have been on large doses of oral narcotics, antidepressants, nonsteroidal anti-inflammatory drugs, and antispasmodics. They usually are bedridden and desperate at this stage of their illness.

a. **Technique.** In general, patients are admitted to the intensive care unit, where they can be monitored and receive test doses of intrathecal morphine. We usually start slowly with 0.5 mg and see if they can tolerate 1 mg over 3 days without severe nausea and vomiting. Many patients start to get pain relief at 15–30 mg/day. Some patients require very high doses of 60–90 mg/day for relief. A few patients have had hyperalgesia secondary to the intrathecal morphine. It has been our observation that patients start diuresing edema fluid 1 to 2 days prior to pain relief.

b. **Complications of the morphine pump** that we have encountered are
   (1) Intractable nausea and vomiting
   (2) Total body numbness
   (3) Chemical meningitis
   (4) Hyperalgesia

c. We have had one patient who has had a spectacular result with the pump but must be maintained on 1 mg/day. If the dose is lowered, she first suffers an edematous leg (the site of her original RSD) and then severe pain. Infection at the site of the pump has been a negligible problem.

2. **Other treatments.** Those patients who require long-term treatment and are not candidates for or who do not want a morphine pump are treated with methadone, antidepressants, and moderate doses of daily nonsteroidal anti-inflammatory agents. Some patients who have seemingly sympathetic independent pain revert to sympathetic maintained pain in former areas of severe involvement and will respond to sympathetic blocks.

References

1. Bej MD, Schwartzman RJ. Abnormalities of cutaneous blood flow regulation in patients with reflex sympathetic dystrophy as measured by laser doppler fluxmetry. *Arch Neurol* 48:912, 1991.
2. Blumberg H, Griesser HJ, Hornyak E. Mechanisms and role of peripheral blood flow dysregulation in pain sensation and edema in reflex sympathetic dystrophy. In Hicks SM, Janig W, Boos RN (eds.), *Reflex Sympathetic Dystrophy: Current Management of Pain.* Boston: Kluwer, 1990.
3. Janig W. Causalgia and reflex sympathetic dystrophy: in which way is the sympathetic nervous system involved? *Trends Neurosci* 8:471, 1987.
4. Schwartzman RJ, Kerrigan J. The movement disorder of reflex sympathetic dystrophy. *Neurology* 40:57, 1990.
5. Schwartzman RJ, McLellan TL. Reflex sympathetic dystrophy. A Review. *Arch Neurol* 44:555, 1987.
6. Bentley JB, Hameroff SR. Diffuse reflex sympathetic dystrophy. *Anesthesiology* 53:256, 1980.
7. DeTakats G. The nature of painful vasodilatation in causalgic states. *Arch Neurol* 50:318, 1943.
8. Schutzer SF, Gossling HR. The treatment of reflex sympathetic dystrophy syndrome. *J Bone Joint Surg Am* 66:625, 1981.
9. Schwartzman RJ. Reflex sympathetic dystrophy. In *Current Therapy in Neurologic Disease.* Philadelphia: B.C. Decker, 1990. Pp. 66–69.
10. Barolat G, Schwartzman RJ, Arias L. Chronic intrathecal morphine infusion for contractable pain in reflex sympathetic dystrophy [abstract]. VI Meeting of the European Society for Stereotactical and Functional Neurosurgery, Basel, Switzerland, June 1–3, 1988.

11. Barolat G, Schwartzman RJ, Woo R. Epidural spinal cord stimulation in the management of reflex sympathetic dystrophy. *Stereotact Funct Neurosurg* 53:29, 1989.
12. Ochoa J. The newly recognized painful ABC syndrome: thermographic aspects. *Thermology* 2:65, 1986.
13. Ochoa JL, Yarnitsky D. Triple cold ("CCC") painful syndrome. *Pain* 5(Suppl):S278, 1990.
14. Blumberg H. Development and treatment of the pain syndrome of reflex sympathetic dystrophy: clinical picture, experimental investigation, and neuropathophysiological consideration. *Der Schmerz* 2:125–143, 1988.
15. Webster GF, Schwartzman RJ, Jacoby RA, et al. Reflex sympathetic dystrophy: occurrence of inflammatory skin lesions in patients with stage II and III disease. *Arch Dermatol* 127:1541, 1991.
16. Bennett GJ, Xie YK. A peripheral mononeuropathy in rat that produces disorders of pain sensation like those seen in man. *Pain* 33:87, 1988
17. Shir Y, Seltzer Z. Effects of sympathectomy in a model of causalgiform pain produced by partial sciatic nerve injury. *Pain* 45:309, 1991.
18. Bausbaum AI, Chi SI, Levine JD. Peripheral and central contribution to the persistent expression of the C-fos proto-oncogene in spinal cord after peripheral nerve injury. In Willis W (ed.), *Hyperalgesia and Allodynia*. New York: Raven, 1992.
19. Beachum WS, Perl ER. Characteristics of a spinal sympathetic reflex. *J Physiol* 173:431, 1964.
20. Dembowsky KP. Factors contributing to the control of sympathetic nervous activity. In Basbaum A, Besson JJ (eds.), *Towards a New Pharmacotherapy of Pain*. Baltimore: Wiley, 1991.
21. Ochoa JL, Torebjork HE. Paresthesia from ectopic impulse generation in human sensory nerves. *Brain* 103:835, 1980.
22. Campbell JN, Raja SN, Selig DK, Belzberg AJ, Meyer RA. Diagnosis and Management of Sympathetically Maintained Pain. In: Fields HL and Liebeskind JC (eds.), *Progress in Pain Research and Management, Vol. 1*. Seattle: IASP Press, 1994.
23. Cline MA, Ochoa J, Torebjork HE. Chronic hyperalgesia and skin warming caused by sensitized C-nociceptors. *Brain* 112:621, 1989.
24. Woolf CJ. Excitability changes in central neurons following peripheral damage role of central sensitization in the pathogenesis of pain. In Willis W (ed.), *Hyperalgesia and Allodynia*. New York: Raven, 1992.
25. Handwerker HO, Anton F, Kocher L, Reeh PW. Nociceptor functions in intact skin and in neurogenic or nonneurogenic inflammation. *Acta Physiol Hung* 69:333, 1987.
26. Campbell JN, Raja SN, Meyer RA, MacKinon SE. Myelinated afferents signal the hyperalgesia associated with nerve injury. *Pain* 32:89, 1988.
27. Treede RD, Raja SN, Davis KD, Meyer RA, Campbell JN. Evidence that alpha adrenergic receptors mediate sympathetically maintained pain. In: Bond MR, Charlton JE, Woolf CJ (eds.), *Pain Research and Clinical Management, Vol 4*. Proceedings of the VI World Congress on Pain. Amsterdam: Elsevier, 1991. Pp 377–382.
28. Hallin RG, Torebjork HE. Studies on cutaneous A and C fiber afferents, skin nerve blocks and perception. In Zotterman Y (ed.), *Sensory Function of the Skin in Primates with Special Reference to Man*. Oxford, UK: Pergamon, 1976. Pp. 137–149.
29. Leipzig TJ, Mullan SF. Causalgic pain relieved by prolonged procaine amide sympathetic blockade. *J Neurosurg* 60:1095, 1981.
30. Walker AE, Nulsun F. Electrical stimulation of the upper thoracic portion of the sympathetic chain in man. *Arch Neurol Psych* 59:559, 1948.
31. Devor M, Janig W. Activation of myelinated afferents ending in a neuroma by stimulation of the sympathetic supply in the rat. *Neurosci Lett* 24:43, 1981.
32. Sato J, Perl ER. Adrenergic excitation of cutaneous pain receptors induced by peripheral nerve injury. *Science* 251:1608, 1991.
33. Roberts WJ, Elardo WM. Sympathetic activation of A-delta nociceptors. *Somatosens Res* 2:33, 1985.
34. Diskenson AH. NMDA receptor antagonists as analgesics. In: Fields HL, Liebeskind JC (eds.), *Progress in Pain Research and Management, Vol. 1*. Seattle: IASP, 1994.
35. Davis SH, Lodge D. Evidence for involvement of N-methylaspartate receptors in "wind-up" of class 2 neurons in the dorsal horn of the rat. *Brain Res* 424:402, 1987.
36. Sugimoto T, Bennett GJ, Kajander KC. Strychnine enhanced transsynaptic degeneration of dorsal horn neurons in rats with an experimental painful peripheral neuropathy. *Neurosci Lett* 98:139, 1989.
37. Sugimoto T, Bennett GJ, Kajander KC. Transsynaptic degeneration in the superfi-

cial dorsal horn after sciatic nerve injury: effects of a chronic constriction injury, transection and strychnine. *Pain* 205, 1990.
38. Wank JK, Johnson KE, Ilstrip DM. Sympathetic blocks for reflex sympathetic dystrophy. *Pain* 23:13, 1985.
39. Hannington-Kiff JG. Intravenous regional sympathetic block with guanethidine. *Lancet* 1:1019, 1974.
40. Herrmann LG, Reineke HG, Caldwell JA. Post-traumatic painful osteoporosis. A clinical and roentgenological entity. *Am J Roentgenol* 47:353, 1942.
41. Simon H, Carlson DH. The use of bone scanning in the diagnosis of reflex sympathetic dystrophy. *Clin Nucl Med* 5:116, 1980.

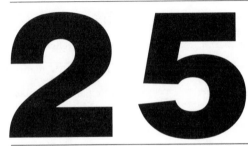

Painful Neuropathies
Alexander Mauskop

I. Diffuse peripheral neuropathies

A. Pain symptoms.
Diagnosis of a diffuse peripheral neuropathy can often be aided by a patient's history. Pain, when present, is often described as tingling, burning, stinging, electric, shooting, and crawling. Pain is typically worse with activity and at night. When sensory loss is present, patients sometimes complain of clumsiness and dropping objects from their hands, rather than numbness. Examination shows impaired sensation in distal parts of the extremities. Signs and symptoms of autonomic dysfunction may be present as well. Sensory loss in the feet always occurs before involvement of the hands.

Allodynia and dysesthesia are often present. Allodynia is defined as pain that is elicited by a nonnoxious stimulus, such as touch. Dysesthesia is a term that indicates presence of an unpleasant sensation that occurs spontaneously or is induced by an external stimulus. Nerve conduction studies can confirm the diagnosis of a peripheral neuropathy in most cases. However, if a characteristic clinical picture is found and the etiology is known, this unpleasant test can be avoided.

B. General approach to treatment

1. To treat painful neuropathies, one must first determine the cause of the neuropathy. Common causes are **diabetes, AIDS, alcohol-related deficiency states,** and **toxic exposure.**

   a. **Diabetic neuropathy.** Diabetes is the most common cause of neuropathies in this country. A high proportion of patients who have had diabetes for a few years will suffer mild to moderate diffuse sensory neuropathy. This neuropathy is often accompanied by painful **paresthesias,** burning, and sharp shooting pain. The presence of pain indicates small-fiber involvement; when only large nerve fibers are involved, the sensory loss is not associated with pain.

   In addition to the general methods of treatment described later in this chapter, good glycemic control is an important prophylactic and therapeutic measure. A clear relation exists between the degree of hyperglycemia and glycosylated hemoglobin levels and the occurrence of neuropathy. Diabetes can cause
   (1) **Cranial neuropathies**
   (2) **Limb and trunk mononeuropathies**
   (3) **Proximal motor neuropathy** (diabetic amyotrophy)
   (4) **Autonomic neuropathy**
   (5) **Sensory or sensory-motor polyneuropathy**

   b. **AIDS-related neuropathy.** Up to 90% of AIDS patients develop a neuropathy. **Symmetric distal sensory neuropathy** is the most common type and often manifests in pain. Drugs that are used for treatment of opportunistic infections and neoplasms in patients with AIDS can cause peripheral neuropathies and complicate the differential diagnosis. Stopping these medications, if it is possible, can help establish the etiology of the neuropathy.

   c. **Alcohol-related and deficiency state neuropathies.** Alcohol alone does not cause peripheral neuropathy. The most likely cause is thought to be a nutritional deficiency. Elimination of alcohol consumption, good nutrition, and vitamin supplementation can lead to full recovery from the neuropathy. Vitamin B_{12} deficiency is common in the elderly and chronically ill. Because the available assays for vitamin B_{12} are unreliable, injections of this vitamin should be given to all patients with an unexplained neuropathy.

Isoniazid can cause **depletion of pyridoxin,** which in turn will result in a peripheral neuropathy. This neuropathy often manifests in painful paresthesias but responds well to pyridoxin supplementation.

Pellagra and **beriberi** are two other deficiency states that can cause a painful neuropathy.

d. **Toxic neuropathies.** Pain is a frequent feature in neuropathies induced by **thallium and arsenic.** Other substances such as lead and mercury usually cause painless neuropathy. Medications listed below rarely cause severe pain, but the sensory neuropathy that can occur is often associated with unpleas; nt paresthesias.

Vincristine
Platinum
Acetazolamide
Misonidazole
Pyridoxine
Thalidomide
Hydralazine
Perhexiline
Gold
Metronidazole
Digitalis
Nitrofurantoin
Disulfiram

2. **Pharmacotherapy** of peripheral neuropathies often involves trials of many different drugs.

a. **Capsaicin** is a topical agent that is available in 0.075% (Zostrix HP) and 0.025% (Zostrix) concentrations. It works by depleting substance P from the small C-fiber nociceptors. It is effective in some patients with postherpetic neuralgia and diabetic neuropathy and may be also beneficial for patients with other types of neuropathic pain. It works better in patients who have superficial burning pain, rather than pain that is deep in location or sharp in quality.

Capsaicin is applied to painful areas 3 to 4 times a day. The patient must be told that the ointment will cause a burning sensation and that pain relief may come only after 2 to 4 weeks. Capsaicin will not be effective with many patients; a lack of any serious side effects, however, may warrant a trial. Capsaicin is especially worth considering in elderly and debilitated patients who often cannot tolerate oral medications. A frequent cause of failure of this treatment is insufficient frequency or duration of applications.

b. **EMLA cream** (eutectic mixture of lidocaine and prilocaine) has a local anesthetic effect and can be effective in some patients. It is used with an occlusive dressing. Caution should be exercised when it is used over large areas because systemic (cardiac and CNS) side effects may occur.

c. **Tricyclic antidepressants (TCAs)** are particularly effective when the pain has a burning or paresthetic quality to it.
   (1) **Amitriptyline** (Elavil) has been studied most extensively of the TCAs.
   (2) **Nortriptyline** (Pamelor), **imipramine** (Tofranil), and **desipramine** (Norpramine), however, are effective and may have fewer anticholinergic side effects and less sedation.
   (3) **If one TCA is ineffective or produces unacceptable side effects, another one should be tried.**
   (4) **The starting dose** for any TCA is 25 mg in a young or middle-aged individual and 10 mg in an elderly person. The average effective analgesic dose, however, is 50 to 75 mg taken once a day in the evening.
   (5) The patients must be told that although these medications are **antidepressants,** they are also used for chronic painful conditions. (When patients find out from other sources that they were given an antidepressant drug, they often become angry and noncompliant, thinking that their complaints were interpreted as depressive symptoms rather than "real" pain.)
   (6) Patients should be warned about possible **side effects** such as dryness of the mouth, drowsiness, and constipation, so that they can take preventive measure against these effects.

(7) Contraindications with TCAs include

(a) Concomitant use of monoamine oxidase inhibitors

(b) Recent myocardial infarction

(c) Cardiac arrhythmias

(d) Glaucoma

(e) Urinary retention

(8) An ECG should be obtained before the treatment of elderly patients.

d. When a patient has mostly lancinating pain, treatment should begin with an **anticonvulsant drug.** Both TCAs and anticonvulsants should be tried in **refractory cases** regardless of the quality of pain. **Anticonvulsants** that are most commonly used for pain relief are **phenytoin** (Dilantin) and **carbamazepine** (Tegretol).

(1) The average dose of phenytoin is 300 mg per day, which can be given once a day if Dilantin brand is used.

(2) The dose of carbamazepine varies from 400 to 1200 mg and more, with the average daily dose of 600–800 mg. Carbamazepine must be given in divided doses every 8 hours.

(3) Blood levels for both medications should be monitored if the average dose is exceeded and if toxicity or noncompliance are suspected.

(4) When using carbamazepine, **WBC and platelet counts must be checked** before treatment, about a month later, and further on with decreasing frequency. This is done for early detection of aplastic anemia and agranulocytosis. An initial drop in WBC is very common after the initiation of treatment and should not be the reason for stopping this drug.

(5) In some patients improved pain relief can be obtained by adding a small dose (1 mg bid-tid) of a phenothiazine such as **fluphenazine** (Prolixin) or **trifluoperazine** (Stelazine).

(6) Opioid analgesics can be effective in neuropathic pain patients. However, their chronic use for nonmalignant pain should be closely monitored.

3. Transcutaneous electrical nerve stimulation (TENS) and acupuncture work in a small number of patients. These are very safe and simple techniques with few side effects and complications. Considering the benign nature of these methods and the chance of a good response, they are worth trying. As with capsaicin, these modes are particularly appropriate for elderly patients and those who do not respond to other therapies.

4. Neural blockade is rarely effective in the treatment of a diffuse peripheral neuropathy.

II. Focal neuropathies

A. Carpal tunnel syndrome (CTS) is one of the most common entrapment neuropathies and often occurs without any obvious external trauma.

1. Causes. Repeated or sustained wrist flexion or hyperextension is a frequent cause of this syndrome. To diagnose it, patients should be questioned about the position of their wrists during driving, sleeping, knitting, typing, filing, etc. There are also systemic conditions that predispose individuals to the development of the CTS. They include **pregnancy, hypothyroidism, acromegaly, rheumatoid arthritis, and diabetes.**

2. Symptoms

a. A typical early symptom is a **painful paresthesia involving the first three fingers** which often wakes patients from sleep. To relieve this pain, many patients shake their hand.

b. As **compression of the median nerve progresses,** the pain becomes worse and can persist throughout the day. The pain often extends to all fingers, the wrist, and the forearm. On examination, sensory loss is easiest to detect at the fingertips.

c. Late in the course of the illness, atrophy of the thenar eminence (opponens pollices and abductor pollices brevis muscles) occurs.

3. Diagnosis

a. Phalen's test involves flexion of both wrists by pressing dorsal surfaces of the hands against each other. Within 1 minute, the patient will experience worsening of the symptoms.

b. Tinel's sign consists of eliciting paresthesias by tapping the carpal tunnel area. Generally, this diagnosis can be made without much difficulty or further testing.

c. If there is any doubt about the diagnosis, **sensory nerve conduction studies** will help to confirm it.

4. Treatment

a. Treatment of mild symptoms begins with wearing a **wrist splint** during sleep.

b. An injection of **corticosteroid** will often provide temporary relief that may last for several months. Frequent and multiple injections, however, should be avoided as they may cause weakening or injury of the tendons. A 2-week course of oral prednisone (20 mg/day) may be effective.

c. The definitive treatment for more severe symptoms is **surgery.** It is relatively simple and involves section of the transverse ligament.

d. When one of the predisposing factors mentioned earlier is present, treatment of that condition usually improves the CTS symptoms. In these patients only **conservative therapy** is suggested pending an improvement in the underlying condition (or in the case of a pregnant patient, the delivery of the baby).

B. Meralgia paresthetica. The term meralgia is derived from the Greek word *meros,* which means thigh.

1. Causes. Meralgia paresthetica often occurs soon after rapid weight gain or loss, including pregnancy and delivery. In many patients, however, no apparent cause is found. The condition often resolves itself spontaneously in a few weeks or months.

2. Symptoms

a. Paresthesias and pain over the lateral anterior surface of the thigh are characteristic symptoms. Low back or buttock pain can be present as well.

b. Standing and walking often aggravate the symptoms.

c. On examination, **sensory loss or hyperesthesia** is found **in the symptomatic area.** This condition is the result of lateral femoral cutaneous nerve entrapment. This entrapment can occur in the psoas muscle, pelvis, and most commonly at the point of attachment of the inguinal ligament to the anterior superior iliac spine.

3. Treatment

a. If symptoms are mild, spontaneous remission is awaited without any treatment.

b. Analgesics and TCAs are often effective for more severe symptoms. Capsaicin has not been tested for treatment of this condition, but it may be worth a trial.

c. A nerve block with a local anesthetic or steroid injection at the anterior superior iliac spine can result in temporary or permanent relief.

d. In severe cases, which do not respond to medications or blocks, nerve decompression or section is performed.

C. Morton's neuroma or Morton's metatarsalgia is a common cause of pain in the foot.

1. Causes. It results from a lesion of the interdigital nerve between the heads of the third and fourth metatarsal bones. Women have this condition much more frequently than men, and high-heeled shoes are often to blame.

2. Symptoms. In addition to pain, patients often experience paresthesias and numbness of the third and fourth toes. Palpation of the space between the heads of metatarsal bones reproduces the symptoms.

3. Treatment

a. Switching to a flat shoe with a soft pad may relieve the problem for a woman.

b. If symptoms persist, **a local steroid injection** may provide relief.

c. TCAs and anticonvulsants can sometimes help.

d. Surgical treatment is very effective and consists of excision of the affected nerve or incision of the deep intermetacarpal ligament.

D. Postherpetic neuralgia. Elderly and immunosuppressed patients are common victims of this disease.

1. Causes

a. The **rash of acute herpes zoster** is often preceded or accompanied by pain. If pain persists for more than a month, the diagnosis of postherpetic neuralgia is made. Because of the characteristic rash, the postherpetic neuralgia diagnosis is made without difficulty.

b. Occasionally, patients with typical pain in dermatomal distribution report never having a rash in the involved area. **Diabetes and other systemic conditions** that cause mononeuritis may affect an intercostal nerve resulting in a pain syndrome similar to postherpetic neuralgia. Search for an underlying systemic condition is necessary when the rash is absent.

2. Treatment

a. Treatment of acute herpes zoster rash within 72 hours of onset with the antiviral drug **famciclovir** (Famvir) results in a significantly shorter duration of postherpetic neuralgia, although the incidence of neuralgia is not affected.

b. Treatment of pain, however, is similar regardless of the cause. After the rash clears, treatment begins with **capsaicin or EMLA cream.**

c. If pain is very severe, add a **TCA** from the start of the treatment unless the pain is tolerable. Reserve TCAs for capsaicin failures.

d. **Anticonvulsants** can be helpful in patients who do not respond or do not tolerate TCAs.

e. In **refractory** cases adding a small dose of a **phenothiazine** such as fluphenazine to the TCA may provide additional relief.

f. **TENS** and **acupuncture** can sometimes be quite effective.

g. There is evidence to suggest that a 2-week course of **prednisone** given in the acute stage can prevent development of postherpetic neuralgia. Start prednisone at 60 mg/day with gradual tapering over the following 2 weeks. Prednisone should not be used in immunosuppressed patients because of possible dissemination of herpes zoster.

h. Many patients are very refractory to all treatments and should be given a trial of opioids. Some patients respond to **oxycodone** (Percocet), while others may require **transdermal fentanyl** (Duragesic) to obtain some relief. The risk of addiction in a patient who experiences severe pain is very small. Constipation and sedation, however, can be a problem.

Selected Readings

Dawson DM, Hallett M, Millender LH. *Entrapment Neuropathies* (2nd ed.). Boston: Little, Brown, 1990.

Steward JD. *Focal Peripheral Neuropathies.* New York: Elsevier, 1987.

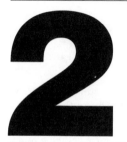

Headaches
Alexander Mauskop

I. **Background.** It is estimated that up to 40 million people in the United States suffer from chronic headaches. Most of these people do not consult doctors because they consider the problem to be too trivial or they think that no treatment is available. Patients who do consult a physician are usually those whose headaches significantly disrupt their lives. Educating the public about available treatments through the media and practicing physicians has increased, but more needs to be done.

II. **History**

A. **Diagnosis of headache type.** Most of the information leading to the diagnosis of the headache type is obtained from the patient's history.

1. **Frequency and duration.** Increasing frequency or duration of headaches indicates the need for a reevaluation of the patient. Daily headaches are often the result of caffeine or medication overuse. In women, headaches that are very brief but intense and frequent (several times a day) suggest the diagnosis of chronic paroxysmal hemicrania, which almost always responds to indomethacin.

2. **Time patterns.** A patient who wakes up with a headache, which then quickly resolves without medications, should be suspected of having a brain tumor or another space-occupying lesion. Tension-type headaches tend to worsen as the day progresses, but it is not unusual to have a headache on awakening as well. Cluster headaches tend to be very regular in their time of occurrence. Typically these headaches wake the patient up from sleep in early morning hours.

3. **Character and location of pain.** Burning occipital pain suggests a focal neuropathy. Unilateral and pulsatile pain is most common in migraine and cluster headaches.

4. **Precipitating factors.** Alteration of sleep patterns, tyramine-rich foods, alcohol, chocolate, and other foods can provoke a migraine attack. Overexertion and emotional stress are among the most common precipitating factors for both tension-type and migraine headaches. Strong sensory stimuli such as loud noise, strong odors, bright and flashing lights can induce a headache in a susceptible individual. Changes in barometric pressure, such as with weather changes, flying, or climbing a mountain, can provoke a headache.

5. **Preceding and accompanying symptoms.** Migraine headaches are often preceded by a visual and other types of aura. Nausea and sensitivity to light, noise, and movement are typical accompaniments to migraine headaches. Agitation, unilateral nasal congestion, and tearing frequently occur with an attack of cluster headache. Dizziness can occur with migraine and cervicogenic headaches.

III. **Physical examination.** A general medical examination is necessary to detect many of the systemic conditions that can lead to headaches. After a detailed history, a neurologic examination is the most important diagnostic step. With few exceptions, this examination should be normal for the types of headache described below. Patients with cluster headaches often have Horner's syndrome that can transiently persist for some time after the attack. Benign intracranial hypertension is accompanied by papilledema and can lead to visual field defects and cranial nerve palsies, especially of the sixth nerve.

IV. **Ancillary tests**

A. If the history or physical examination raises any doubt about benign etiology of headaches, an imaging procedure such as **CT scan** or, preferably, **MRI** should be performed. Concern over a possible brain tumor or another serious condition often makes the headache worse. Negative CT scan or MRI reassures the patient and can reduce headaches.

B. A CT scan or MRI of the brain is routinely performed to **exclude a subdural hematoma,** which in the elderly may develop from a trivial head injury suffered many weeks or months earlier. Up to 40% of elderly patients with a chronic subdural hematoma give no history of a head injury. Conditions such as metastatic brain tumor and cerebrovascular disease are also more common in the elderly than in younger persons.

C. Laboratory tests on patients who have not had any screening blood tests in many months should include a **CBC, thyroid function tests,** and a standard battery of **blood chemistry tests.** These tests may detect anemia, systemic infections, renal insufficiency, hypothyroidism, and other conditions that may cause headaches.

D. An **erythrocyte sedimentation rate (ESR)** must always be obtained in a patient over 60 years of age with a recent onset of headaches. If the ESR is high, a temporal artery biopsy is necessary to confirm the diagnosis of giant cell arteritis.

E. Electroencephalography has traditionally been considered unnecessary in patients with headaches and is still not a part of a standard headache workup. Morning-onset headaches can be the only manifestation of a nocturnal seizure, and an EEG may be diagnostic.

V. Tension-type headaches are described as pressing or tightening in quality, of mild or moderate intensity, bilateral in location, without associated nausea, photophobia, or phonophobia. They are not made worse by routine physical activity as may be the case with migraine headaches. Tension headaches are the most common type of headache and have many precipitating factors.

Removal of identifiable causes and precipitating factors is the ideal way to treat this type of headache. Although the most common precipitating factor—stress—is often difficult to alleviate, reducing the physical effects of stress can be achieved through both nonpharmacologic and pharmacologic methods.

A. Nonpharmacologic treatment

1. Biofeedback is one of the most effective treatments for both tension and migraine headaches. Meditation, yoga, and other mental exercises can help, but biofeedback is a more direct approach aimed at eliminating headaches. Well-trained staff and patient compliance with home exercises are essential for achieving a high success rate. Follow-up studies indicate up to 80% to 90% improvement 5 years after completion of a biofeedback training course. This course usually consists of 30- to 60-minute sessions every week for 6 to 15 weeks. Children can learn to rid themselves of headaches in as few as three to four sessions.

2. Transcutaneous electrical nerve stimulation (TENS) and **acupuncture** can provide fast relief for tension headaches. These methods have a solid scientific basis, but lack clinical studies proving their efficacy. Acupuncture can stop an acute headache or, with a series of treatments, relieve a chronic one.

3. Regular physical exercise is an excellent way to reduce adverse effects of stress on the body.

B. Pharmacologic treatment

1. Abortive therapy. Sporadic attacks of severe tension-type headaches may respond to **analgesics.**

    a. Nonsteroidal anti-inflammatory agents such as **aspirin, ibuprofen** (Motrin, Advil), or **naproxen** (Naprosyn, Anaprox, Aleve) have proved effective.

    b. Codeine or even stronger opioids may be required for a patient with occasional severe attacks. Chronic use of opioid analgesics in the treatment of headaches should be avoided.

    c. Drug combinations are often very effective for infrequent use. Combination of **acetaminophen** or **aspirin** with **caffeine** and a short-acting barbiturate such as **butalbital** is very popular with many patients (Fiorinal, Fioricet, Esgic, Medigesic).

    d. Isometheptene, a sympathomimetic amine with vasoconstrictive properties, is available in combination with **dichloralphenazone,** a mild sedative, and **acetaminophen** (Midrin, Isocom). This combination can be effective in many patients who do not respond to other drugs. Drowsiness is a potential side effect. A limit of 15 to 20 tablets a month is placed on combination drugs or strong analgesics. If a patient takes more than that amount, the medication may begin to worsen the headache through a rebound mechanism. Such patients require prophylactic treatment.

2. Prophylactic therapy

    a. Pharmacologic treatment of severe persistent headaches begins with **nortrip-**

tyline (Pamelor) or another **tricyclic antidepressant** (TCA). Detailed guidelines for the use of TCAs are provided in Chapter 6 on psychotropic adjuvant analgesics and in Chapter 25 on painful neuropathies. Other antidepressants such as fluoxetine (Prozac), sertraline (Zoloft), and paroxetine (Paxil) can be effective with fewer side effects. Young women, who constitute the majority of migraine sufferers, often prefer the latter group because these drugs, unlike TCAs, do not have a potential for weight gain and can even help them reduce weight.

   b. Propranolol, timolol, and other **beta blockers** are much less effective than TCAs in tension headaches but can be tried when other medications fail.

   c. Despite the fact that stress and tension are major causes of tension headaches, use of **tranquilizers should be avoided.** Chronic use of these drugs can lead to addiction and worsening of headaches.

VI. Migraine headaches
A. Nonpharmacologic treatment
   1. Dietary changes can occasionally completely stop migraine headaches, but in many patients they only reduce the frequency of attacks. Some of the foods that can provoke migraine headaches are yogurt, bananas, dried fruit, beans, aged cheese, pickled and marinated foods, and buttermilk. Monosodium glutamate and aspartame should be avoided. Among the alcoholic beverages, red wine and beer are more likely to induce a migraine headache than vodka.

   2. Biofeedback, relaxation techniques, and **regular aerobic exercise** are as effective for prevention of migraine headaches as they are for tension headaches.

B. Pharmacologic treatment
   1. Abortive therapy is used when the attacks are not very frequent.

   a. Nonsteroidal anti-inflammatory agents mentioned above can be effective for migraine headaches as well. Rapid onset of action can be achieved by using an effervescent form of **aspirin** (Alka-Seltzer). Ketorolac (Toradol) is the only NSAID that is available in a parenteral form. It is an excellent analgesic (30 mg of ketrolac IM equals 10 mg of morphine sulfate IM) with a good side-effect profile. Patients can self-inject ketorolac intramuscularly for severe migraine attacks, or it can be given by the physician intravenously.

   b. Combination medications listed in section **V.B.1.c** under tension headaches can be very effective. Addition of codeine to some of the combinations (Fiorinal with Codeine and Fioricet with Codeine) improves their efficacy for severe headaches.

   c. Sumatriptan (Imitrex) is a "designer" drug specifically developed to bind to 5-hydroxytryptamine-1D ($5HT_{1D}$) serotonin receptor, which is operational in the pathogenesis of migraine headaches. Sumatriptan injection relieves both the pain and the nausea and allows the patient to return to normal functioning within 10 to 20 minutes. Sumatriptan is available in an injection that can be self-administered by the patient using an autoinjector. Tablet form of sumatriptan has a slower onset of action. Common side effects are a flushed sensation, paresthesias, and injection-site pain. Sumatriptan is contraindicated in patients with uncontrolled hypertension, ischemic heart disease, and complicated migraines (migraines that are accompanied by a transient neurologic deficit). Sumatriptan and ergots should not be given on the same day.

   d. Dihydroergotamine (DHE-45) is effective for abortive treatment of migraines. This ergot derivative is available only in a parenteral form and can be given subcutaneously, intramuscularly, or intravenously. A dose of 1 mg is sufficient for most patients, but some may require 2 or 3 mg. The starting dose should be 0.5 mg q45min prn. Once a total effective dose is established for a patient, that amount is given for future attacks.

   e. If the headache is accompanied by nausea, an injection of an antiemetic such as **prochlorperazine** (Compazine) or **metoclopramide** (Reglan) 10 mg IM can be effective. These medications can be given with dihydroergotamine.

   f. Ergots alone (Ergomar, sublingual) and with **caffeine** (Cafergot, tablets and suppositories; Wigraine, tablets) are limited in their utility by a relatively high incidence of nausea. Reducing the dose, particularly of Cafergot suppositories, to one quarter or one half of a suppository can avoid nausea and provide effective and rapid relief. Ergots are contraindicated in patients with cardiac or peripheral ischemia and pregnant women.

   g. Opioid drugs can be effective but usually cause sedation. They should be only used in patients with infrequent attacks. Meperidine tablets and injections (Demerol) and oxycodone with acetaminophen tablets (Percocet) are some of the commonly used opioid drugs.

2. Prophylactic therapy

a. **Tricyclic and other antidepressants** can be as effective for migraine headaches as they are for tension-type ones.

b. **Propranolol, timolol,** and other **beta blockers** are good prophylactic drugs. The effective dose for propranolol can be as low as 40 mg/day but is usually 80 to 240 mg. The long-acting preparation of propranolol (Inderal LA) facilitates its use. Contraindications for the use of beta blockers are bronchial asthma, sinus bradycardia, greater than first degree block, congestive heart failure, and diabetes.

c. In some patients who do not respond to either a TCA or a beta blocker alone, use of these two drugs together may stop the headaches. No clinical trials have been published, however, to prove the efficacy of this combination.

d. **Divalproex sodium** (Depakote) can relieve migraine headaches in patients who do not respond to beta blockers or antidepressants. The starting dose is usually 250 mg/day with a gradual increase up to 2000 mg in a divided dose. Potential side effects include nausea, drowsiness, and weight gain.

e. **Calcium channel blockers** are sometimes effective for migraines, but are more likely to benefit a patient with cluster headaches.

f. **Nonsteroidal anti-inflammatory drugs** (NSAIDs) can be given prophylactically with good results.

VII. Cervicogenic headaches

A. **Elderly patients.** Cervicogenic headaches are very common in elderly patients owing to arthritic changes in the cervical spine. Pain described as radiating from the neck or occipital in location suggests this diagnosis. Pain of cervical spine origin, however, can sometimes be felt in the front of the head. Loss of sensation over the occipital area, often on one side, can accompany occipital neuralgia. Neck muscles are tender and frequently in spasm, and their movement can aggravate the pain. **Treatment** is as follows:

1. With many patients, **immobilization by a soft cervical collar** during the night is all that is needed to stop the headache.

2. More often, a combination of an **NSAID with a cervical collar** and regular neck exercises will provide relief.

3. **Local heat application, TENS, and acupuncture** may be effective.

4. If the headache is occipital and has a burning or lancinating quality, greater occipital neuralgia is the likely cause. **Blockade of the nerve** by a local anesthetic is relatively easy to perform and may provide lasting relief. A successful block of this nerve does not have any diagnostic significance as many types of headaches including cluster and migraine will sometimes respond as well.

5. **TCAs** also have a good potential to relieve pain of occipital neuralgia. The starting dose should be only 10 mg every night because of the higher incidence of side effects in elderly patients.

B. **Whiplash injuries,** another frequent cause of cervicogenic headaches, are commonly sustained in car accidents. **Treatment** is as follows:

1. Treatment should include a **soft cervical collar** that the patient wears only at night. Wearing the collar during the day for any length of time may cause atrophy of the neck muscles, which may in turn delay the recovery. If pain is severe, the collar can be worn around the clock for the first few days.

2. An active **exercise program** is started as soon as it is tolerated by the patient. Providing good analgesia allows an early start for such exercises.

3. Analgesics, local heat, trigger point injections, acupuncture, and TENS are effective as a part of the treatment of acute neck pain and the associated headache.

4. When muscle spasm is prominent, a short course (1–2 weeks) of **diazepam** (Valium) 5–10 mg q8h is very effective and carries no risk of addiction.

VIII. Posttraumatic headaches. In many patients posttraumatic headaches will subside in a few weeks or months without any treatment. Chronic posttraumatic headaches in many patients, however, are notoriously hard to treat regardless of the presence or absence of litigation.

A. **Biofeedback, amitriptyline, fluoxetine, propranolol, acupuncture, or TENS** are effective treatments in certain patients.

B. **A supportive and understanding attitude** is important in treating this condition because of the frequent ineffectiveness of treatment and because of the associated neurologic and psychiatric symptoms (memory impairment, dizziness, anxiety, and depression).

IX. **Cluster headaches** are the most intense headaches of all, leading some patients to thoughts of suicide.

A. **Symptoms**

1. Headaches occur in clusters, frequently during the same season each year, with each episode lasting for several weeks or months.

2. The pain often wakes the patient from sleep—sometimes at the same time—every night and usually lasts for 30 to 90 minutes. Such regular occurrence, however, is not always present.

3. The pain is described as retro-orbital, unilateral, and is associated with agitation, nasal congestion, conjunctival injection, and lacrimation.

4. Cluster headaches can be affected by external factors although not to the extent that migraine or tension-type headaches are.

   a. Alcohol consumption during the cluster almost always provokes a headache.

   b. Prolonged excessive emotional or physical stress can occasionally start a new cluster of headaches.

B. **Abortive treatment** of cluster headaches begins with measures designed to reduce the pain of each attack while prophylactic drugs take effect.

1. The most benign and frequently effective treatment is inhalation of **oxygen.** It is done through a mask (not nasal prongs) using 100% oxygen at 8–10 liters/min. It should be used for patients who experience most of their attacks at home. If headaches occur during the day, patients can store another oxygen tank at work.

2. **Ergotamine** (Cafergot, Wigraine, Ergomac) can abort a cluster headache in up to 75% of patients. It is best given by a suppository or sublingually to provide rapid onset of action. **Dihydroergotamine** (DHE-45) is given only by injection and can be self-administered by the patient.

3. **Sumatriptan** (Imitrex) injection is very effective in most patients and has few side effects. It can also be self-administered by the patient using an autoinjector.

C. **Prophylactic treatment**

1. A short course of **prednisone** will frequently stop the cluster. Dosage is started at 60–80 mg daily and then is tapered down over a period of 2 weeks.

2. **Calcium channel blockers** are suggested for patients not responding to a course of prednisone.

   a. **Nifedipine** (Procardia) 40–120 mg/day, **verapamil** (Calan, Isoptin) 120–360 mg/day, and **nimodipine** (Nimotop) 180–360 mg/day have prevented cluster headaches in some patients.

   b. Long-acting preparations of nifedipine and verapamil allow for once-a-day dosage. Nimodipine has to be taken every 4 hours.

3. **Methysergide** (Sansert) in a dosage of 2 mg tid-qid is recommended for patients who fail to get relief from prednisone and calcium channel blockers. Fibrotic complications should not occur because clusters rarely last for more than a few months. However, some reports suggest that this complication is more likely to be idiosyncratic rather than dose-related.

4. **Divalproex sodium** (Depakote) 750–2000 mg/day in divided doses can provide relief for some patients.

5. **Lithium carbonate,** 300 mg bid-qid, is effective within 1 to 2 weeks of therapy. It can work for both episodic and chronic forms of cluster headaches, sometimes transforming chronic into episodic. Adding 2–4 mg of ergotamine a day to lithium may produce remission in patients who do not respond to lithium alone.

6. **Ergotamine** in a dose of 2 mg can provide good relief if taken 2 hours before the expected attack. Regular intake of ergotamine 1–2 mg tid has been reported to be effective in some patients.

X. **Headaches associated with substances or their withdrawal**

A. **Causes**

1. Many prescription medications can cause headaches. The most common offenders are **nitrates, appetite suppressants, oral contraceptives, estrogens, and antihypertensive medications.**

2. Foods can also cause headaches, specifically those containing **nitrites, monosodium glutamate, tyramine, and aspartame.**

3. Other factors that can lead to headaches include excessive intake of **caffeine, analgesics, benzodiazepines, barbiturates, and ergot preparations.**

B. **Treatment**

1. Eliminating offending foods and drugs can occasionally relieve all of a patient's headaches, or reduce their frequency and intensity.

2. The treatment of a patient who is dependent on analgesics, caffeine, or ergot preparations can be very difficult.

   a. In such a patient the headaches, to a great extent, are due to an ongoing withdrawal or rebound from these substances. An abrupt complete cutoff temporarily worsens the pain, and some patients prefer to get off these drugs gradually.

   b. Withdrawal headaches can be treated with self-administration of injectable sumatriptan (Imitrex), dihydroergotamine (DHE-45), or ketorolac (Toradol).

   c. Admission to a hospital is occasionally necessary because of uncontrollable pain. While in the hospital, dihydroergotamine administered intravenously or intramuscularly, opioid analgesics, and prochlorperazine (Compazine) or chlorpromazine (Thorazine) will provide relief or, at least, will sedate the patient.

   d. The prophylactic drugs are started after the withdrawal is completed. These drugs work better after the patient is taken off analgesics and sedatives, and medications that were ineffective while the patient was overusing abortive drugs can become effective.

XI. **Benign intracranial hypertension (pseudotumor cerebri).** This condition should be first treated by removing possible causes such as vitamin A, tetracycline, or nalidixic acid, and by reducing excessive weight.

A. **Acetazolamide** (Diamox) is an effective drug in many patients and is available in a sustained-release preparation. The dose ranges between 250 and 1500 mg daily.

B. For patients with severe persistent headaches, **lumbar punctures** can be performed while other treatments are being tried. These can also be performed during pregnancy. In pregnant women this condition often subsides after the delivery.

C. **Beta blockers and TCAs** can sometimes provide relief of headache.

D. **Prednisone** is useful in reducing intracranial pressure from a brain tumor, but its efficacy in pseudotumor cerebri remains controversial.

E. Regular **visual field testing** is paramount in the management of benign intracranial hypertension. Patients with progressive visual loss should undergo optic nerve sheath fenestration. This operation is the treatment of choice for patients with visual impairment, but it is not consistently effective for the relief of headaches.

F. A **lumbar-peritoneal shunt** is more appropriate for patients with intractable headaches, but it should be used as a last resort because of the potential for complications.

XII. **Headache after lumbar puncture.** The use of a thin or conical spinal needle reduces the incidence of headaches after lumbar puncture. Contrary to popular belief, bed rest following a lumbar puncture does not prevent these headaches.

A. When a patient does develop headaches, bed rest, good hydration, and analgesics will provide relief. Most patients improve within a few days of this regimen.

B. Those who do not improve should receive a blood patch. This procedure involves withdrawing 15–20 ml of the patient's venous blood and injecting it into the epidural space at the same level where the lumbar puncture was performed. This stops the leakage of cerebrospinal fluid that caused the headache.

Selected Readings

Classification and diagnostic criteria for headache disorders, cranial neuralgias and facial pain. *Cephalalgia* 8 (Suppl 7), 1988.

Lance JW. *Mechanism and Management of Headache* (5th ed.). London: Butterworth, 1993.

Olesen J, Tfelt-Hansen P, Welch KMA (eds). *The Headaches.* New York: Raven, 1993.

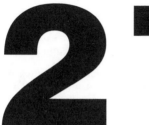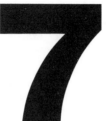

I. History and physical examination
A. History
1. **The chief complaint.** The patient's exact presenting complaint and interpretation of the meaning of that complaint must be ascertained in order to put the diagnosis in perspective. Often a patient with head and neck pain will assume that he or she has an "ear or throat infection," or a patient with headache or midfacial pain will assume that it is caused by a "sinus" problem. Because pain is often mistaken for pressure or fullness, it is very important to determine the location, periodicity, timing, frequency, severity, character, exacerbating factors, remitting factors, previous therapy, and results of that therapy. Record the chronology of the complaint, with specific attention to exact dates.
2. **Related symptoms** that may aid in diagnosis are
   a. **Ear:** itching, drainage or discharge, hearing loss, dizziness or lightheadedness, tinnitus, pressure or fullness, or bleeding
   b. **Nose:** congestion or obstruction, seasonal stuffiness, sneezing, bleeding, loss of smell, itching, or anterior or posterior drainage
   c. **Throat:** difficulty swallowing (dysphagia), pain on swallowing (odynophagia), change in voice or hoarseness, bleeding, dental symptoms, or change in taste
   d. **Neck:** mass, tenderness, or limitation of motion
3. **Medical and surgical history.** A knowledge of the patient's general medical condition and a list of all current and previous medications are vital to a complete history. Is a patient complaining of chronic ear pain diabetic? Does a patient complaining of nasal pain have a past history of syphilis? Does a patient with oral pain have a predisposing reason to be immunosuppressed? Often patients who have had ear surgery as children do not remember it and may need to have their memories jogged.
4. **Family history.** Size of the family, parental and sibling diseases or disorders (i.e., thyroid disease, sinus disease, cancer), and congenital disorders.
5. **Social history.** As there is a positive correlation between tobacco and alcohol use and cancer of the head and neck, this information must be obtained. Drug use and any job-related or environmental exposures to noxious fumes, reactive metals, and wood dust should also be known. Recent travel is also important.
B. Physical examination
1. **Visual examination of the face and neck** begins while obtaining the history from the patient. The presence of asymmetry in the face at rest and with a variety of expressions gives information as to the status of the facial nerve. The presence of scars suggests a history of trauma or surgery. Proptotic eyes can signify thyroid or sinus disease. Patients with allergic rhinitis often have puffy "bags" under their eyes and frequently rub the anterior part of the nose with the forefinger, commonly known as the "allergic salute." Obvious neck masses should be noted, and a thorough examination of the mass, as well as the entire head and neck, should follow.
2. **Examination of the ear**
   a. **Pinna and periauricular areas.** Note any evidence of trauma or congenital malformation. Check for a scar in the postauricular area, which can be evidence of previous ear surgery. A small dimple just in front of the ear could be a preauricular sinus. Examine the skin for inflammation or eczema.
   b. **External auditory canal.** With the otoscope, using slight upward, outward, and backward traction, grasp the pinna and insert the speculum of the

otoscope into the canal. Be sure to select the largest speculum that will fit the ear canal comfortably. After removing any cerumen gently with a curette, irrigation, or a suction catheter, examine the skin of the external auditory canal. Note the color of the skin, as well as any bony outgrowths (exostoses) that block the visualization of the tympanic membrane.

c. **Tympanic membrane.** Examine the tympanic membrane for integrity, color, air fluid levels, and finally, using the pneumatic insufflater, mobility. Note any whitish patches or areas of transparency in the tympanic membrane. This may indicate tympanosclerosis or evidence of a previous perforation, which may be secondary to surgery, trauma, or otitis media.

d. **Hearing.** Tuning fork testing provides a quick and inexpensive evaluation of potential hearing loss. Weber's test is performed by placing a 512-Hz tuning fork on the middle of the forehead or incisor teeth and asking the patient if he or she hears it equally in both ears or whether hearing in one ear is louder than the other. A normal test shows no preference. A person with conductive hearing loss, which indicates an abnormality in the middle or external ear, will hear the tuning fork lateralized to the affected ear. A person with sensorineural hearing loss, implying abnormality in the inner ear or brain, will hear it lateralized away from the affected ear. Weber's test is supplemented by the Rinne test, in which the vibrating tuning fork is placed with the handle on the mastoid tip and the patient is asked to tell the examiner when he or she no longer hears the sound. The examiner then places the fork at the entrance to the ear canal, and if the patient can still hear the sound, it implies that air conduction is better than bone conduction and that the middle ear transformer mechanism is working properly. More extensive audiologic testing can be performed by an audiologist as needed.

3. **Examination of the nose and sinuses**

a. **Nose.** Examination of the nose begins by inspecting the bone and cartilage for evidence of trauma, asymmetry, or dilated blood vessels. Internal examination is performed with a nasal speculum, which is opened in a vertical fashion to avoid uncomfortable pressure against the nasal septal mucosa. The internal nasal examination should include inspection of the vestibule, the mucosa, the nasal septum, the lateral wall of the nose, and the nasopharynx. The vestibule should be examined for evidence of folliculitis and fissures. The nasal mucosa should be assessed next. Normal nasal mucosa appears pink. In allergic conditions it tends to have a pale, gray, or bluish tinge, while in acute or chronic inflammatory conditions it is a deeper red in color. The nasal septum should be in or close to the midline and be reasonably flat on each side. Irregularities of the septum, such as a spur, ridge, or deflection, may cause no disturbance, unless severe enough to obstruct the airway. The lateral wall is then examined from anterior to posterior while observing the position, size, and mucosal covering of the inferior and middle turbinates. Drainage from underneath the middle turbinate may indicate a sinus infection. Also, note any intranasal lesions, masses, polyps, or foreign bodies. In most patients, after use of topical decongestants, the examiner can look through the nose to inspect part of the nasopharynx. The nasopharynx can also be examined with a dental mirror or a fiberoptic nasopharyngoscope.

b. **Sinuses.** Examination of the sinuses is performed more indirectly than other aspects of the physical examination. Information can be gathered, first, by inspection and palpation of the overlying soft tissue; second, by noting secretions draining from the sinuses; and third, by transillumination of the maxillary and frontal sinuses.

4. **Examination of the oral cavity and oropharynx.** Examine the lips by external inspection. Then hold a tongue blade in each hand to allow retraction of the lips for inspection of the intraoral structures. These include the tongue, floor of mouth, teeth and gingivae, buccal mucosa, palate, uvula, tonsils, and posterior pharyngeal wall. Visual inspection is supplemented by palpation. While wearing gloves, palpate the floor of mouth with attention to the submandibular salivary glands, and then the tongue.

5. **Examination of the larynx and hypopharynx.** This examination is classically performed with a laryngeal mirror or with a fiberoptic nasopharyngoscope. The base of the tongue, epiglottis, false cords, true cords, arytenoids, and

glottic opening should be noted. In addition, the pyriform sinuses, which are lateral to the larynx, should be inspected.

6. **Examination of the neck.** After inspection of the neck, palpation should proceed from posterior to anterior bilaterally. The suboccipital and posterior triangles are palpated initially, and the presence of any enlarged lymph glands should be noted. Moving the hands anteriorly, grasp the sternocleidomastoid muscles and gently displace them laterally in order to palpate the lymph glands along the jugular chains. Then check for the presence of carotid pulsations, bruits, or thrills. Avoid excessive pressure on the carotid bulbs as this can cause syncope, particularly in elderly patients. Finally, palpate the anterior structures of the neck, including the hyoid bone, thyroid cartilage, cricoid cartilage, and thyroid gland.

II. **Ear pain (otalgia).** In evaluating otalgia, the clinician must first determine if it originates from the ear itself (otogenic) or from other structures in the head and neck (nonotogenic) that share a common innervation. The ear is innervated by branches of the fifth, seventh, ninth, and tenth cranial nerves as well as the second and third cervical nerves. A careful history and thorough physical examination can provide the basis for this differentiation.

A. **Otogenic causes of ear pain**

1. **Otitis externa** is a bacterial infection of the soft tissue of the external auditory canal. Diagnostic clues that raise the suspicion of external otitis include a previous history of swimming, Q-tip use or other instrumentation of the ear canal, and pain of the external canal, associated with itching and discharge. On physical examination, the auricle is often tender to movement and, in some instances, so painful that the patient will not allow otoscopic examination. The skin of the external auditory canal is erythematous and at times so edematous that the tympanic membrane cannot be visualized with the otoscope.

    External otitis is treated with thorough cleaning of the external auditory canal, and by educating the patient to keep the ear dry and to discontinue Q-tip use. Combination antibiotic and hydrocortisone drops (e.g., Cortisporin Otic suspension) are also used to decrease swelling and pain and eradicate the infection.

2. **"Malignant" otitis externa** is a serious, **life-threatening form of otitis externa,** which is most commonly seen in diabetic or immunocompromised patients. The patient tends to present with severe ear pain and, occasionally, drainage. The characteristic finding of reddish-pink granulation tissue in the floor of the external ear canal assists in establishing the correct diagnosis. As the infection spreads beyond the external auditory canal, involvement of the temporomandibular joint, mastoid, periauricular skin, and parotid may occur. This is a chronic refractory condition that requires intensive antibiotic therapy if further complications are to be avoided. Such complications include intracranial extension, facial nerve paralysis, and death if treatment is not thorough. It is important to have a comprehensive otologic and radiologic evaluation to exclude the possibility of neoplasm or other conditions that may mimic malignant otitis externa.

3. **Otitis media** is inflammation of the middle ear space usually, although not always, caused by a bacterium. Patients with acute otitis media usually have a history of otalgia beginning after an upper respiratory tract infection. Serous otitis media, also called otitis media with effusion, involves a collection of fluid in the middle ear space. The patient often does not complain of severe pain but rather a sensation of the ear being "clogged." Both acute and serous otitis media may be treated with antibiotics. Caution should be exercised in treating persistent serous otitis media in an adult. This condition often signifies the presence of a nasopharyngeal mass that impairs eustachian tube function. Careful examination of the nasopharynx is necessary.

4. **Chronic otitis media** generally follows numerous episodes of inadequately treated acute otitis media, commonly beginning in childhood. The patient may have a chronically draining ear, but without the complaint of pain. The presence of pain is strongly suggestive of an osteitis, which may signal an impending complication, and immediate otolaryngologic referral is then advised.

5. **Bullous myringitis** is a viral infection of the tympanic membrane and must be differentiated from acute otitis media as well as the Ramsay Hunt syndrome

mentioned below. Treatment for bullous myringitis is supportive, generally consisting of analgesic administration. Antibiotics are usually not given unless there is evidence of a secondary bacterial infection.

6. **Cerumen** (earwax) buildup in the external auditory canal can manifest as chronic otalgia. The patient may also have attempted removal with a Q-tip, causing a secondary external otitis. Careful cleaning using a small wire loop and wax curette is the treatment of choice.

7. **Furunculosis**, or infection of a hair follicle, may occur in the most lateral, cartilaginous portion of the ear canal. Initial treatment consists of warm soaks to encourage drainage, and antibiotics. If the patient does not respond to these measures, incision and drainage may be necessary.

8. **Herpetic external otitis.** Herpetic infection of the external ear canal resembles herpetic lesions elsewhere in the body. Small, vesicular eruptions are characteristic of the herpes simplex virus. Symptomatic treatment with lanolin–boric acid ointment is recommended. This must be differentiated from the far more serious geniculate ganglion (Ramsay Hunt) syndrome, which is caused by the herpes zoster virus. Characteristic findings include the above-mentioned vesicles as well as a partial or complete facial paralysis. As the virus attacks the geniculate ganglion, a loss of taste and decreased salivation may accompany the pain and facial paralysis characteristic of the disease. There have been reports of improvement in symptoms following treatment with oral acyclovir.

B. **Nonotogenic causes of ear pain**

1. **Myofacial pain dysfunction (MPD)** is discomfort commonly located in the region of the auricle. When a patient presents with acute or chronic ear pain with no otoscopic abnormalities, a diagnosis of MPD should be entertained. Physical examination may demonstrate crepitus or clicking of the temporomandibular joint on palpation with occasional limitation of range of motion. Intraoral palpation of the pterygoid muscles may elicit the characteristic pain. Symptomatic treatment consists of joint rest, soft diet, warm soaks, and an oral nonsteroidal anti-inflammatory medication.

2. **Recent tonsillectomy or adenoidectomy.** Patients who have recently undergone tonsillectomy or adenoidectomy may complain of persistent postoperative otalgia. The tonsillar fossa is innervated by the glossopharyngeal nerve, a branch of which (Jacobson's nerve) provides sensation to the ear and may be the mechanism for referred pain. Also, edema of the eustachian tube orifice following adenoidectomy may produce acute otitis media with otalgia.

3. **Eagle's syndrome.** A prominent, elongated styloid process may irritate the trigeminal, glossopharyngeal, or vagus nerves causing throat pain or referred pain to the ear. Diagnosis is made by palpation of an abnormally long styloid process while examining the oropharynx. Radiographic studies of the temporal bone and base of the skull should confirm the diagnosis. Definitive treatment consists of transoral resection of the styloid process.

4. **Neoplasia of the upper aerodigestive tract.** Benign or malignant lesions of the nasopharynx, oropharynx, hard and soft palate, and laryngopharynx may present with otalgia as an early symptom. The clinician must be especially suspicious of patients with a history of tobacco and alcohol abuse, as these are prominent etiologic factors in the development of these neoplasms. A thorough head and neck examination is the only method of excluding this diagnosis. If no other source of otalgia is discovered and the head and neck examination is unremarkable, monthly follow-up examinations are necessary so as not to miss these potentially treatable lesions.

5. **Other nonotogenic causes of ear pain.** Glossopharyngeal, vidian, and other neuralgias may present with ear pain. Before diagnosing a neuralgia, other causes of neuropathy (multiple sclerosis, vascular compression, tumor) must be excluded.

III. **Nasal pain.** The nose has a rich sensory supply from the trigeminal nerve. Complaints may involve related structures such as the orbit, cranial cavity, or palate. The history must be directed at associated symptoms such as nasal discharge, as well as a history of trauma or substance abuse. A complete examination of the head and neck and radiographic studies of the paranasal sinuses are often necessary to delineate a specific rhinologic problem. Finally, ophthalmologic examination may provide valuable information about the status of the orbit, which is occasionally involved in nasal or paranasal sinus disease.

A. Chronic and acute rhinosinusitis. Sinusitis, whether acute or chronic, is often manifested by facial pain or pressure, ear pain, or frontal headache. The patient often has a preceding upper respiratory tract infection and fever. Tenderness may be elicited by applying pressure to the areas overlying the frontal and maxillary sinuses with the examiner's thumbs. The decision to treat as an outpatient with oral antibiotics or as an inpatient with intravenous antibiotics depends on whether an imminent complication is suspected.

The patient with chronic sinusitis may have a variety of head and neck symptoms. Drainage of purulent material into the oropharynx and larynx may manifest as halitosis, chronic cough, or a feeling of "always having to clear the throat." Significant physical findings may include nasal polyposis, presence of cloudy nasal drainage or erythema of the mucosa, or a foreign body in the child.

B. Allergic rhinitis. The pain is often accompanied by nasal obstruction, watery discharge from the nose and eyes, and associated itching. Seasonal occurrence of these symptoms clues the practitioner to an allergic etiology. Physical examination reveals "allergic shiners" (chronic edema of the infraorbital area) as well as the patient exhibiting the "allergic salute" (frequent rubbing of the nasal vestibule with the forefinger). The intranasal examination will reveal a pale, gray, and boggy mucosal lining of the nasal cavity. Immediate treatment is directed at relieving symptoms with a systemic nasal decongestant and topical steroid spray. Referral to an allergist for determination of the offending agent and possible immunotherapy is warranted for the patient who is refractory to symptomatic treatment.

C. Vasomotor rhinitis. Patients with this condition complain of a sensation of pain that is actually the sensation of nasal obstruction. The disease consists of a continuing cycle of obstruction and discharge that is secondary to an imbalance between sympathetic and parasympathetic activity. Attacks are brought on by emotional stress or environmental factors that increase parasympathetic discharge. This disease entity should be differentiated from other forms of nasal obstruction such as sinusitis, allergic rhinitis, and rhinitis medicamentosa.

D. Rhinitis medicamentosa is typically found in persons who chronically use or abuse over-the-counter topical nasal decongestants. Prolonged use of these medications produces a "rebound" phenomenon in which the spray actually causes swelling of the nasal mucosa with obstruction rather than decongestion. Treatment consists of tapering of the offending agent (stopping abruptly is difficult for most patients) as well as institution of a topical steroid spray.

E. Wegener's granulomatosis is a potentially life-threatening necrotizing vasculitis of the respiratory tract and kidneys (glomerulitis), which often initially presents with nasal obstruction. The patient may also have systemic symptoms such as night sweats, arthralgias, and fatigue. Prompt pharmacologic treatment is essential.

F. Relapsing polychondritis is a rare disorder characterized by recurrent inflammation of the cartilage of the ear, nose, and joints. The acute attack is painful and may initially respond well to anti-inflammatory agents. Diagnosis is primarily by exclusion.

G. Trauma. Acute trauma to the nose is almost always associated with pain of the soft tissue or bone. Traumatic deformities of the nose may also give rise to chronic pain, as seen in patients with a traumatic septal injury in which the septum touches the lateral nasal wall. Septoplasty may greatly improve symptoms in these patients. Patients who have had rhinoplasty may also complain of chronic nasal pain due to the healing of the osteotomies that are performed to reposition the nasal bones. Pain in the location of the bone and periosteum is not unusual and should not be regarded as a complication of the procedure. Trauma to the paranasal sinuses, especially the frontal sinus, may give rise to a mucocele. This can lead to slowly progressive frontal pain. Diagnosis is by CT scan, and treatment is surgical.

H. Foreign bodies in the nose, almost always found in the young or emotionally disturbed population, characteristically present with a persistent foul-smelling nasal discharge. Treatment is removal and institution of antibiotics.

I. Neoplasms of the nose are mostly skin cancers that involve the external nose. Intranasal and paranasal sinus neoplasms are uncommon, but they must be suspected in a patient with persistent pain, nasal obstruction, epistaxis, and rhinorrhea. The most common neoplasm of the nose is the papilloma, which has been associated with squamous cell carcinoma in approximately 5% of cases.

IV. Oral cavity pain

A. Aphthous stomatitis is characterized by exquisitely painful, ulcerated lesions that appear on the buccal mucosa and gingiva. The lesions vary from less than 1 mm to more than 1 cm in diameter and are surrounded by an erythematous border. They have a propensity to develop after bouts of emotional stress and afflict many people on a recurrent basis. They are commonly known as "canker sores" or "cold sores." There has been an association noted between aphthous ulcers and various systemic diseases such as vitamin B_{12} deficiency, inflammatory bowel disease, and Behçet's syndrome. These lesions usually are self-limited and regress in 1 to 2 weeks. The phenomenon of giant aphthous ulcers (up to 4–5 cm) has been observed in patients with AIDS. Treatment of these lesions is symptomatic with topical steroids and, in more severe cases, with systemic steroids.

B. Pyrosis refers to a nonspecific symptom of a burning tongue. Various systemic abnormalities can give rise to this symptom including vitamin B_{12} deficiency, hyperglycemia, and various forms of anemia. Evaluation consists of identifying a systemic cause as well as ruling out local causes such as lichen planus, candidiasis, or malignant neoplasms.

C. Hairy tongue is characterized by a brown or black, hairlike appearance to the tongue caused by elongation of the filiform papillae located on the anterior two thirds of the tongue. It is associated with antibiotic use, nutritional deficiencies, and poor oral hygiene and is generally not painful. However, the word "pain" may be used by the patient to describe the unpleasant perception of the abnormal tongue. Symptomatic treatment involves frequent brushing of the tongue with a peroxide solution. Attention is directed toward correcting nutritional deficiencies and discontinuing antibiotic use.

D. Trauma. Burns secondary to hot liquids or caustic substances, poorly fitting dental appliances, and lacerations of the tongue or buccal mucosa may produce oral cavity pain. Treatment consists of removing the underlying cause such as poorly fitting dental appliances. Lacerations usually will heal spontaneously without surgical intervention.

V. Throat pain

A. Viral pharyngitis. There is usually a concomitant upper respiratory tract infection with rhinorrhea, headache, and nasal congestion. The degree of throat pain is usually not as severe as in other forms of pharyngitis. In a patient with a persistent sore throat, unresponsive to antibiotics, the diagnosis of infectious mononucleosis must be entertained.

B. Bacterial pharyngitis. There will usually be severe odynophagia and dysphagia, with associated fever and cervical adenopathy.

C. Fungal pharyngitis is usually secondary to *Candida albicans* and generally signifies an underlying abnormality of the immune system. Treatment consists of symptomatic relief and the institution of an oral antifungal wash. Sometimes systemic antifungal treatment is necessary.

D. Noninfectious pharyngitis symptoms include a sore throat in the morning that becomes better as the day progresses. This is often found in smokers and chronic mouth breathers, and treatment is directed at cessation of smoking and examination of the nose and nasopharynx for treatable causes of nasal obstruction.

E. Laryngitis symptoms include pain, hoarseness, and a dry nonproductive cough. The etiology may be infectious or noninfectious and is aggravated by smoking, vocal abuse, and various chemical solvents used in industry. The patient who has gastroesophageal reflux commonly has irritation of the larynx from gastric acid, which produces a bitter taste in the mouth, especially in the morning. Treatment is directed at the underlying cause such as voice rest for vocal abuse, and H_2-blockers or antacids for gastroesophageal reflux.

F. Tonsillitis, although characterized by the same symptom complex as bacterial pharyngitis, can also have the finding of whitish exudates on the tonsils. Special mention should be given to the **potential complications** of an untreatable bacterial pharyngitis or tonsillitis. These involve **deeper infections of the soft tissues** in and around the pharynx and neck. Peritonsillar abscess is perhaps the most common and benign of these "space" infections. The patient has the characteristic symptom complex of pharyngitis with the additional physical finding of unilateral swelling of one tonsillar fossa. Another clue to differentiating peritonsillar abscess from tonsillitis is that the uvula will be midline in the latter condition, whereas in an abscess the uvula will be deviated toward the uninvolved tonsil. Trismus is strongly suggestive of involvement of the pterygoid musculature. Treatment is the same as for any other abscess in the body, namely, surgical drainage followed by administration of antibiotics.

G. **Foreign bodies.** The oropharynx and larynx are common places for the lodgment of foreign bodies. Whether these are blunt or sharp foreign bodies, they generally result in pain that can be localized to the site of the object itself. The patient may still have a foreign body sensation even several weeks after the actual event has occurred. This may be due to a nonhealed laceration of the regional mucosa or to the fact that the foreign body has burrowed submucosally. Full clinical and radiologic evaluations are indicated. In questionable cases endoscopy may be necessary. One must be extremely suspicious when patients present with drooling, inability to swallow solids or liquids, or a change in voice. Although removal of the foreign body can generally be performed by perioral endoscopy, deeper foreign bodies may require neck exploration.

H. **Neoplasms.** Pain is also a common finding with neoplasms of the upper aerodigestive tract. Most throat neoplasms are cancerous and occur in patients who have a history of heavy smoking or alcohol abuse.

I. **Trauma.** External blunt trauma to the larynx is a potentially life-threatening situation that demands immediate evaluation by an otolaryngologist. The long-term complications of laryngeal trauma involve a variety of stenotic lesions. These may be the cause of chronic throat pain or the sensation of a foreign body. Stenotic lesions may also be found in patients who have a history of endotracheal intubation and mechanical ventilation. Treatment is surgical and is designed to restore or preserve the laryngeal functions of protection of the lower airway, respiration, and phonation.

J. **Other causes of throat pain**
  1. **Eagle's syndrome (elongation of the styloid process)** is a frequently unsuspected cause of throat pain, which generally occurs in patients who have had a tonsillectomy. Treatment involves surgery, and a diagnosis is made by intraoral palpation of the throat with identification of the bony prominence as well as reproduction of pain.
  2. **Arthritis.** The larynx contains several synovial joints, and arthritis, particularly of the cricoarytenoid joint, may be demonstrated. Treatment is the same as for other forms of arthritis.
  3. **AIDS.** The incidence of candidiasis, herpetic infections, tuberculosis, and Kaposi's sarcoma of the hypopharynx, larynx, and esophagus related to AIDS is ever-increasing. Treatment is generally directed at eradicating the infection and symptomatically ameliorating the pain.

VI. **Neck pain (anterior)** (Posterior cervical pain, a musculoskeletal disorder, is explained in Chap. 28.)
  A. **Thyroid disorders**
    1. **Thyroiditis**
      a. **Acute**—pain and tenderness at the site of infection along with fever and malaise.
      b. **Subacute**—thought to be viral in origin, the gland is firm and tender with the patient giving a history of a previous upper respiratory infection preceding the onset of the neck pain. Treatment is symptomatic and usually involves the use of anti-inflammatory agents.
    2. Many slowly enlarging **thyroid neoplasms** (whether benign or malignant) are not painful. The onset of pain in the region of a thyroid neoplasm suggests bleeding, local trauma, or infection. When the thyroid gland becomes markedly enlarged, the patient may also experience discomfort owing to compression of the trachea or esophagus.
  B. **Sialoadenitis** is an infection of a salivary gland, usually secondary to obstruction of the gland's duct. Treatment involves hydration, sialogogues (bitter lemon), and oral antibiotics. Surgical removal is the treatment of choice.
  C. **Lymphadenitis** is usually secondary to acute or chronic infection in another area of the head and neck, i.e., tonsil, oropharynx, or the ear. Differentiation from malignant transformation must be made. Tenderness, with a preceding or concurrent infection elsewhere, and a young age (90% of children's nodes are inflammatory) favor the diagnosis of inflammatory lymph nodes. Treatment is directed at the primary source of infection.

D. Infected cysts. Congenital cysts in the head and neck may become acutely or chronically infected. Acutely infected cysts should be treated with antibiotics and surgical drainage. Surgical excision is indicated for all cysts after the infection has subsided.

E. Carotidynia is pain of unknown etiology, elicited on palpation of the carotid artery, usually at the site of the bifurcation. Treatment consists of anti-inflammatory agents and warm soaks. The presence of a neoplasm must be excluded in the patient with previously mentioned risk factors.

F. Trauma to the anterior neck rarely causes chronic pain in the patient, unless the laryngeal cartilages have been involved. Previous fractures to these cartilages may produce a neuralgia. Treatment consists of warm soaks and anti-inflammatory agents. The endolarynx must be examined for the presence of stenoses, which may require eventual surgical reconstruction.

G. Neoplasms. Neoplastic disease in the neck, particularly that involving metastatic spread to lymph nodes, rarely causes pain. The exceptions are when the lesion is secondarily infected or involves one of the sensory nerves in the neck. In patients who have had previous radical neck dissection, transection of these nerves may cause neuromas, which are often confused with recurrent disease. Pain on palpation is suggestive of neuroma, but the only safe way to rule out malignancy is fine-needle aspiration followed by excisional biopsy.

VII. Neurologic causes. Before diagnosing a neuralgia, other causes of neuropathy (multiple sclerosis, vascular compression, tumor) must be excluded.

A. Trigeminal neuralgia is severe, lancinating pain, located in the distribution of one or more divisions of the trigeminal nerve of brief duration (a few seconds to 1 minute). Females are more commonly affected than males, and the disease occurs rarely in individuals younger than 40. Most patients will have an associated "trigger area," which will elicit a painful response when touched. The anticonvulsant carbamazepine is the drug of choice, although it is limited by its often toxic side effects. In patients refractory to a medical regimen, a variety of neurosurgical procedures including trigeminal rhinotomy, trigeminal neurectomy, neurovascular decompression procedures, and gasserian ganglion anesthetic injection have been efficacious. However, complications and recurrence can occur.

B. Glossopharyngeal neuralgia is a sharp, lancinating pain in the distribution of the ubiquitous glossopharyngeal nerve. It can therefore occur in the ear, throat, tongue, or back of the nose. The pain is often "triggered" by the actions of swallowing, chewing, or touching the external ear. Certain spicy foods may also trigger pain in the oropharynx. The pain is rarely found in younger individuals. Initial treatment is with carbamazepine, and surgery is attempted in medically refractory cases.

C. Sphenopalatine neuralgia, also known as **Sluder's syndrome,** is not considered a classic neuralgia because the pain is often not lancinating and may last from hours to days. The pain is commonly located in the hard palate, behind the eyes, and in the back of the nose. Other disorders, especially acute sinusitis, must be ruled out. Treatment is empirical, with some clinicians using topical cocaine and others using surgery.

D. Other head and neck neuralgias are Raeder's paratrigeminal syndrome, occipital neuralgia, postherpetic neuralgia, and reflex sympathetic dystrophy.

Selected Readings

Ballenger JJ. Headache and neuralgia of the face. In *Diseases of the Nose, Throat, Ear, Head, and Neck.* Malvern, PA: Lea & Febiger, 1991. Pp. 158–167.

Bates SR, Fogelson MH. Headache. In Paparella MM, Shumrick DA, Gluckman JL, Meyerhoff WL (eds.), *Otolaryngology.* Philadelphia: W.B. Saunders, 1991. Pp. 841–847.

Cooper BC, Lucente FE. *Management of Facial, Head and Neck Pain.* Philadelphia: W.B. Saunders, 1989.

Dierks EJ. Temporomandibular disorders and facial pain syndromes. In Paparella MM, Shumrick DA, Gluckman JL, Meyerhoff WL (eds.), *Otolaryngology.* Philadelphia: W.B. Saunders, 1991. Pp. 849–864.

Jacobson AL, Donolon WC. Headache and facial pain. The *Otolaryngol Clin North Am* 22, 1989.

Lucente FE, Goldberg JE. Headache and facial pain. In Meyerhoff WL, Rice DH (eds.), *Otolaryngology Head and Neck Surgery.* Philadelphia: W.B. Saunders, 1992. Pp. 119–127.

Lucente FE, Pincus RL. Facial pain and headache. In Bluestone CD, Stool SE (eds.), *Pediatric Otolaryngology.* Philadelphia: W.B. Saunders, 1990. Pp. 680–685.

Lucente FE, Sobol SM. *Essentials of Otolaryngology.* New York: Raven, 1993.

Mann JD, Lundeen TF. Headaches and facial pain. In Baily BJ (ed.), *Head and Neck Surgery–Otolaryngology.* Philadelphia: J.B. Lippincott, 1993. Pp. 761–773.

Phero JL, Katz JA, Raj PP. Evaluation and management of patients with chronic head and neck pain. In Paparella MM, Shumrick DA, Gluckman JL, Meyerhoff WL (eds.), *Otolaryngology.* Philadelphia: W.B. Saunders, 1991. Pp. 817–839.

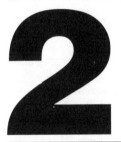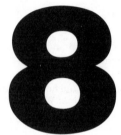

Chronic Pain and Temporomandibular Disorders
Barry C. Cooper

I. Background
A. Definition. Temporomandibular disorders are alterations or abnormalities in the morphology or function of the mandible with respect to the temporomandibular (glenoid) fossa in the skull and the neuromuscular dysfunction associated with that articulation.

B. Differential diagnosis. The complex anatomic and physiologic relationships in the head and neck permit temporomandibular disorders to coexist with or mimic other disease entities. The painful area may be the primary site of disease or may be referred pain.

II. Classification
A. Intracapsular disorders (intrinsic)
  1. Acquired abnormalities
  a. Direct trauma to the joint
  b. Indirect trauma from the mandible
  c. Subtle chronic trauma secondary to dysfunction of the neuromuscular apparatus that postures the mandible, to accommodate either an unhealthy dental occlusion or muscle function—the most common cause of intracapsular craniomandibular disorders because of the unhealthy functional demands placed on the joint structures by an extracapsular process
  d. Inflammation
  e. Infection
  2. Developmental conditions (rare)—aplasia, hypoplasia, hyperplasia of the mandibular condyle

B. Extracapsular disorders (extrinsic) involve the musculoskeletal components of the craniomandibular complex, the craniocervical complex, as well as the cervical musculoskeletal system.[1] Hyperirritability, resulting in pain and limitation in any part of the muscular system of the head and neck, can affect any part of the area's neuromuscular network. The symptoms of pain and limitation of movement result from the accumulation of nociceptive metabolites in fatigued, immobile muscles. These noxious stimuli irritate the nerve endings, and protective muscle "splinting" ensues, further immobilizing the muscles and increasing the buildup of waste metabolites.

  Intracapsular and extracapsular disorders can occur simultaneously and affect each other.

III. Symptoms
A. Pain
  1. Temporomandibular joint (TMJ) pain (static or dynamic)
  2. Headaches, tinnitus, otalgia, and oral or dental pain
  3. Facial, cervical, shoulder, back, and intercostal chest pain

B. Dysfunction
  1. Mandibular movement: limited, deviated, slow, or irregular
  2. Head movement: limited rotation or roll
  3. Ear: muffling, dizziness (nonrotational), conductive hearing loss, clicking
  4. Throat: difficulty in swallowing or in prolonged speech
  5. TMJ: subluxation, closed or open locking; facial asymmetry (torticollis)

C. Self-destructing dentition signs
  1. Attrition or wear on the surface of the teeth (incisal edges of anterior teeth is most common)
  2. Looseness of teeth due to bone loss
  3. Movement of teeth (drifting)

a. **Spreading** of maxillary anteriors
b. **Crowding** of mandibular anteriors

IV. **Anatomy and physiology of the craniomandibular system**

A. **Temporomandibular joints** are formed by the articulation of the condyles of the mandible and the glenoid fossae. They are diarthrodial and synovial,[2] permitting both rotary and translatory movements, and have an interposed fibrocartilaginous disk. The left and right TMJs function simultaneously, to some extent, whenever the mandible moves. Therefore, any functional disturbance in one TMJ or its musculature can affect the function of the contralateral joint and muscles, and symptoms can present bilaterally or migrate from one side of the head and neck to the other.

The TMJ is supported by a ligamentous capsule and surrounded by a complex muscular network. Excessive stretch, compression, or deformation of these tissues as well as the bony structures of the joint can cause pain or dysfunction. The interposed disk, however, is neither innervated nor vascularized and cannot be the source of pain. Fluid accumulation within the joint space (hemarthrosis) can result in degenerative joint disease. Traumatic osteoarthritis and systemic rheumatoid arthritis can affect the TMJ as well.

B. **Musculoskeletal system.** The craniocervical skeletal system is composed of the skull, mandible, hyoid bone, laryngeal cartilages, and cervical vertebrae. The muscular system is composed of the masticatory, facial, and cervical (anterior, lateral, and posterior) muscles.[3]

The movements of the mandible and its posturing in space are the responsibility of the masticatory muscles and other head and neck muscles. There is a direct relationship between the mandibular position and the position of the hyoid bone attached to it by the suprahyoid muscles. The hyoid, in turn, is connected to the cervical vertebrae by fascial attachments and inferiorly by the infrahyoid muscles to the sternum. Abnormal cervical posture, for example, creates tensile pressures on the hyoid bone, which affects mandibular posture.[1,4] This can result in developmental abnormalities in the growing mandible with resultant dental malocclusion. Nasal obstruction during early childhood has been shown to be accompanied by elevation of the skull with extension on the cervical spine. This causes soft tissue stretching from beneath the mandible, resulting in open anterior bites (front teeth do not meet) and increases in mandibular gonial angles.[5] The muscular compromise associated with this developmental aberration can predispose the individual to temporomandibular disorders.

C. **The masticatory muscles**

1. **Elevators of the mandible (mouth closers)—temporalis, masseter, and medial pterygoid muscles.** The temporalis muscle is a broad fan-shaped muscle that attaches to the coronoid process of the mandible, which is anterior to the condyle and the TMJ. It originates from the temporal bone from the area behind the eyebrow and extends across the side of the skull to a position just posterior to the upper portion of the ear. It is the principal elevator of the mandible and is the muscle that postures the jaw "at rest." When the position of maximum dental occlusion (interdigitation) is "overclosed" or posteriorly displaced, the temporalis muscle overcontracts. This can result in fatigue and pain and is a common cause of temporal headaches. The medial pterygoid muscle overcontracts in this condition as well.

2. **Depressors of the mandible (mouth openers)—lateral pterygoid, digastric, and suprahyoid muscles.** The lateral pterygoid is responsible for lateral movement of the mandible toward the contralateral side and for opening the mouth. When both left and right lateral pterygoid muscles are simultaneously contracted, a smooth straight vertical opening movement of the mandible is observed. When one lateral pterygoid muscle is in spasm and the contralateral muscle is relaxed, opening movement is deflected toward the side of the spastic muscle. Mandibular deflection toward the side of dysfunction is also a diagnostic sign of internal derangement within the joint of the affected side. In the latter case, the disk is displaced anterior to the condyle and does not recapture over the condyle upon opening, thereby producing a "closed lock." This may not permit normal translatory movement of the condyle on opening and results in a pivoting around the affected side.

The lateral pterygoid muscle is often found to be in a state of hyperactivity and fatigue in patients with extracapsular temporomandibular disorders. Associated spasm can refer pain to the TMJ area and to the ear.

V. History
A. Precipitating event
1. **Prolonged opening or hyperextension of the mandible,** during dental procedures or medical procedures in or through the mouth (i.e., intubation) or during nontraumatic events such as biting a large food item, yawning, or yelling.
2. **Traumatic head and neck injuries** can result in momentary whiplash and can often cause rapid mandibular flexion and extension as well as "jawlash," with symptoms occurring immediately or weeks later.[6]

B. General medical history.
Inquire about family history, previous similar conditions, former treatments and their effectiveness, as well as any other coexisting pathologic conditions (most importantly in the head and neck).

C. Description of pain—quality, intensity, and course of each pain episode, as well as any precipitating (triggering) or modulating events
1. **Neuralgic**—stabbing, lancinating, often having a typical trigger area; follows neurologic pathways, of very short duration
2. **Myogenous**—more diffuse and of longer duration (hours to days); frequently precipitated by activities such as chewing food, prolonged opening or hyperextension of the mandible, rotation of the head, or stress-induced muscular tension

D. Mental status.
The head and neck are invested with great importance by the brain, and dysfunction or pain in the head and neck can elicit a profound psychosomatic response. Caution must therefore be exercised when differentiating chronic head and neck pain from a primary psychologic disorder with psychogenic pain.

VI. Clinical examination
A. Head posture.
Observe the patient's head posture both frontally and sagittally and note any tilt. Then observe the cervical and shoulder posture and note if a vertical plumb line dropped from the malar process on the face intersects the clavicle. If it falls ahead of the clavicle, the head is postured forward. This can be associated with cervical, muscular, and mandibular abnormalities. Craniocervical and craniomandibular disorder symptoms can also be associated with either of these postural abnormalities.

Observe the patient's face for symmetry. Asymmetry can be secondary to mandibular malposition or bilateral anatomic disparity as well as pathologic conditions that cause swelling.

B. Mandibular movement.
Visualize the opening and closing of the mouth by parting the patient's lips with a gloved thumb and forefinger. Observe the extent and quality of the wide opening-and-closing movement of the mouth and note if it is rapid, fluid, and symmetrical. An opening deflection to one side indicates more dysfunction on the side toward which the mandible is deflected. An S-shaped opening-and-closing movement indicates bilateral dysfunction. Maximum opening of the mouth should range between 35 and 50 mm measured between the incisal edges of the anterior teeth. Staggered, irregular (dyskinetic), or very slow (bradykinetic) movements also indicate temporomandibular dysfunction.

C. Temporomandibular joints
are located immediately anterior to the tragus of each ear. Palpate the two TMJs simultaneously using one's index fingers, asking the patient to indicate anything that causes pain. Pain on palpation indicates inflammation beneath the skin. Pain on opening and closing may also indicate inflammation in the joint capsule, within the joint, or in the muscle system attached to the condyle. As the patient opens and closes, one should normally feel the condyle move (translate) anteriorly beneath one's fingers. No translation indicates dysfunction. One may also be able to feel clicking or crepitus.

D. External auditory canal.
Press the volar portion of one's fifth finger forward against the anterior wall of the patient's external auditory canal and observe whether the patient reports pain. Ask the patient to open the mouth wide and then close on the rear teeth. This maneuver may elicit a painful response, indicating compression of the retrodiskal tissues by the posteriorly displaced condyle accompanying occlusion of the teeth. Be certain that the patient closes with the back teeth fully in occlusion because some patients tend to close more anteriorly. This test of pain upon pressure in the ear canal is a very old clinical test of intracapsular TMJ dysfunction. One may also be able to feel a clicking sensation.

E. Temporomandibular joint sounds.
A stethoscope can be used to listen to TMJ joint sounds, which include
1. **Clicking (popping)** is associated with opening of the mouth and is usually indicative of recapturing of an anteriorly displaced disk. As the mandible

translates anteriorly, it "bumps" into an anteriorly displaced disk and slips under the thickened posterior rim of the disk. On the other hand, clicking that occurs at normal wide opening (50 mm or more) indicates subluxation—that is, a hyperextension of the condyle beyond the eminence of the joint socket.

2. **Crepitus (crackling)** is associated with the rubbing of bones and is observed when the disk has been either perforated or displaced anteriorly and bone-to-bone contact occurs. This represents a more serious stage of disease than clicking and indicates the presence of degenerative changes in the bone, which can include osteophyte formation or flattening of the condylar surface.

3. **The absence of observable sounds** does not rule out joint dysfunction because at certain stages of the illness there are no joint sounds: e.g., severe limitation of opening when the patient previously reported clicking. With limited opening, the point in the condylar movement at which the disk had been recapturable is no longer reached, and the click does not occur. Chronic anteriorly dislocated disks can no longer become recaptured and will not produce a click on opening. Closing clicks indicate that the disk slips off the condyle as the condyle translates posteriorly in the fossa, leaving the disk anteriorly displaced.

F. Extraoral muscle examination

1. **Temporalis muscle** is a common site of headaches. Place one's forefingers on the patient's temples between the eyebrows and the hairline and palpate the entire extent of the muscles bilaterally with fingers reaching the most posterior fibers behind the ear. Ask the patient to report all presently tender areas as well as those that are painful at other times. The differential diagnosis of pain in this area must include temporal arteritis, which is significant as it can result in visual loss if not treated promptly. The patient's age is significant here.

2. **Angle of the mandible.** Palpate the angles of the mandible with four fingers (not the thumb). Wrap the fingers around the back of the angle of the mandible, pressing inward. This area is commonly tender in patients with temporomandibular disorder as it is the crossroads of many muscles, including the medial pterygoid, posterior digastric and stylohyoid muscles, as well as the stylomandibular ligaments.

   Note that the parotid gland is located in this area as well. Parotid disease or obstruction must also be considered in the differential diagnosis of facial and oral pain and is characterized by a history of swelling and pain immediately preceding eating or in anticipation of eating as saliva production increases.

   Moving anteriorly, palpate the submandibular area, which includes the suprahyoid muscles (digastric, hyoglossus) and submandibular salivary glands. This area is usually not tender to palpation in patients with temporomandibular disorders.

3. **Anterior neck muscles.** Palpate the remaining anterior neck muscles (infrahyoid) between the hyoid bone and sternum. Muscle tension here is due to mandibular overclosure occlusion and can be transmitted to the intercostal muscles below. This domino-type phenomenon can also extend to the posterior and lateral cervical muscles. Connections between the cervical muscles, tongue muscles, and deep muscles of the neck can affect swallowing comfort or cause a generalized feeling of tightness in the structures within the neck.

4. **Posterior and lateral cervical muscles.** Palpate these from their origins to their insertions. Posterior cervical, shoulder, and back muscles are tested from the rear of the patient, beginning on the occiput and moving downward to the lower portion of the trapezius. Lateral cervical muscles are palpated beginning at the mastoid and moving downward. Posterior cervical muscles are affected by abnormal head-posturing habits such as cradling a telephone between the head and shoulder. Carrying a heavy handbag on a shoulder strap may also lead to muscle fatigue and complaints of head, neck, or shoulder pain. Fatigue within these muscles can produce "trigger points" in the muscles, which refer pain to "target areas" elsewhere in the head and neck.[7]

G. Intraoral muscle examination

1. **Lateral pterygoids** are the muscles responsible for opening the mouth and for anterior and lateral mandibular movements, and are almost always tender to palpation in patients with a temporomandibular disorder. Use the left forefinger to palpate the patient's left lateral pterygoid and the right forefinger to palpate the right pterygoid. Press a gloved index finger diagonally across the patient's mouth, behind and above the last maxillary molar, upward and

laterally toward the external ear. During this maneuver one is actually pressing on fibers of the medial and lateral pterygoids. The medial muscle fibers run vertically and are superficial to the deeper lateral pterygoid muscle fibers, which run in an oblique horizontal direction.

   2. The **medial pterygoid** is a mandibular elevator, together with the temporalis. It postures the mandible at rest and brings about occlusion of the teeth. To palpate the medial pterygoid, move the forefinger downward beside the tongue where it attaches to the inner aspect of the angle of the mandible. Both medial and lateral pterygoids will usually be tender to palpation in patients with myogenous temporomandibular disorder, which is diagnostic for this illness.

   3. The **masseter muscle** is also a mandibular elevator. It is not a posturing muscle, but rather is responsible for generating pressure when the teeth are in occlusion or in contact with a bolus of food. Dysfunction of the masseter results from clenching or grinding (bruxing) the teeth together. It is palpated by compressing it between the examiner's thumb inside the mouth and forefinger on the outside, from its zygomatic attachment to its attachment on the superficial surface of the angle of the mandible. Although not usually tender to palpation, the masseter is often tender in patients who grind or brux during sleep or while awake. Night bruxers may be aware of a tightness of their jaws upon awakening in the morning but may not be aware of their clenching during sleep.

   4. **Mylohyoid muscles** are next palpated in the anterior floor of the mouth. Not usually tender in patients with temporomandibular disorder, the mylohyoid can serve as a control to differentiate between tender and nontender muscles on palpation.

H. **Intraoral examination.** Many symptoms of temporomandibular disorders involve the teeth. Ask patients to bite together fully on the back teeth in their natural swallowing closure position. If a severely deep overbite is observed (the upper anterior teeth almost covering the lower teeth), the mandible has usually overclosed. This is accompanied by a distal displacement of the condyle in the TMJ. It is often associated with anterior displacement of the disk and stretching of the retrodiskal fibers, which create an unhealthy relation among the components within the TMJ. Overclosure of the mandible occurs when the mandibular elevator muscles (temporalis, masseter, and medial pterygoid muscles) overcontract and the mandibular depressor muscles (lateral pterygoid and suprahyoid muscles) are stretched beyond their resting lengths. Hence, the occlusal position also affects muscle function and can create muscle fatigue.

Observe whether the patient has a full complement of teeth in the maxillary and mandibular dental arches. Normally, the interdigitation of the teeth in occlusion serves to protect the TMJ against excessive loading. Missing upper or lower posterior teeth, unilaterally or bilaterally, creates pressure within the TMJs. Patients who have complete or partial dentures should be questioned about whether they wear the dentures 24 hours a day. If they do not wear replacement teeth, they should be advised to do so.

Severe abrasion or wearing of the surface of the teeth is an indication of prolonged excessive biting or grinding activity. This is most easily detected on the edges of the upper and lower anterior teeth. It is caused either by a centrally mediated behavioral muscle activity or by a specific muscle activity pattern attempting to wear away surface detail on the teeth. Such irregularities in the tooth detail or prematurities in contact may prevent the mandible from coming into a muscularly comfortable stable occlusal position.

VII. **Diagnosis and treatment of extracapsular disorders**

A. **Computerized electronic testing instruments** provide precise objective measurement of mandibular function and associated masticatory muscle function.[8] Quantitative measurements are made of mandibular movement (electronic jaw tracking), muscle activity (electromyography), and TMJ sounds (sonography). Utilized before treatment to determine the state of function or dysfunction, they are aids in diagnosis and treatment planning. Utilized after treatment, they provide quantification of outcome results and assist in long-term treatment design.[9,10]

B. **Transcutaneous electrical nerve stimulation (TENS)** provides relaxation of the masticatory muscles, which are in a state of hyperactivity. Applied bilaterally to the sides of the face between the TMJ and the coronoid process of the mandible, it transmits a painless, subtle, low-voltage, low-frequency electrical stimulus through the skin and soft tissues to the mandibular division of the trigeminal nerve.[11] This nerve innervates all of the masticatory muscles as well as the tensor tympani muscle in the middle ear and the tensor veli palatini muscle, which opens the eustachian tube in the oropharynx. Relaxation of the masticatory muscles permits the mandible to achieve its true rest position rather than the accommodated, incompletely rested position that predisposes to muscle fatigue.[12]

C. Orthotic appliances. Covering the posterior mandibular teeth, the orthosis provides a new occlusal surface that interdigitates with the maxillary teeth in occlusion and improves mandibular and muscular function.[9,13]

D. Dental procedures. Reconstructive and orthodontic procedures attempt to establish a durable neuromuscular occlusion that is synchronized with healthy masticatory muscle function. The prognosis is good. For some patients a form of long-term therapy is required.

VIII. Treatment of intracapsular disorders. Further diagnostic and therapeutic procedures may be indicated for those patients who have intracapsular TMJ disease that does not respond to the conservative extracapsular treatments described above.[14-17] These include arthroscopic or open joint surgery with postoperative physical therapy and open surgery of the TMJ, which is utilized when it is absolutely necessary to restore function.[18] The prognosis of these procedures is guarded, however, and they should be instituted only after noninvasive, reversible therapies have been attempted and have not effected a sufficient resolution.

References

1. Rocabado M. Biomechanical relationship of the cranial, cervical and hyoid bones. *J Craniomandibular Pract* 1:62–66, 1983.
2. McNeill C. *Temporomandibular Disorders: Guidelines for Classification, Assessment and Management.* Chicago: Quintessence, 1993. Pp. 42–61.
3. Goss CM. *Grey's Anatomy* (29th American ed.). Philadelphia: Lea & Febiger, 1973.
4. Hairston LE, Blanton PL. An electromyographic study of mandibular position in response to changes in body position. *J Prosthet Dent* 49:2, 1983.
5. Solow B, Kreiborg S. Soft tissue stretching: a possible control factor in craniofacial morphogenesis. *Scand J Dent Res* 85:505–507, 1977.
6. Kinnie BH. From the outside looking in. Presented at the American Academy of Dental Radiology, Atlanta, October 19, 1984.
7. Travel J, Rinzler SH. The myofascial genesis of pain. *Postgrad Med* 11:425–434, 1952.
8. Jankelson B. Measurement accuracy of the mandibular kinesiograph: a computerized study. *J Prosthet Dent* 44:656–666, 1980.
9. Cooper BC. Neuromuscular occlusion: concept and application. *NY State Dental J* 56:24–28, 1990.
10. Cooper B, Cooper D, Lucente F. Electromyography of masticatory muscles in craniomandibular disorders. *Laryngoscope* 10:150–157, 1991.
11. Jankelson B, Sparks S, Crane P, Radke JC. Neural conduction of the myomonitor stimulus: a quantitative analysis. *J Prosthet Dent* 34:245–253, 1975.
12. Cooper BC, Alleva M, Cooper DL, Lucente FE. Myofacial pain dysfunction: analysis of 476 patients. *Laryngoscope* 96:1099–1106, 1986.
13. Kawazoe VA, Kotani H, Hamada T. Relations between integrated electromyographic activity and biting force during voluntary isometric contraction in human masticatory muscles. *J Dent Res* 58:140, 1979.
14. Katzberg RW, Dolwick M, Helms, CS, et al. Arthrography of the temporomandibular joint. *Am J Radiol* 134:995–1003, 1980.
15. Manzione JV, Katzberg RW, Brodsky G, et al. Internal derangements of the temporomandibular joints. *Radiology* 150:111–115, 1984.
16. Katzberg RW, Shenck J, Roberts D, et al. Magnetic resonance imaging. *Oral Surg* 59:322–325, 1985.
17. Schelhas KP, Wildes CH, Omlie MR, et al. Temporomandibular joint imaging: practical application of available technology. *Arch Otolaryngol Head Neck Surg* 113:744–748, 1987.
18. Dolwick MF, et al. Criteria for TMJ meniscus surgery. Presented at the Ad Hoc Study Group of TMJ Meniscus Surgery of the American Association of Oral and Maxillofacial Surgeons, Chicago, November 1984.

Selected Readings

Cooper BC. Craniomandibular disorders. In Lucente F, Sobel S (eds.), *Essentials of Otolaryngology* (3rd ed.). New York: Raven, 1993.

Cooper BC. Myofacial pain dysfunction: cause, clinical appearance, current therapy. *Primary ENT* 3:2–7, 1987.

Cooper BC. Nasorespiratory function and orofacial development. *Otolaryngol Clin North Am* 22:413–441, 1989.

Cooper B, Cooper, D. Recognizing otolaryngologic symptoms in patients with temporomandibular disorders. *J Craniomandibular Pract* 11:260–267, 1993.

Cooper B, Cooper D. A multidisciplinary approach to the management of facial, head and neck pain. *J Prosthet Dent* 66:72–78, 1991.

Cooper BC, Lucente FE. *Management of Facial, Head and Neck Pain.* Philadelphia: W.B. Saunders, 1989.

Cooper BC, Mattucci KF. Myofacial pain dysfunction: a clinical examination procedure. *Int Surg* 72:165–169, 1985.

Cooper BC, Rabuzzi D. Myofacial pain dysfunction: a clinical study of asymptomatic subjects. *Laryngoscope* 94:68–75, 1984.

Costen JB. A syndrome of ear, nose and sinus symptoms dependent upon disturbed function of the temporomandibular joint. *Ann Otol Rhinol Laryngol* 43:1–5, 1934.

Garry JF. Early iatrogenic orofacial, muscle, skeletal and TMJ dysfunction. In Morgan, House, Hall, Vamvas (eds.), *Diseases of the Temporomandibular Apparatus* (2nd ed.). St. Louis: C.V. Mosby, 1987. P. 65.

Gervais R, Fitzsimmons G, Thomas N. Masseter and temporalis electromyographic activity in asymptomatic, subclinical and temporomandibular joint dysfunction patients. *J Craniomandibular Pract* 7:52–57, 1989.

Hickman D, Cramer R, Stauber W. The effect of four jaw relations on electromyographic activity in human masticatory muscles. *Arch Oral Biol* 38:261–264, 1993.

Ishigaki S, Bessette R, Maruyama T. A clinical study of temporomandibular joint (TMJ) vibration in TMJ dysfunction patients. *J Craniomandibular Pract* 11:7–13, 1993.

Kuwahara T, Bessette R, Maruyama T. Chewing pattern analysis in TMD patients with unilateral and bilateral internal derangement. *J Craniomandibular Pract* 13:167–172, 1995.

Lefkowitz M, Goldstein S, Lebovits A. Management of chronic pain of the head and neck: an anesthesiologist's perspective. In Cooper B, Lucente F (eds.), *Management of Facial, Head and Neck Pain.* Philadelphia: W.B. Saunders, 1989.

Lunn RH, Cooper BC, Coy RE, et al. Principles, concepts and practices in the management of craniomandibular diseases. In *Compendium,* vol. 20. Chicago: American Equilibration Society, 1987. Pp. 180–227.

Milhaib MA, Rosen M. History and etiology of MPD. *J Prosthet Dent* 44:438, 1980.

Moss ML. The functional matrix concept and its relationship to temporomandibular joint dysfunction and treatment. *Dent Clin North Am* 27:445–455, 1983.

Okeson JP (ed.). *Bell's Orofacial Pain* (5th ed.). Chicago: Quintessence, 1995.

Thomas M, Cooper BC. Recognition of craniomandibular disorders: a legal and professional responsibility. *NY State Dental J* 55:26–28, 1989.

Tsolka P, Fenion M, McCullock A, Preiskel H. A controlled clinical, electromyographic and kinesiographic assessment of craniomandibular disorders in women. *J Orofacial Pain* 8:80–89, 1994.

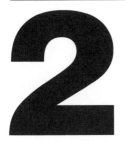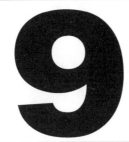

29

Trigeminal Neuralgia
Jyoti Patel-Silvera
David J. Wlody
Mathew Lefkowitz

I. Background. Trigeminal neuralgia (tic douloureux) is a pain syndrome that can usually be diagnosed on clinical grounds alone. Although there are many causes for facial pain, the symptomatology of trigeminal neuralgia is distinctive. The differentiation of tic douloureux from other facial pain syndromes is essential because it is **amenable to specific treatment** in the great majority of patients.

II. Pathophysiology

A. The trigeminal nerve arises from sensory and motor nuclei in the pons. The sensory root travels from the ventrolateral surface of the pons to the petrous portion of the temporal bone, where it expands into the gasserian ganglion, which is located within Meckel's cave. The nerve then divides into three divisions: the **ophthalmic,** which passes through the superior orbital fissure; the **maxillary,** which traverses the foramen rotundum; and the **mandibular,** which passes through the foramen ovale. These three divisions provide sensory innervation for the face.

B. In the vast majority of patients with trigeminal neuralgia, **compression of the nerve by a vascular structure** can be demonstrated within the posterior fossa. The segment of the nerve that is compressed will determine the division in which pain is perceived. Thus, pain in the second or third division is associated with compression of the rostral and anterior portion of the nerve, whereas pain in the first division is associated with compression of the caudal and posterior portion of the nerve.[1] Patients with multiple sclerosis are at increased risk of developing trigeminal neuralgia, and commonly have a demyelinated plaque in the retrogasserian portion of the nerve. It is not known, however, whether neuralgia appears as a result of the plaque, or whether the plaque is a result of nerve compression.

III. Signs and symptoms

A. The onset of trigeminal neuralgia usually occurs between the ages of 50 and 70; approximately 60% of cases are seen in females.

1. The onset of pain is **not associated with trauma or surgery.**

2. Pain is **often triggered by a minor stimulus,** such as shaving or brushing the teeth. As such, patients with trigeminal neuralgia may avoid normal activities of self-care, and can present a dishevelled and unkempt appearance.

3. Typically, patients with trigeminal neuralgia will report **unilateral, lancinating facial pain** that is limited to a single division of the fifth cranial nerve or to a combination of two divisions. The most common distributions are the second division (20%), third division (15%), and second and third division in combination (35%).[1]

4. Bilateral pain is possible, but never during a single attack; more typically, development of contralateral pain **will occur years after the initial episode.**

B. The pain is typically **crescendo in character,** and the interval between attacks can range from minutes to months or even years. Importantly, pain is completely absent between attacks, and there are no demonstrable sensory changes between attacks.

IV. Differential diagnosis

A. Unfortunately, there are no specific studies that will lead to an unequivocal diagnosis of trigeminal neuralgia. However, the history is so typical that **the diagnosis is seldom in doubt.** Nevertheless, a skull x-ray and CT scan or MRI should be used to rule out a neoplastic etiology for the symptoms. Other causes of facial pain that should be considered include

1. Atypical facial neuralgia

2. Postherpetic neuralgia
3. Cluster headache
4. Glossopharyngeal neuralgia
5. Myofascial pain
6. Temporomandibular joint (TMJ) syndrome
7. Neoplasm
8. Temporal arteritis
9. Sinusitis
10. Migraine
11. Tension headache
12. Eagle's syndrome (stylohyoid syndrome)
13. Dental pathology

B. **Atypical facial pain** can be **misdiagnosed as trigeminal neuralgia.** This disorder is more frequently associated with a constant burning or aching pain. Unlike trigeminal neuralgia, there is often a region of hypesthesia. A trigger point is unusual, but when present it is usually within the area of pain.[1]

V. **Pharmacologic treatment.** The principal treatment of trigeminal neuralgia is pharmacologic. The anticonvulsants **carbamazepine** and **diphenylhydantoin** have been used with great success. The antispasmodic agent **baclofen** has been introduced as an alternative to the anticonvulsant agents. Surgery should be considered only in those patients failing such treatment. In the event that pharmacologic therapy fails, gangliolysis, peripheral neurectomy or neurolysis, microvascular decompression, rhizotomy, or medullary trigeminal tractotomy can be attempted.

A. **Carbamazepine (Tegretol)**

1. The standard initial treatment of trigeminal neuralgia, carbamazepine is effective in approximately two thirds of patients. The initial therapy is 100 mg daily and should be increased by 100 mg every 2 days until a total daily dose of 600 mg is reached. This should be administered on a q8h schedule.
2. If there is insufficient response to this regimen after 1 week, the total dose should be increased by 200 mg. The daily dose can be increased by 200 mg every week, until a total dose of 1800 mg is reached. There is little utility to increasing the dose beyond this level.[1]
3. Gastric irritation is not uncommon; less frequently, myelosuppression may occur. For this reason, a CBC should be obtained monthly for the first year of treatment, and every 3 months thereafter.
4. Although many patients receiving carbamazepine will display mild leukopenia, it is necessary to stop therapy only if the WBC falls below 3500 cells/mm.[1] Finally, excessive somnolence may require cessation of therapy.

B. **Diphenylhydantoin (Dilantin)**

1. In those patients whose response to carbamazepine is limited, or in whom the side effects are unacceptable, treatment with diphenylhydantoin is frequently successful.
2. The typical dose is 300–400 mg daily, in divided doses given bid. Plasma levels should be monitored, and the drug should be stopped if a therapeutic response is not seen after plasma levels of 15–25 μg/ml have been achieved for 3 weeks.
3. As with carbamazepine, excessive sedation may require cessation of therapy, although this side effect can be related to excessive drug levels, and may respond to a lower dose of the drug.

C. **Baclofen (Lioresal)**

1. The skeletal muscle relaxant baclofen has been used successfully in the treatment of trigeminal neuralgia.[2] It is typically added to the primary agents because it appears to act synergistically with them.
2. The initial dose is 10 mg at bedtime for 2 days, after which the dose is increased to 10 mg bid. The total daily dose is increased by 10 mg every week, until a total dose of 80 mg is reached.
3. Baclofen may cause somnolence, ataxia, and confusion. Overdosage may produce seizures. **Abrupt termination** of therapy may lead to auditory and visual hallucinations and **should be avoided.**[3]

VI. **Neurolytic procedures**

A. **Gasserian gangliolysis**

1. Destruction of the gasserian ganglion **should be reserved for patients who have failed an adequate trial of pharmacologic therapy.** Initially, neurolysis was performed with chemical agents such as phenol, but recently radiofre-

quency thermal destruction has become a more common technique. Strictly speaking, the ganglion is not destroyed; the site of the lesion is within the retrogasserian portion of the nerve.

2. Gangliolysis is performed percutaneously and **does not require general anesthesia,** although sedation is required at several points during the procedure. Stimulation of the nerve allows the determination of those fibers responsible for the patient's pain. This permits selective destruction of those fibers, which allows the retention of normal sensation in divisions that are unaffected. In general, the treated division becomes analgesic, but otherwise retains normal sensation. This is a significant advantage of this procedure over peripheral neurectomy, in which pain relief is achieved at the cost of losing normal sensation in the treated division. This is of particular concern in cranial nerve V_1, where loss of corneal sensation can lead to the development of keratitis.

3. Radiofrequency gangliolysis leads to immediate pain relief in 99% of patients. At an average follow-up of 8 years, 14% of patients had recurrence of their pain; however, **repeat gangliolysis is equally as effective as the initial procedure.** Of those patients not demonstrating a recurrence, 92% rated their result as good or excellent; 5% rated their result as fair, primarily due to persistent dysesthesias.[4]

B. **Peripheral neurectomy or neurolysis.** Surgical and chemical destruction of peripheral branches of the trigeminal nerve have been used to treat trigeminal neuralgia for many years. Peripheral destructive procedures are reserved for those patients with little relief after percutaneous gangliolysis who are felt to be poor candidates for intracranial decompressive procedures. These procedures are much less frequently used since the advent of gasserian gangliolysis because

1. Pain relief seldom lasts longer than 1 year, and repeated procedures are likely to give even shorter periods of relief.

2. These peripheral procedures produce dense anesthesia, and as such are much more likely to lead to the development of dysesthesias and anesthesia dolorosa.

VII. **Intracranial procedures**

A. **Microvascular decompression**

1. Microvascular decompression of the trigeminal nerve is **commonly reserved for those patients with a poor response to gasserian gangliolysis.** However, in particularly expert hands, the results of decompression are so impressive and morbidity so low that the procedure may be a valid initial treatment in healthy patients who have failed medical therapy.[5]

2. The success of this procedure is due to the **high incidence of vascular compression of the nerve,** and is secondary to atherosclerotic changes in the intracranial vessels, which causes them to elongate and compress the nerve. This compression is probably further exacerbated by age-related sagging of the brain within the posterior fossa.

3. Decompression is performed via a **retromastoid craniectomy** under general anesthesia. Brain stem auditory-evoked response monitoring is helpful in preventing damage to the auditory nerve. When the compressing vessel is identified, it is mobilized and held away from the nerve with a Teflon pledget.

4. This procedure can be expected to produce complete relief of pain in 80% to 85% of patients. Another 10% will have partial relief of their pain, which is usually then well controlled with carbamazepine. In the 10% of patients with little relief after surgery, reexploration is usually indicated. The great majority of **patients retain normal sensation in the face** after decompression, which is a significant advantage over the neurodestructive procedures.

5. The recurrence rate is reported to be 7% in patients who did not undergo a previous destructive procedure, versus almost 50% in those who did undergo such a procedure. This would argue for a more widespread use of microvascular decompression, but only by those surgeons who have demonstrated a low rate of complications.

B. **Retrogasserian neurotomy** is section of the trigeminal nerve proximal to the gasserian ganglion.

1. It is generally reserved for those patients

a. Without obvious compression of the nerve at the time of an initial attempted decompressive procedure

b. Who have a poor result after decompression

2. Selective section of the root fibers should allow retention of normal sensation in the unaffected area of the face. Procedural risks include

   a. Unwanted anesthesia of the first division, leading to the potential of developing corneal injury

   b. The development of anesthesia dolorosa, which is a significant possibility due to the dense sensory loss in the affected region

   c. Loss of motor function

C. **Subnuclealis caudalis dorsal root entry zone (DREZ) lesions** of the subnuclealis caudalis have been shown to give good relief of postherpetic neuralgia in the trigeminal distribution, but only partial and short-lived relief in the treatment of trigeminal neuralgia.[6]

D. **Medullary trigeminal tractotomy,** section of the nucleus caudalis of the fifth cranial nerve and the overlying fibers of the descending spinal tract, will selectively interrupt pain sensation of the head and face, while preserving somatic sensation and motor function. Although there is not much experience in the use of this procedure for trigeminal neuralgia, it has been recommended as a secondary treatment for the disorder, particularly in patients with contralateral corneal anesthesia or trigeminal motor weakness, as these complications are unlikely to occur after tractotomy.[5]

VIII. **A stepwise treatment plan**

A. **The initial treatment** of trigeminal neuralgia **should be pharmacologic.** In stepwise fashion, **diphenylhydantoin** and **then baclofen** should be **added to carbamazepine** if pain relief is not achieved with maximum recommended dosages or at therapeutic plasma drug levels. Of course, unacceptable side effects should lead to the cessation of the offending drug.

B. **Gangliolysis** is frequently recommended for those patients whose pain is unrelieved by drug therapy, and it is certainly appropriate for those patients felt to be high-risk candidates for intracranial surgery. However, in view of the high success rate of microvascular decompression and its low mortality in skilled hands, it may be the procedure of choice in otherwise healthy patients failing drug treatment.

C. In patients with poor relief after gangliolysis, **microvascular decompression** is a logical next step. Should such a patient be considered to be at an unacceptably high risk to undergo craniotomy, peripheral neurolysis of the affected branches should be performed.

D. Patients without obvious compression of the trigeminal nerve at craniotomy are candidates for **retrogasserian neurotomy.** Similarly, patients with inadequate pain relief after decompression should undergo reexploration, as the compression of the trigeminal nerve may have recurred; if such recurrence cannot be demonstrated, retrogasserian neurotomy is indicated.

E. In those patients with persistent pain after craniotomy and reexploration, **trigeminal tractotomy** should be considered. Obviously, this highly aggressive procedure requires a degree of surgical experience and skill that may be available in only a very few centers.

References

1. Loeser J. Cranial neuralgias. In Bonica JJ (ed.), *The Management of Pain* (2nd ed.). Philadelphia: Lea & Febiger, 1990.
2. Fromm GH, Terrence CF, Chattha AS. Baclofen in the treatment of trigeminal neuralgia: double blind study and long term follow-up. *Ann Neurol* 15:240, 1984.
3. Cedarbaum JM, Schleifer LS. Drugs for Parkinson's disease, spasticity, and acute muscle spasms. In Gilman AG, Rall TW, Nies AS, Taylor P (eds.), *The Pharmacological Basis of Therapeutics.* New York: Pergamon, 1990. P. 480.
4. Loeser JD, Sweet WH, Tew JM, van Loveren H. Neurosurgical operations involving peripheral nerves. In Bonica JJ (ed.), *The Management of Pain* (2nd ed.). Philadelphia: Lea & Febiger, 1990. Pp. 2056–2059.
5. Jannetta PJ, Gildenberg PL, Loeser JD, et al. Operations on the brain and brain stem for chronic pain. In Bonica JJ (ed.), *The Management of Pain* (2nd ed.). Philadelphia: Lea & Febiger, 1990. Pp. 2082–2089.
6. Rosomoff HL, Papo I, Loeser JD. Neurosurgical operations on the spinal cord. In Bonica JJ (ed.), *The Management of Pain* (2nd ed.). Philadelphia: Lea & Febiger, 1990. P. 2079.

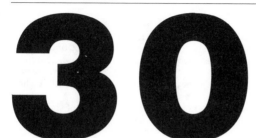

Intraoral Pain

Barry C. Cooper

I. **Background. Intraoral pain** can emanate from teeth, their supporting structures, and from the tissues lining the mouth, and can be acute or chronic. It can be localized or nonspecific and may be referred from elsewhere, or be an oral manifestation of a systemic disease.[1,2]

II. **Dental pain. Tooth pain** a superficial somatic type of pain, is readily reproducible by provocation and eliminated by local anesthetic application. It can be provoked by thermal stimuli (hot or cold), chemical stimuli (sweets), and palpation (biting pressure). It can be chronic or acute, spontaneous or only present on provocation.

Pain may emanate from a single tooth, from several teeth, or from a diffuse area,[3] and is most often unilateral and restricted to a single arch, maxillary or mandibular. If dental or periodontal disease is rampant, however, it can cause pain throughout the mouth. When the pain comes from teeth in the most posterior part of the mouth, the differentiation between maxillary and mandibular sites is sometimes difficult. For example, pain due to erupting mandibular third molars (wisdom teeth) may be felt throughout the mandible and oropharynx.

A. **Pulpal disease**

1. **Hyperemia.** The dental pulp contains nervous tissue and a blood supply. The initial reaction to any trauma to the dental pulp is hyperemia. In its earliest stage, hyperemia causes diffuse pain in several teeth in the area of the damaged tooth. As disease progresses, the pain becomes more localized, and in its mildest form, there is sensitivity to touch, including biting, and sensitivity to extreme temperatures, both hot and cold. Sensations are usually brief, lasting only as long as the noxious stimulus is applied, and subside after removal of the stimulus.

2. **Degeneration.** If hyperemia is allowed to progress, pulpal degeneration can ensue secondary to the compression of the engorged tissues within the rigid pulp canal inside the tooth. When the pulp has terminally necrosed, the tooth is exquisitely sensitive to touch, and the necrotic debris can be painfully expanded by the application of heat. In this stage, the sensitivity can last longer than the time the provoking stimulus is applied, or the pain may occur spontaneously without provocation. The application of cold (with ice), however, contracts the debris and relieves the pain.

   This type of pulpal disease is irreversible, although it can be successfully treated by scrupulously removing the debris and sterilizing the pulpal canal within the root and filling it with an inert material (root canal therapy). The diagnosis of this stage is made by determining whether the tooth is painful upon the application of heat or pressure and is selectively relieved by cold. Radiographs are also helpful if the disease process has caused a loss of calcium in the bone around the root apex. Whether the tooth will eventually heal or further degenerate depends on the magnitude and duration of the noxious stimulant as well as the extent of pulpal reaction to the stimulus.

B. **Etiology.** A combination of mechanical, chemical, thermal, and bacterial irritants can elicit an inflammatory response within the dental pulp.

1. **Functional trauma.** Traumatic occlusion can cause mechanical irritation to the pulp.[4] New dental restorations can traumatize the pulp by promoting malocclusion. Defective restorations can cause sensitivity to chemical agents such as sweets and thermal irritants.

2. **Fractures.** Fractured teeth are sensitive to temperature and to touch because the exposed dentin, the layer immediately beneath the noninnervated enamel, is exposed to noxious irritants. Vertically split teeth are also sensitive to

biting and even to touch[5] secondary to irritation of nerve structures within the dental pulp or in the periodontal surrounding structures. Incomplete fractures can cause chronic sensitivity. These are often not diagnosable until either part of the tooth can be moved with an examination instrument, or pulpal damage progresses to the terminal degenerative state producing radiographic findings of translucency around the roots as well as the classic thermal response.

3. **Other Trauma.** Trauma that does not break the continuity of the tooth's structure can still cause a hyperemic response and progress to degeneration. A history of trauma to the mouth is important in discovering the cause of this condition. A blow to the face or a hyperextension-flexion injury (whiplash) during which the mandibular teeth are momentarily flung into the maxillary teeth can cause damage to the teeth, temporomandibular joints, and masticatory musculature.[6] Subtle trauma can occur from hitting a coffee cup against the front teeth or unintentional biting directly on a fork while eating.

4. **Noxious habits.** Clenching, grinding, and frequent biting on objects such as pens, pipes, and fingernails can also irritate dental pulpal tissues causing pulpal hyperemia.

5. **Eruption.** The natural erupted position of teeth can cause traumatic occlusion, as can tooth migration. Erupting teeth can cause pain as they irritate the gingival tissues as well.

6. **Impaction** of teeth can cause pain in the gingival tissues and may cause pain within the alveolar bone.[7] Exfoliating deciduous (primary) teeth in children may also press against the intact gingiva with their sharp undersurface. This can occur over a prolonged period of time, sometimes lasting for months. Retained portions of teeth beneath the gingival surface can cause pain if active infection exists.

7. **Tooth decay** can cause pulpal hyperemia by acting as a chemical irritant. It is also important to remember that teeth can become nonvital with or without the introduction of bacteria into the pulp tissue.

C. **Diagnosis**
   1. **Clinical examination.** Note any bilateral asymmetry or missing parts of teeth that may have been fractured off. Nonvisable fractures can be more readily seen by transilluminating the tooth with a bright light. Note any tooth decay that appears initially chalky and later as a dark brown substance.

   Tooth movement indicates loss of supporting structure or fracture and can be felt by rocking the tooth between two rigid instruments and not with two fingertips, which are themselves compressible. Percuss single teeth with a blunt-ended rigid instrument and have the patient bite on a tongue blade to determine if individual teeth are sensitive to pressure.

   2. **Radiography** shows tooth decay, the status of dental restorations, integrity of tooth structure, root fractures, alveolar supporting bone levels, and disease within the bone adjacent to the teeth.[8] Radiolucency at the root apex of a tooth indicates pathology beneath the tooth caused by pulpal hyperemia, pulpal degeneration, or extension of periodontal disease. Panoramic radiographs visualize the entire dental apparatus and can reveal fractures, impacted teeth, and disease within the teeth as well as the maxilla and mandible. Lateral and frontal plane films can also be used to visualize disease in the hard structures of the oral cavity.

D. **Treatment**
   1. **Trauma with loss of structure.** Start conservatively with rest by elimination of occlusal contact. This is done judiciously by the removal of a minute amount of occlusal enamel to eliminate contact with the antagonistic teeth. This is a temporary measure as natural eruption of the tooth will return it to a functional position within several days.

   2. **Displacement.** If one or more teeth have been loosened or displaced, they can be gently manipulated into their proper place in the dental arch and fixed to adjacent firm teeth with composite restorative material. Teeth can be left splinted in this manner for several months.

   3. **Evulsion.** An evulsed tooth should be kept moist, gently cleaned, reimplanted quickly,[9,10] and stabilized by bonding it to adjacent teeth. It may eventually become devitalized, however. Endodontic treatment (root canal therapy) should be performed within 2 weeks.

   4. **Fractured teeth.** Restoration is possible if the fracture line does not extend

below the attachment of the gingival tissue to bone. If a gingival attachment is lacking, however, the stage is set for periodontal invasion by food and bacteria. Periodontal inflammation and abscess formation can follow thereby compromising the support of the tooth. A fracture that exposes the pulp or causes the pulp to undergo necrosis requires endodontic therapy prior to reconstruction. Teeth that have lost the entire coronal portion of their structure, that portion normally exposed in the mouth, can be restored, but a vertically fractured tooth must be extracted because the pulp chamber cannot be isolated and sterilized to permit successful root canal therapy.

5. **Defective restorations**—replacement
6. **Gingival recession**—desensitize the area or coat the surface of the root.
7. **Impacted teeth** are frequently extracted. They also can be surgically uncovered and have orthodontic appliances attached bringing them into proper position.
8. **Erupting mandibular third molars (wisdom teeth)** are frequently the cause of pain in the mandible, throat, and ear for a period of days at a time. The discomfort may reoccur frequently or intermittently over a prolonged period of time, even years. Gingival swelling associated with erupting teeth (pericoronitis) can occur after the tooth breaks through the gingiva and is only partially exposed. Ameliorative therapy consists of frequent rinses with hot salt water, which shrinks the swollen tissues and washes away food from under the gingival hood that partially covers the erupting tooth.
9. **Periodontal disease.** Inflamed or infected areas around the affected teeth[11] are first debrided and treated with antibiotics if necessary. Further periodontal surgery, including tooth extraction, may be necessary in more advanced cases.

III. **Soft and hard tissue diseases**
   A. **Symptoms.** Pain, burning,[12] anesthesia, chemical or thermal sensitivity, as well as swelling and pressure.[13,14]
   B. **Etiology.** Pain can emanate directly from the oral cavity or be referred from elsewhere. Direct painful disease processes include infection, neoplasia, and connective tissue, developmental, and nutritional disorders. Examples of referred symptoms include cardiac pain, causing discomfort in the mandibular molars, and the pain associated with trigeminal neuralgia, which can affect the second or third division of that nerve.[15]

   The oral cavity can be subjected to minor and major trauma, which can injure its soft tissue lining and deeper bony structures. Sharp or abrasive foods, nonfood objects such as pencils, caustic chemicals, hot beverages, and solid foods can traumatize the oral mucosa. Deep penetrating gunshot wounds and pointed objects can thrust through the mucosa into the bone. The highly innervated oral tissues will remain painful until healing is complete.
   C. **History.** Inquire about systemic diseases that might present with oral manifestations or oral pain.
   D. **Clinical examination.** After palpating the external head and neck structures, begin the intraoral examination.
      1. **Buccal mucosa.** With adequate light examine the cheeks visually and manually. Note any swelling, inflammation, induration, ulceration, or break in the normal continuity of the buccal mucosa. Begin on one side of the mouth and compare for bilateral symmetry. With a gloved hand, place the thumb on the inside of the mouth and the forefinger on the outside of the face opposite the thumb and palpate the buccal muscles (masseter and buccinator) and the parotid gland between the fingers. Observe the opening of the parotid gland's duct. Obstruction of that gland's orifice or its duct can cause pain and swelling at the time of eating owing to accumulation of saliva. Observe the tissues of the cheeks while continuing upward to the depth of the fold of the mucosa above the maxillary teeth as it reflects onto the gingiva. In a downward direction observe the oral mucosa of the cheek through the depth of the fold beneath the mandibular teeth as it reflects up onto the gingiva. Moving anteriorly, examine the inner surfaces of the upper and lower lips and the anterior gingiva.

      Scrutinize any white lesion or ulceration. Raised discrete white lesions are more likely to be manifestations of more serious disease than flat indiscrete lesions. Commonly occurring hyperkeratosis resulting from chronic irritants in the mouth, such as smoking, should be differentiated from neoplastic or precancerous lesions. All white lesions in the oral cavity should be suspect until a definitive diagnosis is made.[16,17]

2. **Palate.** Examine the palate beginning behind the anterior teeth and ending as far back in the oropharynx as possible. Note any interruptions in the normal pink glistening palatal mucosa, inflammation, swelling, ulceration, or white lesions.

Occasionally there is a bony projection (flat or raised) in the midline of the palate usually covered with normal pink mucosa, which may become traumatized and secondarily inflamed or ulcerated. This is a bony exostosis, called the **torus palatinus,** and is not a disease process.

Examine the anterior palate immediately behind the anterior teeth for it is commonly traumatized by physical, thermal, and chemical irritants. A slough is frequently observed after drinking very hot beverages or eating pizza. The area is extremely painful as it overlies the incisal foramen through which the palate's sensory nerves exit from the bone.

3. **Tongue and floor of the mouth.** Ask the patient to protrude the tongue then grasp it with a gauze sponge. Examine its lateral borders noting any white lesions, ulceration, or induration. This is a common location of oral neoplasia, as is the floor of the mouth beneath the tongue, which can be visualized as the tongue is moved to the opposite side of the mouth. Traumatic injuries are also common in this area. Note any scalloped contours on the lateral surface. This is not pathologic but indicates a long-standing pressure of the tongue against the lingual (inner) surfaces of the teeth. It is a sign of prolonged tongue-assisted mandibular posturing and is a soft tissue accommodation to overclosure of the mandible in occlusion which can predispose to temporomandibular disorders. A red or white pattern may be observed on the surface of the tongue also. Called geographic tongue, because of its maplike appearance, the pattern changes within a few days. It is a nonpathologic inflammatory condition, which should be monitored until it disappears.

4. **Canker sores.** A common lesion, in any soft tissue of the mouth, is an ulcerated canker sore. Although preceded by a vesicular state, it is usually not noticed by the patient until the vesicle breaks leaving a painful gray slough surrounded by a pink halo. The illness is self-limiting, healing within 14 days. Multiple lesions of various sizes may exist and are very painful, especially when foods are placed in the mouth.

5. **Gingiva.** Examine the gingiva on the outer and inner sides of both dental arches. Note any inflammation, bleeding, purulence, foreign objects (including pieces of teeth and dental restorations), food debris, or broken off pieces of calculus (tartar).

E. **Other diagnostic modalities.** Dental radiographs are helpful in diagnosing oral infection, neoplasm, fracture, cyst formation, foreign body, or erupting teeth. They are excellent for a general overview and provide precise clarity of detailed structures. CT scans and MRI are also utilized to visualize the craniomandibular structures. Bacterial cultures[18] and histologic examination of biopsy specimens can also contribute to the diagnosis of soft and hard tissue disease. When noninvasive diagnostic techniques have failed to make a definitive diagnosis, exploratory surgery can be undertaken.

Consultation with other health care providers[19] may be necessary to fully diagnose and treat a patient complaining of intraoral pain, especially when complaints include pain in other head and neck areas and no physical cause of the pain is discernible.

F. **Treatment.** Remove local irritants if they are disrupting soft tissues, employ antibiotics if indicated, and utilize warm saline, hydrogen peroxide, and special chemical rinses for the management of inflammation (gingivitis).

To ameliorate superficial somatic pain, apply topical anesthetics. This is an excellent technique for differential diagnosis to discriminate between superficial somatic pain (eliminated with local anesthetic) and deep somatic pain, neurogenous pain, and psychosomatic pain with superficially referred manifestations, which are not eliminated with local anesthetic application.

Surgical removal of diseased tissue and cysts, which often cause pressure on teeth, can be employed as can periodontal treatment. The latter always includes debridement of the affected tissues and sometimes soft and hard tissue surgery to restore healthy periodontal architecture.

Inflammatory soft tissue diseases, such as pemphigus vulgaris, are treated with systemic and local medications. Neoplasia within the oral tissues may be treated with a combination of surgery, chemotherapy, and radiotherapy. Canker sores can be palliatively treated with medications that coat the lesions with a waterproof salve containing topical anesthetics.

IV. **Prognosis**

    A. **Periodontal disease.** Therapy is successful on a long-term basis if the amount of bone loss around the teeth is not excessive and a stringent home care regimen is maintained.

    B. **Necrotic pulpal tissue and periapical disease.** Endodontic treatment is very effective in providing a long-term cure.

    C. **Tooth evulsion.** Reimplantation has a guarded prognosis.

    D. **Chronic intraoral inflammatory disease (i.e., pemphigus).** Pharmacologic therapy has a variable prognosis, sometimes maintaining long-term comfort rather than eliminating the disease process.

    E. **Neoplasia.** Variable prognosis depending on characteristics of neoplasm and a patient's response to therapy.

V. **Neurogenous pain.** The severing of a dental nerve, as occurs during endodontic treatment or tooth extraction, can result in a deafferentation phenomenon producing a chronic pain of neurogenous nature.[20] If complaints of anesthesia, paresthesia, hyperesthesia, and hypoesthesia are offered, the possibility of neurogenic pain should be entertained. This pain cannot be treated superficially.

References

1. Glick DH. Locating referred pulpal pains. *Oral Surg* 15:613, 1962.
2. Matson MS. Pain in the orificial region associated with coronary insufficiency. *Oral Surg* 16:284, 1963.
3. Mitchell D, Tarpley R. Painful pulpitis. *Oral Surg* 13:1360, 1960.
4. Landay MA, Seltzer S. The effects of excessive occlusal force on the pulp. *Oral Surg* 32:623, 1971.
5. Cameron C. Cracked tooth syndrome; additional findings. *J Am Dent Assoc* 93:971, 1976.
6. Kinnie BH. From the outside looking in. Presented to the American Academy of Dental Radiology, Atlanta, October 19, 1984.
7. Tanner HA, Kitchen RN. An effective treatment for pain in the eruption of primary and permanent teeth. *J Dent Child* 31:289–292, 1964.
8. Hensen BF. Clinical and roentgenologic carries detection. *Dentomaxillofacial Radiol* 9:34–36, 1980.
9. Edgerton MT. Emergency care of maxillofacial injuries. In Zuidema GD, Rutherford RB, Ballinger WF II (eds.), *The Management of Trauma* (3rd ed.). Philadelphia: W.B. Saunders, 1979.
10. Braham RL, Roberts MW, Morris ME. Management of dental trauma in children and adolescents. *J Trauma* 17:857–865, 1977.
11. Catalgo E, Santis H. Response of the oral tissue to exogenous foreign materials. *J Periodontol* 45:93, 1974.
12. Gruskka M. Burning mouth: a preview and update. *Ont Dent* 60:56–61, 1983.
13. Kreisberg MK. Atypical odontalgia: differential diagnosis and treatment. *J Am Dent Assoc* 104:852, 1982.
14. Sicher H. Problems of pain in dentistry. *Oral Surg* 7:149, 1954.
15. Roberts AM, Person P. Etiology and treatment of idiopathic trigeminal and atypical facial neuralgias. *Oral Surg* 48:298, 1979.
16. Shafer WG, Hine MK, Levey BM. *A Textbook of Oral Pathology* (4th ed.). Philadelphia: W.B. Saunders, 1983.
17. Zegarelli EV, Kutscher AH, Hyman GA. *Diagnosis of Diseases of the Mouth and Jaws* (2nd ed.). Philadelphia: Lea & Fibeger, 1978.
18. Kannangara DW, Thadepelli H, McQuinter JL. Bacteriology and treatment of dental infections. *Oral Surg* 50:103, 1980.
19. Feinman C. Psychogenic facial pain: presentation and treatment. *J Psychosom Res* 27:403–410, 1983.
20. Okeson, JP. *Bell's Orofacial Pains* (5th ed.). Chicago: Quintessence, 1995.

Selected Readings

Andreasen JO. *Traumatic Injuries of the Teeth.* St. Louis: C.V. Mosby, 1972.

Bender IB, Seltzer S. The effect of periodontal disease on the pulp. *Oral Surg* 33:458, 1972.

Bender IB, Seltzer S, Soltanoff W. Endodontic success—a reappraisal of criteria. *Oral Surg* 22:780, 1966.

Bernick S. Vascular and nerve changes associated with the healing of the human pulp. *Oral Surg* 33:983, 1972.

Bhaskar SN, Rappaport HM. Dental vitality tests and pulp status. *J Am Dent Assoc* 86:409, 1973.

Blair HA. Relationships between endodontics and periodontics. *J Periodontol* 43:209, 1972.

Kruger G. *Textbook of Oral and Maxillofacial Surgery* (5th ed.). St. Louis: C.V. Mosby, 1979.

Lozada F, Silverman S, Cram D. Pemphigus vulgaris: a study of six cases treated with levamisole and prednisone. *Oral Surg* 54:161, 1982.

Lubke RG, Glick DH, Ingle JI. Indications and contraindications for endodontic surgery. *Oral Surg* 18:97, 1964.

Morris ML. Diagnosis, prognosis and treatment of the loose tooth. *Oral Surg* 6:957–964, 1963.

Seltzer S, Bender IB, Zionty M. The interrelationship of pulp and periodontal disease. *Oral Surg* 16:1474, 1963.

Shklar G. The oral lesions of pemphigus vulgaris. *Oral Surg* 23:629, 1967.

Trapnell DH, Bowerman JLE. *Dental Manifestation of Systemic Disease.* London: Butterworth, 1973.

31

Pelvic and Low Abdominal Pain
John S. McDonald

I. **Background.** Pain in the gynecologic patient is often difficult to diagnose for many members of the health care team. **Gynecologic pain** may be expressed as **either pelvic or abdominal** pain. The differentiation is elusive, and often pelvic and abdominal pain can be interchanged because of the location of the pelvic viscera in the lower abdominal cavity. Consultation for pain limited to the pelvic area often occurs only after significant agony is endured by the patient. This is partly because the patient is loath to seek medical advice regarding her sexual organs unless the pain is either unbearable or not manageable with over-the-counter drugs. This discussion will focus on the differential diagnosis of the various etiologies of acute and chronic abdominal and pelvic pain. Table 31-1 summarizes the characteristics of many of the abdominal and pelvic pain syndromes.

II. **Acute disorders**
   A. **Common pelvic pain problems**
      1. **Introital glandular problems**
         a. **Bartholinitis.** Pain, tenderness, and dyspareunia are the three chief complaints of this disease process. The diagnosis is easily made with visualization of the Bartholin's glands, which lie in the posterior aspect of the lower part of the labrum magus on each side. Infection is usually the problem, and once the gland has been infected, inflamed, and finally purulent, the only choice is for surgical opening along the inner aspect of the labia with finger dissection of the multiple cystic ductal dilatations that often occur. Appropriate antibiotic therapy based on culture results is an essential adjunct to surgery.
         b. **Skene's urethritis.** Skene's glands lie just at the urethral orifice and usually suffer from an inflammatory process. Again, culture and use of appropriate antibiotics are the keystone of management.
      2. **Viral infections**
         a. **Herpes virus** is present in the cervix of asymptomatic women and in the urethras and prostates of asymptomatic men. The cycle is predictable and almost self-diagnostic. The incubation period after infection is short, generally lasting from 2 to 7 days, followed by tingling and itching, which occur just before painful vesicular eruptions occur. Dysuria, dyspareunia, and groin pain due to lymphadenopathy may develop. Treatment consists of generous applications of acyclovir (Zovirax) cream, which dry up the vesicular eruptions relatively quickly. This treatment does not eradicate the virus from the sacral sensory ganglia; thus, recurrence months or years later is common. Postherpetic neuralgia can also occur.
         b. **Condyloma acuminata,** the common venereal wart, is flat and takes many forms. It is often but not always void of painful stimulus. The larger lesions may have to be eradicated with fulguration, cryotherapy, or even surgical excision. The early phases of the disease process can also be treated with 5-fluorouracil.
      3. **Mucous membrane problems**
         a. **Vaginitis.** It is common for vaginal problems to be associated with itching, burning, discharge, or even vaginal pain. In the sexually active female the most common symptom often becomes dyspareunia. There are many bacterial and viral causes; candidiasis also looms as a causative agent. The most common protozoal cause is *Trichomonas*. The diagnosis is made by visual inspection of the mucous membrane through a careful speculum examination.

Table 31-1. Abdominal and pelvic pain

	Appendicitis	Diverticu-litis	Mesenteric thrombosis	Acute salpingitis	Ruptured ectopic	Corpus luteum cyst
Age	Any	20–40	40–60	16–40	25–35	14–21
Onset	Gradual	Gradual	Sudden	Gradual	Sudden	Sudden
Profile	Colicky-constant, general area-McBurney	Dull ache LLQ radiates umbilicus and pubes	Severe, knifelike epigastric-general	Dull ache iliac fossae, radiates low back	Severe, sharp, stabbing, unilateral, iliac fossae with radiation back	Brief, severe illness
Symptoms	N/V, rigidity, constipation or diarrhea (less)	Constipation, N/V, tenderness and rigidity LLQ	History of vascular disease, collapse, abdominal tenderness, melena	History of sexual promiscuity, vaginal discharge dysuria, rigidity lower abdomen	History of amenorrhea, other symptoms of pregnancy, collapse, tenderness, anemia, cul-de-sac masses and ovarian	Patient mid-cycle, nausea, tenderness with rigidity, vaginal bleeding
Temperature (°F)	99–100	99–100	98 or lower	100–103	99–100	99
WBC	10,000–18,000	10,000–15,000	10,000–12,000	12,000–25,000	10,000–12,000	10,000–12,000
Pelvic exam	Clear right ovary and parametrium Rectal exam confirms right-sided pain	Clear pelvic structures bilaterally Rectal exam produces diffuse discomfort poorly localized	Clear pelvic structures bilaterally Rectal exam negative	Acute tenderness in area location; slight cervix movement causes exquisite pain	Palpable mass with tenderness on involved side Rectal exam confirmatory	Confirm mass on involved side with or without tenderness, may detect peritoneal pain if cystic rupture Rectal exam confirmatory

LLQ = left lower quadrant; N/V = nausea and/or vomiting.

   b. **Vaginismus** was first described as an involuntary disorder of the supporting musculature of the vagina including the levator ani, pubococcygeus, and perhaps the deep transverse perineal muscles.[1]
      (1) **Symptoms.** It can cause significant sexual dysfunction because of the physical effects, which prevent vaginal entry by extreme muscle spasm, and the psychological effects, which elicit overt associated pain behavior.
      (2) **Diagnosis.** On examination, the patient is often found to be anxious and distressed about undergoing pelvic examination. The doctor must reassure the patient that she can be examined without undue pain with slow, careful, single-digit exploration before any attempted speculum insertion. Often these patients have attempted speculum examinations before which have proved to be disastrous for both the patient and the examiner. The psychological impact of such a scenario only reinforces in the patient the idea that she has something seriously wrong with her anatomy.
      (3) **Causes.** Congenital, infectious, traumatic, or psychogenic etiologies are

Table 31-1. Continued

Twisted ovary	Renal colic	Pyelitis/ cystitis	Dysmenor- rhea	Endometri- tis	Fibroids	Uterine inversion
18–40	45–70	30–70	17–37	20–40	30–50	40–60
Sudden	Sudden	Gradual	Sudden	Gradual	Gradual	Sudden
Sharp and stablike in iliac fossa radiating to lower back	Severe, colicky renal region, radiates hip or thigh ipsilateral	Dull, ache in bladder, radiates ureters	Aching, griping, colicky, supra- pubic pain	Soreness and cramps, low back pain	Dull, dragging sensation	Violent pain
History of pelvic mass collapse, iliac tender- ness, pelvic mass	Tenderness in renal area, rigidity, hematuria or pyuria	History of renal problems, dyuria, pyuria, chills, fever, tender renal areas	1–3 Days of constant cramplike pain with also referred backache, associated loose stools	Chills, fever, tender abdomen, malaise	Pelvic pressure, dull ache, sensation constant	Sudden violent constant pain
98.6	98.6–100	101–104	98–99	101–103	98	98
10,000– 12,000	10,000– 12,000	15,000– 25,000	8,000– 12,000	10,000– 18,000	8,000– 12,000	8,000– 12,000
Detecting of mass and tenderness on involved side Rectal exam confirma- tory	Clear pelvic structures Rectal exam confirma- tory	Clear pelvic structures Rectal exam confirma- tory	Diffuse uterine tender- ness; otherwise, negative Rectal exam negative	Severe uterine tender- ness, no para- metrial tenderness Rectal exam, possible rectovagi- nal tender- ness	Some tender- ness, may detect irregular masses Rectal exam confirma- tory	Obvious uterine inversion

possible. There may be many varied reasons for psychogenic vaginismus, such as sexual avoidance due to childhood or even adulthood trauma or marital sexual adjustment problems.

(4) **Treatment.** Any approach must gain the confidence of the patient so that she can understand that her condition can usually be successfully treated. Along with the use of mechanical vaginal dilators, treatment should provide reassurance and support through repeated psychotherapy sessions aimed at the psychogenic aspect of the disease process. Over time the therapy sessions will help the patient regain confidence and realize that she is "healthy." Similarly, she will gradually begin to experi- ence the physical capacitance she thought not possible owing to her own careful manipulation of the mechanical dilators. It is important to involve the partner very early in the diagnosis and treatment so that the patient does not feel isolated and does not have to hide the treatment methods. Therapy should continue until the patient and her partner begin to experience success with both the physical and psychological aspects of

the problem. Treatment of this disorder illustrates the importance of a multidisciplinary approach. The gynecologist, the psychologist or psychiatrist, and perhaps a marital counselor should work closely to ensure complete and long-lasting relief from this disorder.

c. **Cervicitis.** Lymphatic drainage and the tendency for superficial infections to occur can lead to low back pain. Except for dilatation, the cervix is remarkably devoid of pain sensation. Significant excoriations and crypt formations are often found through a colposcopic examination without any real complaints of pain from the patient. A very common sign of cervicitis, however, is discharge which may become malodorous. Again, diagnosis is made via a visual examination of the cervix, with colposcopy added for definition and mapping. Treatment usually consists of actual destruction of the superficial involved areas by cautery, cryotherapy, or surgical excision by performing a conization of the cervix.

4. **Myofascial disease of the pelvic floor** has been called pyriformis syndrome, coccygodynia, or levator ani spasm syndrome, among others. Effective therapy includes local injection of the pelvic floor muscles in spasm and relaxation exercises.[2]

5. **Uterine pathology**
   a. **Acute dysmenorrhea**
      (1) **Symptoms.** The pain is usually sharp, intermittent, and cramping and may begin just before the onset of menstruation and become gradually progressive until it reaches incapacitating levels.
      (2) **Treatment.** Nonsteroidal anti-inflammatory compounds such as **indomethacin, ibuprofen,** and **mefenaminic acid** are effective. Use of **progestational drugs** has also been popular because of their effectiveness in suppressing prostaglandin levels during the menstrual periods.
   b. **Endometriosis** is another significant cause of pain in menstruating women. The working **diagnosis** of endometriosis is suggested by **dysmenorrhea, dyspareunia, dysfunctional uterine bleeding, and infertility.** Traditionally, confirmation was by laparotomy or laparoscopy; currently it is mostly by **laparoscopy.** In a 1977 surgical study, both dyspareunia and dysmenorrhea were improved in the surgery group.[3]
   c. **Endometritis.** With this disorder, pain occurs after a term delivery or when there is an early delivery or abortion. The pain is usually characterized by lower abdominal tenderness and an abrupt temperature rise to 101–103°F. Pelvic examination reveals exquisite tenderness with minimal movement of the cervix, which in turn moves the uterus and parametrial structures. Again, local cultures and blood cultures should be obtained for identification of the causative agent and institution of appropriate antibiotics. A probe should be placed through the cervical canal to ensure proper drainage.[3]
   d. **Uterine fibroids** are the most common tumors of the uterus. They are often asymptomatic, but can become painful with age and degeneration. Fibroids are not fibrous tissue but smooth muscle tumors, rich with blood supplies.[4] Although they usually occur in the fundus, they may grow in the cervix and even in the round and broad ligaments. Pain can occur due to torsion and occlusion of the local blood supply. Unusually, pain has also been caused by subserous fibroids attaching to nearby organs, such as the liver, which subsequently simulates cholecystitis during involution of the fibroid stalk attachment. Recent innovation in surgical approaches to submucous fibroids have allowed effective alternatives to laparotomy.[5]
   e. **Uterine inversion** is a rare but serious problem that can occur during abortion or delivery of a placenta. The uterine cavity becomes partially or completely involuted because of strenuous pushing or pulling, with resultant immediate and violent pain and serious bleeding. The diagnosis is made by speculum examination or is readily apparent if the uterus is completely inverted and extruding from the introitus. The patient may or may not have to be anesthetized, and the uterine corpus should be carefully replaced while trying to avoid rupture.[6] Immediate detection and treatment quickly must follow one another when this problem occurs.[7]

6. **Fallopian tube and ovarian pathology**
   a. **Acute salpingitis.** An acute infection process of the fallopian tubes presents the following symptoms:

(1) Acute onset of **pain** in both lower abdominal quadrants with rebound tenderness
(2) Fever
(3) A **discrete tenderness** on movement **of the cervix**
(4) On bimanual examination, there is also point **tenderness along the pathway of the tubes** from the midline out to the pelvic brim bilaterally. On occasion there may be small palpable masses present, indicative of pyosalpinx or hydrosalpinx.

b. Ruptured ectopic pregnancy. Many gynecologic conditions can be confused with ectopic pregnancy. The most frequently misdiagnosed disorders are a corpus luteum cyst, urinary tract disease, appendicitis, and salpingitis.[8] Hemorrhage is the chief concern in this process and is responsible for a large number of deaths. It is important to quickly diagnose and treat this problem so that hemorrhage and rupture do not occur. Ultrasound will confirm the diagnosis.

c. Corpus luteum cyst. Pain from this cyst occurs gradually and unilaterally, progressing to severe tenderness over the affected ovary. There may or may not be a palpable mass depending on the size of the cyst. Even small cystic bleeds can produce exquisite pain and tenderness. The menstrual period is often delayed as in ectopic pregnancy, with which it is often confused. Laparotomy may be indicated because of brisk bleeding secondary to a vessel rupture along the margin of the cyst. Early detection and treatment can prevent life-threatening hemorrhage just as in ruptured ectopic pregnancy.

d. Twisted ovarian cyst can be any type of ovarian-based cyst that grows to a size that causes local vascular embarrassment. It is this embarrassment that causes the pain and demands immediate attention. Most often, the only symptoms from ovarian cysts are a sense of pelvic ache or heaviness, which does not always occur in the early stages. It is not until torsion or twisting that the pain, often sharp and stabbing, radiates into the iliac fossa and low back, prompting the individual to seek medical attention.

B. Common abdominal pain problems

1. Vascular origins of pain: mesenteric thrombosis. Pain occurs suddenly and is located in the epigastrium rather than the lower abdomen. The pain is severe and knifelike, and the abdomen is tender and may be rigid owing to the effect of free peritoneal blood.[9] Nausea and vomiting may occur early with hyperactive bowel sounds progressing to a quiet abdomen.

2. Bowel pathology

a. Diverticulitis. Small outpouchings in the large intestine result in weakened wall structures and isolation from the main lumen of the bowel by a narrowed neck structure. These can become inflamed and may rupture with severe consequences indicative of localized peritonitis. The onset is usually gradual but eventually moves from a dull ache with left lower quadrant radiation to more generalized abdominal tenderness and even rigidity.[10]

b. Appendicitis. Anorexia, nausea, and vomiting occur with mild to moderate abdominal pain that is somewhat generalized at onset, eventually localizes to the periumbilical area, and then, finally, in classic form to the right lower quadrant. It occurs more frequently in persons under 30 years of age. The differential diagnosis becomes difficult when ectopic pregnancy, ovarian or cystic torsion, or acute salpingitis are considered. A careful pelvic examination should rule out pathology in the ovarian and tubal structures of the right side if they can be palpated separately on bimanual examination. Furthermore, rectal tenderness and pain on hyperextension of the pelvis and lower spine should elicit typical pain patterns. More recently, ultrasound has been used as a very effective tool in differential diagnosis.[11]

3. Urinary tract pathology

a. Pyelitis or cystitis. Early symptoms include frequency of and a constant burning pain with micturition. Often there is a dull ache in the lower abdomen over the central portion of the pubic bone. There may be cloudy, foul-smelling urine as an added complaint. The patient often complains of lassitude and perineal heaviness and pressure.[12]

b. Renal colic results in pain that is sudden, episodic, and agonizing; it is widely considered to be comparable to the pain of childbirth. It is located in the costovertebral angle and flank area with radiation to the lower quadrant of the abdomen.[13] It may be associated with urinary frequency and urgency and hematuria. The pain is typically and diagnostically episodic in nature owing to peristaltic wave generation in the ureter and may be accompanied by severe nausea and vomiting.

III. Chronic disorders

A. Vulvodynia

1. **Diagnosis**
   a. Lack of therapeutic responsiveness usually means that patients are seen by several health care providers including gynecologists, dermatologists, psychologists, and psychiatrists. Six **initial parameters** of vulvodynia were established by Dodson and Friedrich:[14]
      (1) It is chronic.
      (2) It is idiopathic in etiology.
      (3) Sexual inactivity plays a large role.
      (4) There are multiple physician visits.
      (5) Allergy is often blamed as a major culprit.
      (6) Psychophysiologic etiology is usually entertained only as a last resort.
   b. **Physical examination** often reveals redness and early chronic epithelial changes. The differential diagnosis must include **vestibulitis, candidiasis, neuralgia, human papillomavirus, lupus, lichen scleroses, and plasma cell vulvitis.** Biopsies should be able to rule out and differentiate between lupus, lichen scleroses, and plasma cell vulvitis.

2. **Psychological factors**
   a. Vulvodynia is a disorder with significant **psychological aspects** because of its associated sexual dysfunction. Important psychological features include:[15]
      (1) Depression
      (2) Anger directed at medical care
      (3) Obsessive behavior
      (4) Nonsexual intimacy
   b. Most patients are **dissatisfied with their sexual relationship.** Younger patients suffering from vulvodynia are usually sexually active because of established patterns. Dysfunction sets in early with a major impact upon sexual behavioral patterns such as frequency, foreplay, and sexual habit.
   c. Women with chronic pelvic conditions tend to have **major problems with marriage, psychosexual interactions, and interpersonal interactions.**[15,16] Vulvodynia is an example of a disease process whose respondent factors influence and help develop operant behavior. Many patients have minimal or moderate changes in the vulva. When present, the cracking and fissuring may be due to trauma secondary to difficult and forceful penile entry in face of vaginismus and absence of adequate lubrication. Over time this type of respondent behavior results in the development of obvious operant behavior. Despite significant emotional distress, most patients may refuse to obtain professional counseling, and many decline the use of suggested antidepressant medication.

B. Pelvic congestion
is also associated with psychological as well as somatic factors. Many investigators have attempted to elucidate the primary causative factors. Beard and associates found that improvement was only obtained when psychotherapy was used.[17] In a Swedish study, 15 women with chronic pelvic pain with demonstrated left-sided varicosities had extraperitoneal resection of the left ovarian vein.[18] Their 8-year follow-up revealed that eight women were cured, three had some pain relief, but four women were not helped at all. The authors proposed that patients receive renal phlebography as a final resort to detect pathology in an otherwise negative workup.

C. Genitofemoral pain.
Afflictions of the genitofemoral nerve are responsible for causing much pain and distress in both females and males. Although this pain can present in many different ways, it typically occurs in the **inguinal area** and the **upper inner thigh** and is **exacerbated with activity.** The **spinal cord segments** of various peripheral nerves, **with area of innervation** of the lower abdomen and upper thigh, are as follows:

1. **Iliohypogastric** T12 and L1
2. **Ilioinguinal L1**
3. **Genitofemoral L1 and L2**
4. **Lateral femoral cutaneous L2 and L3**

Table 31-2. Results of presacral neurectomy

Group	No pathology	Pathology
Dysmenorrhea		
Success	5	24
Failure	3	8
Dyspareunia		
Success	4	22
Failure	0	8

Source: Adapted from Lee RB, Stone K, Maglessen D, et al. Presacral neurectomy for chronic pelvic pain. *Obstet Gynecol* 68:517, 1986.

D. Chronic dysmenorrhea

1. Dysmenorrhea of a chronic nature **accounts for a large number of office gynecology visits.** A study of dysmenorrhea revealed a high incidence and a large number of identified severe cases.[19] The incidence in this study group of 2621 was 72.4%, and 15.4% were severe cases. The etiology has been ascribed to increased contractility, decreased menstrual flow, family history, and nicotine inhibition.

2. **Treatment.** There is much variation in the therapeutic approach, including analgesics for 38% of patients, physician visits for 21%, and other therapeutic trials for 41%. Dysmenorrhea is a disease process that typifies the idea that pain can only be appreciated by the affected patient who, try as she may, cannot express adequately the extent of her pain or suffering.

   a. Despite the wide spectrum of pain therapies, the common goal should be **maximum pain relief with minimum medication.**

   b. Recently, use of the **nonsteroidal anti-inflammatory drugs** such as mefenamic acid, naproxen, and ibuprofen (which reduce endometrial prostaglandin E_2 or $F_{2\alpha}$) have been effective additions to the treatment of dysmenorrhea.

   c. The general consensus for action of **acupuncture** suggests that combined visceral-cutaneous, visceral-visceral, and cutaneous-visceral inputs affect impulses traveling on A fibers that prevent the slower-transmitting A delta and C fibers from passing their information on to the CNS. In addition, there is the well-known increase in endogenous endorphin levels. A 1987 study evaluated the efficacy of acupuncture in the treatment of dysmenorrhea and found it to be an effective treatment for many patients.[20]

   d. When the first lines of defense for dysmenorrhea, using antiprostaglandins and ovulation suppression, have not been effective, and when other opioids have not been adequate, one could consider **presacral neurectomy.** One surgical study of presacral neurectomy included two groups with success and failures as shown in Table 31-2.[21] The authors of this study concluded that presacral neurectomy should be considered as an alternative treatment only in women with dysmenorrhea or dyspareunia for whom medical treatment has failed.

IV. Psychological issues

A. **Somatization disorder.** This diagnosis depends on recognition of a physician-shopper with multiple vague symptoms void of physical cause. These patients use their symptoms as a way to communicate emotions. Despite a chaotic, often violent struggle in their personal lives, these patients display numerous physical symptoms rather than anxiety or depression. Physicians who are not oriented to recognize this tend to repeatedly pursue organic possibilities with multiple tests, procedures, and medications, and even operative procedures.[22]

B. **Concurrent diagnoses and symptoms.** Walker et al. found that chronic pelvic pain sufferers had greater incidences of lifetime major depressive illnesses.[23] There were marked percentage differences of other diagnoses as well between a group with pain as the chief complaint and a group of gynecologic patients without pain (Table 31-3). Also, somatic symptoms were significantly different in these two groups of patients (Table 31-4).

C. **Onset of psychological dysfunction**

1. It is often not possible to determine the onset of psychological dysfunction in

Table 31-3. Depressive illness in patients suffering from chronic pelvic pain

	Pain group	Standard gynecologic patients
Depression	64%	17%
Drug dependency	52%	20%
Dyspareunia	52%	7%
Sexual dysfunction	56%	24%

Source: Adapted from Walker E, Katon W, Harrop-Griffiths J, et al. Relationship of chronic pelvic pain to psychiatric diagnoses and childhood sexual abuse. *Am J Psychiatry* 145:75, 1988.

Table 31-4. Somatic symptoms in patients suffering from chronic pelvic pain

Symptom	Pain group	Standard gynecologic patients
Abdominal pain	52%	10%
Dysmenorrhea	60%	20%
Shortness of breath	24%	3%
Dizziness	28%	7%
Weakness	36%	3%
Abnormal periods	32%	1%

Source: Adapted from Walker E, Katon W, Harrop-Griffiths J, et al. Relationship of chronic pelvic pain to psychiatric diagnoses and childhood sexual abuse. *Am J Psychiatry* 145:75, 1988.

relation to pain. A large proportion of patients with pelvic pain reveal little or no psychological component on initial or follow-up visits. Many physicians refer their pelvic pain patients for psychological examination because all tests have proved negative. Anxiety and depression may act as facilitators of nociception and actually enhance the pain experience.[24] Stress may serve as a stimulator that unleashes a local-tissue pain reaction. Patients' refusal to accept psychological factors as a major cause of their problem prevents them from obtaining successful treatment. The psychologist therefore should be introduced to the patient early in the treatment process.

2. Child sexual abuse and adult sexual adjustment problems are often reported by patients with chronic pelvic pain. Walker et al. found that 64% of women with chronic pelvic pain had experienced some type of sexual abuse at or before the age of 14, whereas the standard gynecologic patients had a 23% incidence of childhood sexual abuse.[23] The study results suggest that chronic pelvic pain in the adult female is associated with a lifetime history of depression and early childhood abuse. Chronic pelvic pain in the adult may result from conflicts about sexuality and intimacy during childhood that are repressed until regular sexual activity begins later in adulthood.

D. **Minnesota Multiphasic Personality Inventory.** Rosenthal et al. studied 103 consecutive chronic pelvic pain patients who were tested with the Minnesota Multiphasic Personality Inventory (MMPI).[25] A physical cause for pain was found in 75% of the women, but 75% of that group also had evidence of psychopathology on the MMPI. Although the MMPI can be used to identify the presence of psychological problems, it is best used as a supportive tool in the diagnostic workup of the patient. MMPI scores support the fact that patients with chronic pelvic pain have high levels of anxiety, depression, and neuroticism.

E. **Multidisciplinary approach.** Management of chronic pelvic pain should be based on a multidisciplinary approach. Centers specializing in pelvic pain usually are staffed by gynecologists, anesthesiologists, and psychologists who have expertise in physical and pelvic examinations as well as in conducting comprehensive psychosexual history workups. Most successful regimens in pain center settings use trigger point injections or acupuncture, biofeedback, psychotherapy, and relaxation techniques.

References

1. Sims JM. *Clinical Notes on Uterine Surgery with Special Reference to Management of the Sterile Condition.* New York: William Wood, 1966. P. 326.
2. Sinaki M, Merritt JL, Stillwell GK. Tension myalgia of the pelvic floor. *Mayo Clin Proc* 52:717, 1977.
3. Garcia GR, David SS. Pelvic endometriosis: infertility and pelvic pain. *Am J Obstet Gynecol* 129:740, 1977.
4. Friedman AJ. Vaginal hemorrhage associated with degenerating submucous leiomyomata during leuprolide acetate treatment. *Fertil Steril* 52:152, 1989.
5. Cowan BD, Knobloch RP, Meeks GR, Weems WL. Transvervical resection of submucous uterine fibroids: an alternative approach to management. *J Miss State Med Assoc* 30:1, 1989.
6. Gudgeon CW. Inversion of the uterus. Replacement without general anaesthesia. *Med J Aust* 2:434, 1979.
7. Brar HS, Greenspoon JS, Platt LD, Paul PH. Acute puerperal uterine inversion. New approaches to management. *J Reprod Med* 34:173, 1989.
8. Khoiny FE. Pelvic inflammatory disease in the adolescent. *J Pediatr Health Care* 3:230, 1989.
9. Clinical conference. A 55-year-old woman with abdominal pain, mucous stools, shock and polycythemia vera. *Chin Med J (Engl)* 102:72, 1989.
10. Wehmann TW, Rongaus VA. Diverticular disease in young adults. *J Am Osteopath Assoc* 89:791, 1989.
11. Fa EM, Cronan JJ. Compression ultrasonography as an aid in the differential diagnosis of appendicitis. *Surg Gynecol Obstet* 169:290, 1989.
12. Loghman-Adham M, Tejero HT, London R. Acute hemorrhagic cystitis due to *Escherichia coli. Child Nephrol Urol* 9:29, 1988.
13. Sinclair D, Wilson S, Toi A, Greenspan L. The evaluation of suspected renal colic: ultrasound scan versus excretory urography. *Ann Emerg Med* 18:556, 1989.
14. Dodson MD, Friedrich EG. Psychosomatic vulvovaginitis. *Obstet Gynecol* 51:23, 1977.
15. Lynch PJ. Vulvodynia: a syndrome of unexplained vulvar pain, psychologic disability and sexual dysfunction. *J Reprod Med* 31:773, 1986.
16. Beard RW, Belsey EM, Lieberman BA, et al. Pelvic pain in women. *Am J Obstet Gynecol* 128:566, 1977.
17. Beard RW, Highman JH, Pearce S, Reginald PW. Diagnosis of pelvic varicosities in women with chronic pelvic pain. *Lancet* 2:946, 1984.
18. Sichlau MJ, Yao JS, Vogelzang RL. Transcatheter embolotherapy for the treatment of pelvic congestion syndrome. *Obstet Gynecol* 83:892–896, 1984.
19. Andersch B, Milsom I. An epidemiologic study of young women with dysmenorrhea. *Am J Obstet Gynecol* 144:655–660, 1982.
20. Helms JM. Acupuncture for the management of primary dysmenorrhea. *Obstet Gynecol* 69:51, 1987.
21. Lee RB, Stone K, Magelssen D, et al. Presacral neurectomy for chronic pelvic pain. *Obstet Gynecol* 68:517, 1986.
22. Quill TE. Somatization disorders. One of medicine's blind spots. *JAMA* 254:3075, 1985.
23. Walker E, Katon W, Harrop-Griffiths J, et al. Relationship of chronic pelvic pain to psychiatric diagnoses and childhood sexual abuse. *Am J Psychiatry* 145:75, 1988.
24. Slocum JC. Neurological factors in chronic pelvic pain: trigger points and the abdominal pelvic pain syndrome. *Am J Obstet Gynecol* 149:536.
25. Rosenthal RH, Ling FW, Rosenthal TL, McNeeley SG. Chronic pelvic pain: psychological features and laparoscopic findings. *Psychosomatics* 25:833–841, 1981.

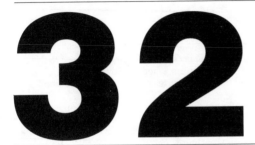

Phantom Limb Pain
Robert A. Marini
Alan M. Levine

I. **Background.** The pain management team plays a crucial role in the treatment of phantom limb pain. Phantom limb, in itself, is a natural consequence of amputation that rarely presents a therapeutic problem. However, the phantom limb can become a site for severe unrelenting pain representing a major obstacle in the rehabilitation process of the amputee. Both preoperative and postoperative intervention may help minimize the development of a potentially debilitating pain syndrome. There is no clear etiology for phantom pain, nor is any one specific treatment modality totally effective. More study is needed specifically in the prevention and treatment of phantom limb pain.

II. **Definition.** It is important to distinguish among various postamputation syndromes so that proper treatment is initiated.

   A. Phantom limb—sensation referred to the missing limb except pain. Virtually all amputees describe a phantom limb sensation. The phantom sensation usually fades after 1 year.

   B. Stump pain—pain occurring at the amputation site. The pain may be diffuse or localized, and is often palpable at the amputation stump.

   C. Phantom limb pain—chronic painful perception referred to the missing limb.

III. **Incidence.** The pain associated with phantom limb can present as a minor problem or can consume the patient's life. There is a higher incidence of those acknowledging the existence of a phantom limb, than those actually suffering from phantom limb pain. The incidence of pain ranges from 0% to 80% depending on the study reviewed, but appears to be independent of the medical or traumatic predisposing circumstance of the amputation. Phantom limb pain is rarely found in the patients who have congenital absence of a limb or underwent amputation before age 6.

   A longer preoperative duration of limb pain correlates with an increased probability of postoperative pain. Many patients experience a similar quality of pain immediately postoperatively as they did preoperatively. The quality continues to change for 6 months to 2 years, after which it becomes more or less constant.

IV. **Pathophysiology.** The cause of phantom limb pain is not well understood, and several hypotheses may explain the etiology.

   A. Central mechanisms

   1. As described by Melzack (1993), the **neuromatrix theory** proposes the existence of neuron networks extending through widespread areas of the brain. Located between the thalamus, cortex, and limbic systems, this complex integrates all sensory inputs from the body into a pattern called the **neurosignature**. The neurosignature represents a continuous outflow from the neuromatrix to the **sentient neural hub** in the brain stem, which traduces the flow of neural patterns into a flow of awareness.

   2. The **gate-control theory** of Melzack and Wall (1965) describes an intact engram receiving neural input from peripheral nerves. When these nerves are severed, there is decreased inhibition at the reticular activating system, increased central neural input, and a higher perception of pain.

   B. Spinal mechanism. Evidence supporting the origin of pain at the spinal level includes changes in neurochemical activity of dorsal horn cells and spinal cord neurons occurring after amputation. Atrophy of spinal cord cells also takes place.

   C. Peripheral mechanism. This theory hypothesizes that pain is caused by persistent sensation from nerve endings at the amputation stump. Peripheral pain origin is evidenced by the following:

   1. The effectiveness of various treatments such as trigger point injections and transcutaneous electrical nerve stimulation (TENS)

2. Decreasing temperature of the affected limb associated with burning, throbbing, and tingling pains, which are preceded by decreases in blood flow
3. Cramping or shooting pains associated with stump muscle spasm
- **D. Psychological factors.** Most do not attribute psychological factors as being the sole cause of phantom limb pain; however, certain studies regard emotional factors as risk factors predisposing to this phenomenon.
  1. As with other chronic pain states, **human behavior influences the phantom pain state.** Stress and depression, for example, increase pain.
  2. Although there is no increased incidence of psychopathology in those with phantom limb pain, the existence of **psychopathology** in a given patient **will exacerbate the pain.**
- **V. Signs and symptoms**
  - **A. Acute pain** often occurs immediately after the operation, may be continuous or paroxysmal, may occur daily, and involves the distal limb segment. Many patients describe a shooting or stabbing pain. Patients who perceive a "knife" in the phantom limb postoperatively may complain of burning pain at 6 months.
  - **B. Intensity** of pain varies dramatically with each patient. Most patients admit that attention and emotional states influence pain intensity. Pain intensity can be classified into four groups:
    1. **Mild** intermittent pain and paresthesia
    2. **Moderate** intermittent pain and paresthesia
    3. **Severe** paresthesia debilitating to the patient
    4. **Chronic** severe pain that grossly impairs lifestyle
  - **C. Abnormal spatial sensations,** such as the feeling that the leg is being twisted, the foot is pointed posteriorly, or the limb is fixed in space, can occur. These sensations (like the incidence of pain in general) are less frequent after 6 months. The likelihood of successful treatment is reduced if pain-free intervals do not occur in the first 6 months postoperatively.
  - **D. Telescoping,** which is the sensation of shrinkage of the phantom limb, occurs in approximately 50% of patients, and is more common in amputations of the upper extremity. It is usually seen in painless phantom limbs.
  - **E. Fading** represents the progressive disappearance of the phantom. The completion of this process may take 6 to 12 months.
  - **F. External stimuli,** such as hitting the stump, weather changes, pain from other parts of the body, and poor prosthetic fit, may exacerbate the pain. Pain relief occurs after rest, stump elevation, hot or cold compression, and other treatments.
- **VI. Differential diagnosis** of phantom limb pain is achieved through the process of eliminating the following:
  - **A. Localized process**
    1. Neuromas
    2. Infection
    3. Bone spurs
    4. Vascular insufficiency
    5. Nerve compression entrapment
    6. Poor-fitting prosthesis
    7. Elevated flap
  - **B. Diffuse process**
    1. Sympathetic dysfunction
    2. Myofascial disease
- **VII. Treatment.** Many different treatments have been tried, but no single treatment is considered definitive. In a survey, the success rate for pain relief after treatment rarely exceeded a placebo response of 30% (Sherman and Sherman, 1985). Surgical intervention appears to be the least effective treatment and is not recommended except when infection or a neuroma is present in the stump. Similarities in pain quality between phantom pain and preoperative pain have been noted. A beneficial reduction in phantom limb pain as a consequence of preoperative treatment has been demonstrated.
  - **A. Preoperative management**
    1. **History and physical examination**
    2. **Behavioral counseling**
       a. How to accept the loss of the limb
       b. Encouraging the patient to express what the loss means to him or her
       c. Warning of the likelihood of postoperative pain
    3. **Epidural anesthesia** treats and diagnoses preoperative pain of the lower

extremities. Patients receiving continuous epidural infusion with complete pain relief using morphine or bupivacaine 72 hours before surgery were less likely to complain of phantom limb pain for a year after the operation.

B. Postoperative management

1. Oral medications

a. Nonsteroidal anti-inflammatory drugs (NSAIDs)

(1) An initial trial of NSAIDs and acetaminophen should be considered. Trials of various NSAIDs are recommended because of the variable individual response to different agents. Patients should be monitored with blood tests for side effects to treatment. Special observation is advised if NSAIDs are used persistently. **Caution is advised in patients with renal insufficiency, liver disease, coagulation disorders, and coronary heart failure.** Peptic ulcer disease may be a relative contraindication to the use of NSAIDs. There are synergic effects in combining different NSAIDs. NSAIDs are not recommended in combination with an acetyl salicylic acid (ASA) due to increased side effects and decreased NSAID blood levels.

(2) Drug dosage

(a) ASA 650 mg PO q3–4h with simethicone (Mylanta)

(b) Acetaminophen 650 mg PO q3–4h (not an anti-inflammatory drug; use with ASA or NSAID)

(c) Ibuprofen 400–600 mg PO q6h with meals

(d) Naproxen (Naprosyn) 250–500 mg PO q12h with meals

(e) Indomethacin (Indocin) 25–50 mg PO q8h with meals

(f) Piroxicam (Feldene) 20 mg PO daily with meals

(g) Nabumetone (Relafen) 500 mg PO q12h with meals

b. Narcotics

(1) Narcotics may be prescribed over long periods without addiction. Drug abuse is rare when the patient is under medical supervision. If the predominant component of pain is not psychological, undermedication should be avoided. Methadone (Dolophine) and morphine (Ms Contin) should be tried before the pain becomes resistant. Fentanyl transdermal patches (Duragesic) may also be tried to provide continuous delivery of narcotics. If, however, the patient requires high doses and functional activity has not improved, other treatment modalities should be considered.

(2) Drug dosage

(a) Oxycodone 5–10 mg PO q6h. (Percocet contains oxycodone 5 mg and acetaminophen 325 mg. Percodan contains oxycodone 5 mg and ASA 325 mg.)

(b) Morphine (Ms Contin) 10–30 mg PO q12h.

(c) Methadone 5–20 mg q8h.

(d) Fentanyl transdermal patch 25–100 μg every 3 days

c. Antidepressants reduce narcotic requirements, improve the patient's ability to sleep, and treat psychiatric problems if they exist. Psychiatric consultation is indicated if psychopathology is suspected. **Tricyclic antidepressants** are contraindicated when the patient is taking monoamine oxidase inhibitors. The most commonly used tricyclic is **amitriptyline** (Elavil) 25–100 mg PO at bedtime. Its action blocks neuronal uptake of norepinephrine and serotonin, potentiating their inhibition of spinal neurons involved in pain perception. Amitriptyline should be used with caution in patients with a history of seizures, arrhythmia, hyperthyroidism, urinary retention associated with prostatic hypertrophy, angle closure glaucoma, and increased intraocular pressure. **Nortriptyline** (Pamelor) has a more pharmacodynamic profile with less orthostatic hypotension and fewer sedative effects. Its mechanism of action is similar to that of amitriptyline. A phenothiazine such as **fluphenazine** 1 mg tid may be added in conjunction with the antidepressant.

d. Neuroleptics, such as **carbamazepine** (Tegretol) 100–200 mg PO tid and **phenytoin** (Dilantin) 50–200 mg PO tid, have been used to treat the lancinating pain arising from phantom limb pain; however, results are not promising.

e. Antispastics. Complaints of cramping pain associated with muscle spasms and muscle tension headaches warrant a trial of **baclofen** (Lioresal). Its role in phantom limb pain is unclear, and it has been used predominantly in spasticity. The recommended dosage is 5–40 mg PO tid.

f. Beta blockers. Propanolol 40–80 mg has been shown to be effective in a small percentage of patients.

g. Calcitonin has been shown to relieve pain 3 hours after intravenous injection of 100 IU over 5 minutes. Pain relief lasted as long as 3 months after injection. Calcitonin has been thought to exert its effects on serotoninergic pathways independent of opiate receptor mechanisms. Allergic response to the protein may occur and previous skin testing is recommended. Although no cases have been reported, hypocalcemic tetany could possibly occur, so parenteral calcium should be available. Calcitonin should not be used during pregnancy or given to nursing mothers. Nausea after injection may be an unwarranted effect.

2. Regional anesthetic block

a. Epidural block

(1) **Local anesthesia** will relieve lower extremity pain temporarily, and serial blocks (total of five, each 2 to 3 days apart) break the cycle of pain and may relieve chronic pain. Injection of approximately 6 ml of 0.25% bupivacaine into the epidural space at L3–4 after a test dose yields adequate sensory block.

(2) **Narcotics** (fentanyl 100–500 mg diluted in 10 ml normal saline) may relieve pain for 4–6 hours. Subarachnoid fentanyl has been used to provide immediate relief of phantom limb pain for a few days.

(3) **Epidural and spinal local anesthetics** have been reported to exacerbate phantom limb pain. This pain should be treated with one dose of epidural or intrathecal narcotics. It is suggested to leave the epidural catheter in place after surgery in an amputee, so narcotics can be given in the event of exacerbation of pain.

(4) Infusion of 0.125% bupivacaine with fentanyl 5 μg/ml at 6–10 ml/hr in the postoperative period can help reduce the development of phantom limb pain.

b. Sympathetic blockade

(1) Patients with decreased stump temperature may benefit from vasodilatation and increased blood flow produced by sympathetic block. Sympathetic denervation of the upper extremity is achieved by **stellate ganglion blockade.** Local anesthetic is injected to block the middle cervical to third and fourth thoracic ganglion. Denervation to the lower extremity requires anesthetic blockade to the **lumbar sympathetic chain** as well as the lowest two thoracic ganglia.

(2) If pain relief is obtained after initial block, a **series of five blocks** 2 to 3 days apart may provide long-term relief.

(3) **An increase in blood flow and limb temperature must be demonstrated before sympathetic block is abandoned** as unsuccessful.

c. Trigger point injections

(1) Effective when pain can be reproduced with palpation

(2) The muscle knot of the affected area is injected with 3–5 ml of 0.25% bupivacaine

3. Neuroelectrical stimulation

a. Transcutaneous electrical nerve stimulation is thought to stimulate large-diameter fibers (mechanoreceptor) that close the "gate" to sensory input into the spinal cord. TENS has been shown to acutely reduce pain in as many as 50% of patients with phantom pain. Application of TENS to the contralateral extremity demonstrated relief of phantom limb pain, which indicates that the sensory cortex may not distinguish the origin of pain. However, long-term relief appears minimal, with patients demonstrating no improvement in pain scores over those of control subjects.

b. Dorsal column stimulation appears to be the most common form of electrical stimulation in patients with intractable chronic pain, and has been in practice for approximately 20 years. In some studies reviewed, initial pain reduction was observed in 50% to 100% of patients; however, long-term effects with intermittent dorsal column (spinal cord) stimulation diminished after 1 to 2 years.

c. Deep brain stimulation. The brain's **periaqueductal** and **periventricular** gray matter have been stimulated to relieve phantom pain, with varying results. When sensory **thalamic** stimulation was implemented, phantom limb pain responded better than with stimulation to the periaqueductal sites.

4. Neurosurgical ablative procedures

a. Peripheral procedures

(1) Stump revision is mainly limited to stump pain resulting from a localized pathologic process or formation of painful neuroma. When the stump is revised to treat pain other than pathology occurring at the amputation site, the rate of treatment failure is high. **Neurotomy** and **spinal dorsal rhizotomy** obtain their effects by denervation between the spinal nerve roots and the amputation stump. These procedures have been abandoned because of their inability to maintain long-term pain relief.

(2) Sympathectomy has been somewhat effective with patients whose pain has been described as "burning," similar to that of causalgia. Most studies reveal the effects to be temporary. When intravenous guanethidine is administered in conjunction with sympathectomy, short-term and long-term results have been promising.

b. Spinal cord procedures

(1) Anterolateral cordotomy has produced conflicting reports. Sustained relief from phantom pain appears to diminish because peripheral networks of interconnecting fibers assume the role of the major spinal tract in relaying pain impulses.

(2) The **dorsal root entry zone (DREZ)** lesion is the preferred neurosurgical technique. The operation is based on destroying the pain-integrating areas of laminae I, II, and V in the dorsal column. Pain relief was produced in 67% of patients with phantom limb pain when compared with stump pain.

c. Brain stem procedures, such as **cortical ablation, midbrain lesions,** and **prefrontal lobotomies,** do not prove to be very useful. Stereotactic lesions created in the thalamus, subthalamus, and mesencephalon resulted in pain relief in 20% of patients in isolated studies; however, long-term effects have not been described.

5. Physical therapy. The application of physical modalities in the rehabilitation process is an important adjunct in the treatment of the amputee with phantom limb pain. There are conflicting data on their efficacy; however, these treatments present few complications.

a. Massage, vibratory, and percussion treatment have been used with some success; 100-Hz stimulation with moderate pressure over a large area (800-cm probe) yields the best results when applying vibratory stimulation.

b. Ultrasound, iontophoresis, and the application of **ice and** superficial **heat** have been claimed to be beneficial in a small percentage of patients.

c. Immediate postoperative prosthesis (IPOP) and **early prosthetic fitting** may decrease the incidence of phantom limb pain. They exert their effects peripherally by reducing stump edema and promote healing after surgery.

6. Psychological techniques. There is no definitive evidence that amputees suffering from chronic phantom limb pain have existing psychopathology or maladaptive psychological profiles. Patients with chronic phantom limb pain are affected by stress, anxiety, and depression similarly to those who experience chronic pain syndromes. The following psychological techniques all have been used with limited success:

a. Hypnosis

b. Psychotherapy

c. Behavioral modification

d. Biofeedback

e. Relaxation therapy

Selected Readings

Bach A, Noreng MF, Tjellden NV. Phantom limb pain in amputees during the first 12 months following limb amputation, after preoperative lumbar epidural blockade. *Pain* 3:297, 1988.

Carabelli RA, Kellerman WC. Phantom limb pain: relief by application of TENS to contralateral extremity. *Arch Phys Med Rehabil* 66:466, 1985.

Engkvist O, Wahren LK, Torebjork E, Nystom B. Effects of regional intravenous guanethidine block in posttraumatic cold intolerance in hand amputee. *J Hand Surg* 10:145, 1985.

Finsen V, Persen L, Lovlien M, et al. Transcutaneous electrical stimulation after major amputation. *J Bone Joint Surg* 70:109, 1988.

Jacobson L, Chabar C. Prolonged relief of acute postamputation phantom limb pain with intrathecal fentanyl and epidural morphine. *Anesthesiology* 71:984, 1989.

Jaeger H, Mailer C. Calcitonin in phantom limb pain: a double-blind study. *Pain* 48:21, 1992.

Jensen TS, Krebs B, Nielsen J, Rasmussen P. Immediate and long-term phantom limb pain in amputees: incidence, clinical characteristics, and relationship to preamputation limb pain. *Pain* 21:267, 1985.

Kessel C, Worz R. Immediate response of phantom limb pain to calcitonin. *Pain* 30:79, 1987.

Krainick JU, Thoden U, Riechert T. Pain reduction in amputees by long-term spinal cord stimulation. *J Neurosurg* 52:346, 1980.

Ludenberg J. Relief of pain from a phantom limb by peripheral stimulation. *J Neurol* 232:79, 1985.

Marsland AR, Weekes J, Atkinson RL, Leong MG. Phantom limb pain: a case for beta blockers? *Pain* 12:295, 1982.

Melzack R. Pain: past, present and future. *Can J Exp Psychol* 47:615, 1993.

Melzack R, Wall P. Pain mechanisms: a new theory. *Science* 150:971, 1965.

Mundinger F, Neumuller H. Programmed transcutaneous (TNS) and central (DBS) stimulation for control of phantom limb and stump pain. In Siegfried J, Zimmerman M (eds.), *Phantom and Stump Pain*. New York: Springer-Verlag, 1981. Pp. 167–178.

Nashold BS, Ostadhl R. Dorsal root entry zone lesions for pain relief. *J Neurosurg* 51:59, 1979.

Raj PP. Practical management of pain (2nd ed.). St. Louis: Mosby–Year Book, 1992. Pp. 505–516.

Rasmussen P, Jensen TS. Phantom pain and phenomena after amputation. *Adv Pain Res Ther* 10:167, 1992.

Saris SC, Iacomo RP, Nashold BS. Dorsal root entry zone lesions in post-amputation pain. *J Neurosurg* 62:72, 1985.

Sherman RA. Stump and phantom limb pain. *Neurol Clin* 7:249, 1989.

Sherman RA. Published treatment of phantom limb pain. *Am J Phys Med* 5:59, 1980.

Sherman RA, Sherman CJ. A comparison of phantom sensations among amputees whose amputations were of civilian and military origins. *Pain* 21:91, 1985.

Sherman RA, Sherman CJ, Bruno GM. Psychological factors influencing chronic phantom limb pain: an analysis of the literature. *Pain* 28:285, 1987.

Siegfried J, Cetinalp E. Neurosurgical treatment of phantom limb pain with intrathecal fentanyl and epidural morphine. *Anesthesiology* 71:984, 1989.

Urban BJ, France RD, Steinberger EK, et al. Long term use of narcotics/antidepressant medication in the management of phantom limb pain. In Siegfried J, Zimmerman M (eds.), *Phantom and Stump Pain*. New York: Springer-Verlag, 1981. Pp. 148–153.

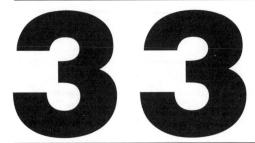

Pain Related to Sickle Cell Disease

Barbara S. Shapiro

I. **Background.** The treatment of patients with sickle cell disease who have vaso-occlusive pain can be uniquely difficult and challenging. Although the pain is usually acute, it can recur frequently, and so must be managed as both an acute and chronic pain condition. The best pharmacologic approaches, if used alone, will be unsatisfactory in the long run. It is crucial that pain management be based on an understanding of the biologic, psychological, and social context of the pain and illness.

II. **Natural history**
   A. **Definition.** A painful episode or "crisis" is an episode of pain, usually unpredictable, occurring anywhere in the body, lasting an indeterminate length of time, and followed by a return to the usual baseline state.
   B. **Pathophysiology.** An inherited alteration of hemoglobin structure results in deformed, **sickle-shaped RBCs** that impede normal arteriolar flow. If collateral flow is also blocked, the occlusion produces tissue hypoxia and infarction, which is called a vaso-occlusive crisis, or painful episode.
   C. **Incidence.** Sickle cell disease is most commonly found in people of African ancestry, although it is also seen in other ethnic groups originally from malaria-endemic areas. There are more than 50,000 people with sickle cell disease in the United States. Pain is the most common problem for these patients and is the most frequent reason for emergency room and inpatient admission.
   D. **Pain characteristics**
      1. **Location.** A painful episode can occur in any tissue or structure supplied with blood vessels, where infarction produces pain. It can involve single or multiple areas of the body and can migrate or change during an episode.
      2. **Temporal factors.** Although the average length of a painful episode is 4 days, it may last from several minutes to several weeks. The onset and resolution of the pain can be rapid or gradual, with children generally having shorter episodes than adults. Pain can occur daily.
      3. **Character.** The pain is usually nociceptive, but patients may also develop neuropathic pain syndromes.
      4. **Severity.** The pain can be mild, moderate, or severe.
      5. **Provocative factors.** Most episodes occur with no identifiable cause. Known precipitating factors are cold, dehydration, infection, menses, stress, and fatigue.
      6. **Variability.** The number, intensity, length, and location of the episodes vary considerably among persons afflicted with sickle cell disease. About 30% of these individuals never or rarely experience sickle-cell-related pain. Half of them may have only one severe episode each year, or may suffer frequent milder episodes. By contrast, the remaining 20% have frequent and severe pain, accounting for a high number of emergency room and inpatient admissions. The pain in most patients will follow an idiosyncratic repetitive pattern of frequency, length, intensity, and even location. The variability in disease severity among patients is largely determined by **physiologic factors,** such as disease subtype and proportion of fetal hemoglobin. The manner in which the disease affects the patient, however, is influenced by the psychosocial context and the patient's coping skills.

III. **Issues affecting treatment**
   A. **Nature of the pain.** Patients who are severely affected by painful episodes have acute pain repeatedly. When viewed in isolation, the syndrome is similar in many respects to other acute pain problems. However, this pain is a recurring symptom

of a lifelong, potentially life-threatening disease. Because of the pain's chronic nature, patients often become depressed, and responses to the pain become integrated into the daily life of the patient and the family. The impact of the pain's unpredictable pattern and severity on the patient is often similar to the learned helplessness seen in laboratory animals. The important issues of control versus helplessness and responsibility versus passivity affect the patient's coping skills and therefore the approach to treatment.

B. **Nature of the disease.** The majority of patients with sickle cell disease can expect to live through at least middle-age, although death from various disease-related causes may occur at any time. Even though the pain can be as intense as cancer-related pain, the patient and the pain must be treated in a manner conducive to a normal lifestyle. One of the aims of treatment is to de-emphasize, as much as possible, the crisis nature of the episodes.

C. **Cultural issues.** The majority of health professionals come from socioeconomic and ethnic backgrounds different from those of many sickle cell patients. This can result in problems with communication and trust. In the management of patients with chronic intractable pain problems, a good relationship between the care providers and the patient is crucial for effective treatment.

D. **Structure of care.** Many patients with sickle cell disease are cared for in tertiary care centers that are part of large academically based medical centers. In such centers, the patient may not have a primary physician during outpatient and inpatient encounters. The pain may be managed in different ways by different physicians. Lack of continuity of care adds to the unpredictability of the pain and creates problems with trust.

E. **Development.** Adults with sickle cell disease are often managed in centers different from those for children. If there is a lack of communication between the staff at these centers, the graduation from one center to another (during the often troublesome years of late adolescence) can create problems.

F. **Home-versus-hospital management**
   1. Pain episodes can be managed at home or in the hospital. Most episodes are managed at home, and may not come to the attention of medical staff. Very severe pain usually demands admission for parenteral analgesia. However, **patients base their decision** on whether to come to the hospital **on a variety of factors,** such as
      a. **Past experience with the hospital**
      b. **Pain coping skills**
      c. **Psychosocial factors**
      d. **Home environment**
      e. **Provision by the care providers of instruction in and support for home management**
   2. **Management at home is not always preferable** to management in the hospital. The severity of the pain may be too great, and it may be unrealistic to expect a patient without supportive and available family members to manage even moderate pain at home. However, a multidisciplinary management program, including instruction in coping skills, can significantly decrease the number of admissions for pain management.

G. **Frequently admitted patients.** A minority of the patients account for the majority of hospital admissions—some patients are admitted more than 40 times each year. Despite the severity of a patient's pain experience, optimal treatment does not involve hospital admission at this great a frequency. Following are suggestions for the treatment of patients with very frequent admissions:
   1. **Optimize the use of nonopioid analgesics** and **nonpharmacologic methods of pain control.**
   2. **Manage pain in a pharmacologically sound manner** in all patients, including known substance abusers. Undermedication leads to behavior aimed at convincing physicians and nurses of the pain severity in an attempt to obtain pain relief. Likewise, medicating on an as-needed basis should be strictly avoided.
   3. **Maintain and review records of emergency room and inpatient admissions and opioid prescriptions for all patients.** A high or increasing frequency of use may indicate a physiologic problem, poor pain coping skills, overutilization for psychosocial reasons, or psychological dependence.
   4. **Provide good continuity of care.**
   5. **Develop a contract** drawn up by both the patient and involved health profes-

sionals that specifies conditions for admission and pain management in the hospital.

6. **Provide education about pain and its management.**
7. **Teach pain coping skills** (relaxation and self-hypnosis, distraction, biofeedback).
8. **Provide psychotherapy** and family therapy if indicated.
9. **Provide accessible telephone support.**
10. **Treat depression** if it is present.

IV. **Assessment**
  A. The assessment of pain in a patient with sickle cell disease is similar to an assessment involving other pain syndromes.
   1. **Patients can be taught a rating scale,** such as a numerical or categorical scale, to communicate pain intensity.
   2. **Parents can be taught how to observe the behavior of infants and very young children.**
   3. **Immediate assessment of pain is necessary** to appropriately tailor pharmacologic intervention.
   4. For emergency room and inpatient care, **sequential ratings of pain intensity, response to analgesia, and sedation should be part of the medical record.**
  B. **It is important to distinguish between sickle-cell-related pain and pain that indicates other problems** such as infection, pneumonia, or cholecystitis. Fever, usually low-grade, is sometimes present during an uncomplicated painful episode, but an infectious process may mimic or precipitate vaso-occlusion. Patients, including children, can usually tell the difference between their typical sickle cell pain and pain from other causes.
  C. **Assessment of psychosocial status and pain coping skills is important for all patients.**
   1. **Acute episodes.** During an acute episode an assessment of the patient's psychosocial status and pain coping skills should be approached after analgesia has been instituted, and the patient has had time to rest. Evaluation of mood during the acute episode can be misleading, as mood alterations are often secondary to the pain and the consequent interruption of normal activities.
   2. **Frequent episodes.** Assessment of the patient with frequent painful episodes must be completed when he or she has returned to baseline. Ideally, this is accomplished during an outpatient visit. Some patients, however, rarely come to the outpatient clinic. If a patient has difficulty keeping scheduled visits, the day of discharge can be used for a full assessment and discussion of future management.

V. **Treatment.** The treatment methods for painful episodes have not changed over the past 20 years; they include **hydration** and the use of **nonopioid and opioid analgesics.** Given the paucity of specific data regarding sickle cell pain management, it is necessary to extrapolate from the research available regarding the treatment of similar pain problems.
  A. **Pharmacologic approaches.** The stepwise approach suggested by the World Health Organization for the control of cancer pain is useful in treating sickle cell pain.
   1. **Mild pain** can be managed with nonopioid analgesics, such as acetaminophen and aspirin as needed.
   2. **For moderate pain,** the nonopioid analgesic is taken around the clock, with the addition of a mild opioid as needed or on a regular schedule.
   3. **For severe pain,** a strong opioid is added to the nonopioid analgesic for severe pain, and both are taken around the clock.
  B. **Nonopioid analgesics. Acetaminophen, aspirin,** and the **nonsteroidal anti-inflammatory drugs** are useful in the treatment of many pain syndromes, including sickle cell pain. They provide analgesia (650 mg of acetaminophen or aspirin has approximately the same analgesic potential as 30 mg of codeine) and have an additive effect when combined with opioids. The site of action and the side effects are different from those of the opioids. The nonopioid analgesics generally do not produce sedation, and tolerance does not develop.
   1. **Acetaminophen** and the other nonsteroidal anti-inflammatory drugs are the backbone of pharmacologic therapy and should be used unless there are specific contraindications. The choice of agent depends on the patient and the clinical situation. Acetaminophen is commonly available, both alone and

in fixed-dose combinations with codeine and oxycodone. It is generally well tolerated, and has no gastric or hematologic side effects. However, frequent administration is required, and caution is suggested in case of hepatic failure. In addition, there is a possible correlation between long-term daily acetaminophen use and renal failure. Until more is known about this effect, patients should be cautioned to limit the number of days on which this medication is taken, as well as the cumulative daily dose.

2. **Aspirin** is widely available, well studied, and available in fixed-dose combinations with oral opioids. However, frequent administration can be problematic owing to gastric and hematologic effects.

3. **Other anti-inflammatory agents** can be administered at longer intervals, and may be better tolerated by some patients. Choline magnesium trisalicylate is less likely than the other drugs to cause GI intolerance and platelet dysfunction. It is not known whether the precise health benefits in treating cancer bone pain with nonsteroid anti-inflammatory drugs can be achieved treating sickle cell pain. Specific effects, however, can be postulated, especially when bony infarction is present.

C. **Opioids** are the mainstay of pharmacologic therapy for moderate to severe pain.

1. **Oral agents.** Recommended oral opioids include codeine, oxycodone, hydromorphone, and morphine.

   a. **Codeine** and **oxycodone** are useful for moderate pain, and are available alone and in fixed-dose preparations with acetaminophen or aspirin.

   b. Strong opioids such as **hydromorphone** and **morphine** are useful for patients with severe pain, especially when home management is a goal. Support and supervision are necessary when strong opioids are used at home. Morphine is available in sustained-release and immediate-release forms. The dose for oral morphine must be 3 times that given intravenously for equal analgesia. If a patient responds to morphine 5 mg IV, a reasonable home maintenance dose could be sustained-release morphine 30 mg PO q8h or q12h for 24 hours, or immediate-release morphine 15 mg PO q3–4h.

   c. **Methadone** is difficult to titrate and is not recommended. **Pentazocine,** an agonist-antagonist preparation available in oral form, has a significant incidence of psychomimetic side effects and is also not recommended.

2. **Parenteral agents**

   a. **Morphine** and **hydromorphone** can be used when parenteral administration is necessary. Morphine is the best-characterized drug and should be used for most patients. Hydromorphone is valuable for the patient who experiences unmanageable side effects such as nausea or pruritus with morphine.

   b. **Meperidine** is widely used but has significant disadvantages, namely, a long-acting metabolite, normeperidine, which can cause seizures. In addition, when used for more than 24 hours, meperidine has been associated with jitteriness and dysphoria. Compared with other readily available opioids, meperidine has no advantages and, except for special circumstances, is not recommended.

      (1) **Drug switching.** Patients who have been managed for many years with meperidine, however, may resist a change to another agent. Also, insisting on the use of an alternative drug may impede the development of trust between patient and care provider, especially when the patient's energy is occupied by the intense pain.

      (2) **Drug addiction.** The patient or the patient's family may believe that meperidine is less addicting than morphine, and that the switch to morphine represents a leap into drug dependence. This concern can usually be relieved through education after a trusting relationship has been established with the care provider.

   c. **Nalbuphine,** an agonist-antagonist, and **buprenorphine,** a partial agonist, can be used for sickle cell pain. The relative advantages and disadvantages of these drugs over opioid agonists are not clear. Further research is necessary before recommendations can be made. Because the agonist-antagonists cause less spasm of the sphincter of Oddi and lower increase in intrabiliary pressure than the agonists, they are useful in treating pancreatitis or cholecystitis. The agonist-antagonist drugs can produce withdrawal symptoms in patients who have been using opioid agonists for more than a few days.

3. **Route of administration.** The route by which opioids are given depends on the clinical situation.
    a. **Severe pain** is more easily controlled, at least initially, with an **intravenous opioid.**
    b. **Oral administration** may avoid the need for an intravenous line, which is not only uncomfortable but if inserted frequently, may lead to difficulties in obtaining intravenous access. A patient with severe pain may be able to avoid hospitalization with the use of strong oral opioids for a few days.
    c. **Intramuscular injection** is the usual route for parenteral management of pain. Repeated intramuscular administration, however, is painful and may lead to sterile abscesses and myofascial fibrosis. Intramuscular injection, therefore, should not be used repetitively. However, changes in patient care should be made slowly and sensitively. Many patients associate pain relief with an injection, and so would be concerned about changing to an alternative method.
4. **Schedule.** The principles of scheduling analgesia for sickle cell pain are similar to those for other acute pain syndromes.
    a. Mild pain can be managed with **analgesia as needed.**
    b. For severe pain, **time-based** (not pain-contingent) **dosage intervals must be used.** Around-the-clock administration gives smooth control of the pain and avoids a cyclical return of pain and anxiety. In addition, the patient does not develop a repertoire of pain behaviors designed to convince the medical and nursing staff that another dose of medication is indicated.
    c. An alternative to around-the-clock dosage intervals is **flexible dosage** or "reverse prn" scheduling. With this method, the patient is given a choice at regularly scheduled intervals of a milder or a stronger analgesic or no analgesia. The medication, if any is chosen, must be given immediately.
    d. Intravenous opioid analgesia may involve **intermittent rapid boluses, a constant infusion** with so-called rescue boluses, or **patient-controlled analgesia.**
        (1) **Intermittent boluses** are recommended in the emergency department, but may be suboptimal for continued inpatient management. In some patients, the bolus's peak effect may be accompanied by side effects, such as profound sedation. In addition, the pain may return before the next dose is administered. More frequent administration may provide smoother control. A morphine bolus, for example, may have to be scheduled every 2 or 3 hours rather than every 4 hours.
        (2) **An alternative to bolus administration is the intravenous infusion.** To determine the rate of an infusion, analgesia, sedation, and the duration of action of the initial bolus must be assessed.
            (a) **An initial bolus.** Because an infusion reaches steady state in 8 to 12 hours, it must be preceded with a bolus to provide immediate analgesia. Overestimation of the rate of an infusion may lead to profound sedation (which is not clinically apparent for many hours).
            (b) **Combined with rescue boluses.** An infusion can be combined with "rescue" boluses, which are offered every 2 hours when the patient is awake. With this method, the infusion can be started at a conservative dose, while providing control for breakthrough pain. For example, a patient who responds to 5 mg of morphine with reasonable pain relief (lasting 3 hours) and minimal sedation could be started on an infusion of about 1.2 mg/hr with a "rescue" dose of about 1.5 mg q2h. After 8 to 12 hours, if the pain has not been relieved, the "rescue" doses are summed and the infusion is increased by about this amount.
        (3) **Patient-controlled analgesia.** Some physicians use patient-controlled analgesia to treat painful episodes. In this method, the patient must take responsibility to help manage the pain. Self-control and responsibility are crucial coping skills and, combined with intervention, serve as the basis for a multidisciplinary treatment program.
5. **Drug doses**
    a. **The correct dose.** Sickle cell pain severity varies with each episode and for each person. Patients with frequent, severe pain (who use opioids) are often tolerant of opioids and their side effects. Those with equally severe but less frequent episodes, however, are not tolerant. As with other pain

syndromes requiring the use of parenteral opioids, the correct dose is the dose that **works without producing intolerable and uncontrollable side effects.**

b. **Addiction.** Many clinicians worry about using opioids in patients with sickle cell disease. **This concern is unfounded.** Moreover, withholding or giving inadequate doses of opioids for moderate or severe pain not only does not prevent addiction, but also makes the patient crave and sometimes beg for medication. Adequate control of pain, within a multidisciplinary framework and a good physician-patient relationship, prevents this cycle.

c. **Tolerable pain.** The objective of adequate analgesia is to make the pain tolerable to the patient. **Elimination of pain is not a reasonable goal** of pharmacologic treatment in this context. Many components of the pain may not be responsive to analgesics, no matter how high the dose.

D. Adjuvants

1. **Tricyclic antidepressants.** There is little research available on the use of tricyclic antidepressants for sickle cell pain. In chronic pain, the analgesic effect of these agents requires continued use. Given what is known concerning the beneficial effects of tricyclic antidepressants on a variety of chronic pain syndromes (and as adjuvants in cancer pain), it is reasonable to give patients with severe and frequent painful episodes a course of tricyclic drugs. Assessment of patient response is essential.

2. **Stimulants**
   a. **Dextroamphetamine, methylphenidate,** and **caffeine** can be useful adjuvants for the control of cancer pain. But, unlike the treatment objectives for cancer pain, the goals of sickle cell pain management are
      (1) To render the pain tolerable
      (2) To minimize hypoxia (which could perpetuate intravascular sickling)
      (3) To facilitate a rapid return to normal life activities
   b. If used to minimize sedation (which could be accompanied by hypoxia), stimulants should be used around the clock. This would, however, disturb normal sleeping patterns. In addition, patients often see these medications as a form of drug abuse. The complexity of the regimen increases as more drugs are added, which makes patient education and control more difficult. Overall, **stimulants** are useful in certain clinical situations, but, without further research, **cannot be recommended routinely.**

3. **Benzodiazepines.** Anxiety is secondary not only to pain but also to concerns about being believed and receiving appropriate medication. The anxiolytics provide no analgesia and may increase respiratory depression.

4. **Side-effect control.** Nausea and vomiting, pruritus, and constipation can be as bothersome as pain. The use of a phenothiazine is usually sufficient to control opioid-induced nausea.
   a. The **nauseated** patient should be asked at regular intervals whether an antiemetic is needed.
   b. **Vomiting** tends to be treated more aggressively than nausea.
   c. **Pruritus** can be controlled with hydroxyzine or diphenhydramine.

E. Cognitive-behavioral and psychological interventions

1. Cognitive-behavioral and psychological interventions **should be integrated into the program of care** along with the medical approach. Patients can be taught cognitive-behavioral coping skills and given individualized pharmacologic approaches for home management.

   The physician and mental health professional should work together because some patients are resistant to psychological intervention unless it is explained and prescribed by the trusted primary care physician. Continued communication between the physician and the mental health worker can ensure optimal integration.

2. **Relaxation, self-hypnosis,** and **biofeedback** are helpful for patients with sickle cell disease. These approaches have no side effects, are relatively easily taught, and can enhance the perception of self-regulation and control. Because of their benefits and minimal risk, these techniques are used extensively in other pain syndromes, and should be part of the treatment plan.

3. **Contracts** are used in a variety of medical situations, especially when issues of adherence, trust, and predictability are important. A contract is an agreement, written or verbal, between a patient (or family) and the medical care providers. Changes are permissible only with mutual agreement. A

perception of control, predictability, and structure reduces the need for repeated and often unproductive negotiations. Without a contract, these repeated discussions may occur during every admission, sometimes with a different outcome each time. For a contract to be successful, pharmacologic management of pain must be adequate.

4. **Family psychotherapy** and **individual psychotherapy** are indicated for specific problems. To be most effective, this approach should be integrated with medical care, the teaching of cognitive-behavioral techniques, and perhaps with the use of a contract.

F. **Physical intervention**
1. **Splints** and **slings** can be useful when a specific part of the body is in pain. If a patient has pain in one arm, splinting the extremity and placing it in a sling can provide stabilization. This will facilitate normal movement and activity, and consequently decrease the need for pharmacologic intervention.
2. **Application of heat**, in the form of heating packs or hot baths, works very well for some patients. The application of cold usually makes sickle cell pain worse. However, an occasional patient responds well to local cold application.
3. **Movement** and **exercise** (within the tolerance of the individual) are effective, especially in patients with prolonged painful episodes. This therapy may include simple maneuvers, such as having the patient sit in a chair at regular intervals, and physical therapy in bed.
4. **Transcutaneous electrical nerve stimulation (TENS)** is an intervention that works especially well in some patients with myofascial pain and certain neuropathic pain syndromes. As far as is known, it has no side effects, does not produce sedation or respiratory depression, and enhances patient control.

G. **Medical intervention**
1. **Hydration,** either oral or intravenous, is used, although there are no confirming studies. Dehydration is a factor known to precipitate vaso-occlusion, and patients often become dehydrated because of vomiting or limited intake due to severe pain.
2. **Oxygen** is often used in the management of sickle cell pain. Once intravascular occlusion has occurred, however, there is no evidence that oxygen will reverse the process or shorten the episode. The administration of oxygen to a patient who is not hypoxemic can reduce the production of erythropoietin. Oxygen should be used only in patients who are hypoxic.
3. **RBC transfusions,** given regularly, can be used as prophylaxis. However, the considerable risks of transfusion include alloimmunization, infection, and iron overload. Transfusions should be used only in those exceptional situations when multidisciplinary intervention has failed.
4. **Epidural analgesia** is occasionally used. Analgesics administered via a catheter placed in the epidural space are commonly used in the management of postoperative and cancer-related pain. This method can produce excellent analgesia with low opioid doses. Its use may be limited because of the risk of producing fibrosis (or other problems) due to the frequency with which catheters must be placed in the epidural space.
   a. For patients with frequent episodes, it is not logical to manage one episode with epidural analgesia (with perhaps excellent results) and then manage several subsequent and equally severe episodes with parenteral opioids. This violates two general principles:
      (1) **Maintaining continuity of care and predictability**
      (2) **De-emphasizing the crisis nature of the condition**
   b. However, if a patient has a particularly severe episode (perhaps an acute chest syndrome) and administration of an optimum dose of opioids does not produce adequate analgesia or produces intolerable side effects, peridural opioids are recommended.

VI. **Outpatient management**
A. Crucial to effective pain management at home is education about
   1. **Assessment** of pain intensity
   2. **Recording** of pain and medications used
   3. **Knowledge of side effects** of medication
   4. **Telephone access** to medical care providers
B. **An individualized stepwise approach** to the management of mild, moderate, and severe pain can be established with the patient and recorded for home reference. The approach should be simple and specific: doses should be listed as number of

tablets and milligrams, and the amount of fluid necessary for adequate hydration should be in glasses of a specific size. Include criteria for emergency room visits.

VII. Emergency room management. The emergency department provides the interface between family-controlled management at home and medically determined management in the hospital. Competent and caring intervention by emergency room staff helps to ensure successful treatment at home or at the hospital. Timely provision of appropriately aggressive pain control can substantially decrease patient anxiety, which, in turn, increases the patient's coping skills and optimism.

A. Continuous care and patient turnover. One of the major challenges in emergency management is providing continuity of care for frequently seen patients. Another problem is the need for rapid patient turnover. Holding areas, where aggressive pain management can be provided for 12 to 24 hours, can decrease the need for inpatient admission. Many patients can manage pain at home after a short period of parenteral opioids and hydration.

B. Initial assessment involves gathering detailed patient information.
   1. The intensity and location of pain
   2. The duration of pain
   3. The pattern of pain (short or long, and whether it was easy to treat)
   4. At-home experience. To determine treatment and disposition, the care provider must understand the patient's home pain management experience:
      a. The patient who comes to the hospital after aggressive and persistent home management has failed is more likely to require admission.
      b. The dates of recent episodes and the patient's history of opioid use (for the most recent 2 months) are helpful in determining the initial opioid dose. The patient who frequently requires opioids is likely to be tolerant to opioids and to require higher starting doses.
   5. Previous hospitalization. The patient with frequent pain requiring hospital-based management is likely to know the doses and medications that have proved most effective. In chronic illness, patients should be encouraged to take a responsible role in their care. A detailed knowledge of past treatment usually reflects an active involvement. Requests for medications and doses that have worked in the past should not be considered malingering or drug-seeking behavior.
   6. The rest of the history and physical examination should focus on the detection of **signs of infection and other problems.**

C. Stages of emergency room opioid management
   1. An initial starting dose is determined and given.
   2. Analgesia and sedation are assessed at the time of peak effect. If analgesia is not adequate, an incremental dose titration is performed.
   3. After adequate analgesia is achieved, disposition of the patient is decided in collaboration with the patient and the family.
   4. Analgesia is maintained, either orally or parenterally.

D. Opioid management
   1. Respiratory complications. As pain is relieved, the respiratory rate may decline to normal. Sedation is often observed when providing adequate analgesia because patients may be sleep-deprived.
      a. If the dose is too large, however, the respiratory rate may fall significantly. This should not occur if titration proceeds with care.
      b. If significant depression without respiratory arrest occurs, small doses of naloxone may be infused. A starting dose of naloxone for a patient with severe pain could be approximately 1 μg/kg of body weight. If there is no response in a few minutes, the dose is doubled and repeated. Meanwhile, respiration can be increased by physical and verbal stimulation. Subsequent doses may be required at intervals of about 20–30 minutes. This dose is considerably below that given to the patient with coma of unknown etiology. However, large doses of naloxone will produce extreme pain, can result in pulmonary edema and other side effects, and make subsequent provision of opioid analgesia difficult until excreted.
      c. In the case of **respiratory arrest with no response to stimulation,** resuscitation includes the use of larger doses of naloxone, along with life support measures.
   2. Starting doses of opioids should be based on
      a. What has worked in the recent past
      b. The intensity of the pain

Table 33-1. Guide to intravenous dose titration

	Analgesia		
Sedation	None	Partial	Adequate
None	Repeat half to full dose	Repeat quarter to half dose	Observe duration of analgesia
Moderate	Repeat half dose	Repeat quarter dose	Observe duration of analgesia
Profound	Reassess patient Monitor Maximize nonopioid intervention	Monitor patient Maximize nonopioid intervention Decrease subsequent dose	Monitor patient Decrease subsequent doses

Analgesia and sedation are assessed 15 to 30 minutes after the initial intravenous dose.

     c. The estimated degrees of opioid tolerance

     d. Adequacy of home management. Adequate home management for moderate and severe pain is defined as the use of a nonopioid and an opioid analgesic at appropriate doses and intervals for several doses. If adequate home-based pain management has failed, the initial opioid dose in the emergency room should offer 2 to 3 times the analgesia given at home. For example, the addition of codeine or oxycodone can approximately double the analgesic efficacy, if only a nonopioid analgesic has been used at home. If the patient has been taking 60 mg of codeine, then the use of hydromorphone 5 mg PO (or morphine 20 mg PO) or morphine 6 mg IV will approximately double the analgesia. It is reasonable to achieve 3 times the home analgesic effect for a patient who is opioid-tolerant and is in very severe pain. A patient who has not used opioids within 2 months should not be considered tolerant of opioids, and traditional doses should be used for the first dose. In contrast, the patient who uses opioids frequently at home, or who is often admitted for pain management, is tolerant to opioids and may require much higher initial doses. Cross-tolerance between opioids may not be complete. Thus, a patient who has been using only oxycodone is not necessarily tolerant to hydromorphone or morphine.

  3. Management after initial dose. The peak effect for oral opioids occurs 45–60 minutes after the dose. The peak effect for intravenous opioids occurs within several minutes of infusion—soon after the dose crosses the blood-brain barrier.

     a. Because the peak effect occurs so rapidly, intravenous doses can be repeated in small increments at very frequent intervals until adequate analgesia is achieved. This dose titration can consist of doses repeated every 10 to 15 minutes.

     b. After the initial dose is given, analgesia and sedation should be assessed during peak effect.

     c. Subsequent dose titration based on that assessment is shown in Table 33-1. The lower ranges are recommended unless the physician is highly experienced in pain management.

  4. Maintenance of analgesia. For the patient with moderate or severe pain who is sent home, scheduled doses are suggested for at least the first 24 hours. Follow-up should be provided, and opioids should be prescribed to maintain the patient until he or she can be seen by the primary care provider. Some patients may be held in the emergency room for a few hours or more. As analgesia subsides, another dose will be required. Analgesia duration will last from half an hour to several hours depending on

     a. The severity of the pain

     b. The individual

     c. Pharmacokinetics

     d. The dose given. The patient should receive another dose of analgesia before the pain becomes severe. If the pain is so severe that the patient requires admission to the hospital, an extra dose of medication before transport may be helpful as movement may exacerbate pain.

VIII. **Inpatient management.** As in the emergency room, there are several phases of management:

A. **Assessment and determination of mode of management.** This phase follows the general principles outlined in section **V.A** on pharmacologic treatment. If the patient has previously been successfully managed with a particular route and schedule, this should probably be continued. If at all possible, the route to be used throughout the acute phase should be introduced immediately; otherwise, the patient must make adjustment to changes in management.

B. **Dose titration.** See section **VII.C** on emergency room treatment.

C. **Maintenance of analgesia.** Assessment of pain, response to analgesia, and sedation should be assessed at regular intervals. During the maintenance phase, the patient should be encouraged to use other techniques of pain control as supplements to pharmacologic therapy.

D. **Weaning** can cause discord between the patient and the medical caretakers.

  1. Precipitous or forced weaning may result in reinstitution of more aggressive therapy. It is far better to wean in a controlled manner, so that there is no necessity to backtrack. The patient will then view the process with optimism rather than with anxiety.

  2. The dose, rather than the interval, should be changed to prevent the recurrence of severe pain. A decrease of about 20–25% per day is reasonable, although for patients with rapid resolution of pain, a much more rapid decrease is necessary.

  3. Substitution of oral for parenteral medication can take place when the dose has been decreased to about one half of the starting dose. It is crucial that patient control and responsibility be emphasized during the weaning process.

  4. For patients on patient-controlled analgesia, it is often sufficient to stop the basal infusion and substitute an oral opioid to be taken at scheduled intervals. The patient-controlled dose can be continued. However, most patients spontaneously decrease and then stop using the medicine. For others, it may be necessary to gradually decrease the patient-controlled dose.

  5. During hospitalization, the nonopioid analgesic should be continued unless the pain stops entirely. The patient can be discharged when the pain is manageable for both the patient and the family.

Selected Readings

Benjamin LJ, Nagel RL. The comprehensive sickle cell day hospital: an alternative to the emergency room for the management of acute sickle pain [abstract]. Presented at the Sixteenth Annual Meeting of the National Sickle Cell Disease Program, Mobile, Alabama, 1991.

Carr DB, Jacox AK (eds.). *Acute Pain Management: Operative or Medical Procedures and Trauma.* Washington, DC: Agency for Health Care Policy and Research, Public Health Service, U.S. Department of Health and Human Services, 1992.

Charache S, Moyer M. Treatment of patients with sickle cell anemia—another view. *Prog Clin Biol Res* 98:73–81, 1982.

Payne R. Pain management in sickle cell disease. *Ann N Y Acad Sci* 565:189–206, 1989.

Serjeant GR. *Sickle Cell Disease.* Oxford, UK: Oxford University Press, 1985.

Shapiro B. Management of painful episodes in sickle cell disease. In Schechter NI, Berde CB, Yaster M (eds.), *Pain in Infants, Children, and Adolescents.* Baltimore: Williams & Wilkins, 1993.

Shapiro B, Cohen D, Howe C. Patient-controlled analgesia for sickle cell related pain. *J Pain Symptom Manage* 8:22–28, 1993.

Vichinsky EP, Johnson R, Lubin BH. Multidisciplinary approach to pain management in sickle cell disease. *Am J Ped Hematol Oncol* 4:328–333, 1982.

Weissman SJ, Schechter NL. Sickle cell anemia: pain management. In Sinatra RS, Hord AH, Ginsberg B, Prebble L (eds.), *Acute Pain: Mechanism and Management.* St. Louis: Mosby–Year Book, 1992. Pp. 508–516.

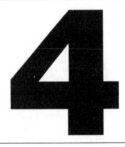

Herpes Zoster and Postherpetic Neuralgia

David J. Wlody

I. Background. Herpes zoster and postherpetic neuralgia are among the most common pain syndromes encountered in clinical practice. The incidence of both zoster and postherpetic neuralgia increases with age, and as Loeser points out, the shift of the age distribution in the United States will inevitably lead to an increase in the incidence of both disorders.[1] The importance of these disorders is that **early treatment of herpes zoster may prevent the subsequent development of postherpetic neuralgia.** As postherpetic neuralgia can be both intensely painful and extremely difficult to treat, the early recognition and aggressive therapy of herpes zoster can be of enormous benefit to patients.

II. Herpes zoster

  A. Definition and incidence

    1. Herpes zoster, also known as **shingles,** is an acute viral infection manifested by the appearance of vesicular lesions in a single dermatome or several contiguous dermatomes. **The causative agent is varicella zoster,** the same DNA virus that produces chickenpox during childhood.

    2. Herpes zoster is **rare in children** and is seen with **increasing frequency in the elderly.** There is an increased incidence of zoster in patients with malignancies (particularly lymphomas) and in patients who are iatrogenically immunosuppressed. There is some evidence of an increased incidence in patients with AIDS.[2]

    3. Herpes zoster is a **self-limited process.** In 10–50% of patients with zoster, however, pain may persist long after healing of the vesicular lesions in a syndrome known as postherpetic neuralgia (see section **III**).

  B. Pathology

    1. The **initial varicella infection in childhood** produces a viremia that leads to the characteristic skin lesions of chickenpox. Retrograde axonal transport carries the virus to the cells of the dorsal root ganglion, where it can remain quiescent for years.

    2. With impairment of the normal immune response, **the virus can be reactivated,** transported via the sensory nerve to the skin, and there produce the characteristic vesicular lesions in a dermatomal distribution.

    3. Herpes zoster never represents a primary infection; it is only seen in patients with a previous varicella infection.

  C. Clinical presentation

    1. Herpes zoster presents with pain and paresthesias limited to a single dermatome or several contiguous dermatomes. This is followed in several days by vesicle formation. The vesicles typically crust in 1 week and heal in approximately 1 month, leaving regions of hypopigmentation. **During the acute stage** of zoster, **pain may be severe** and aggravated by touch or movement.

    2. The **most common site** of involvement **is the thoracic region, but any site may be involved.** Involvement of the geniculate ganglion can produce the Ramsay Hunt syndrome consisting of Bell's palsy, vertigo, and lesions of the external ear and auditory canal. Involvement of the trigeminal ganglion can produce corneal lesions and pupillary disturbances.

    3. Constitutional symptoms including fever, headache, malaise, lymphadenopathy, and nausea are not uncommon.

    4. A localized herpes simplex infection in a single dermatome can be confused with zoster. **Viral cultures** can distinguish the two disorders.

    5. It is particularly important to distinguish herpes simplex keratitis from ophthalmic herpes zoster. **Corticosteroid therapy, which is appropriate for ophthalmic zoster, is contraindicated in herpes simplex.**

D. Treatment of herpes zoster

1. One could argue that the self-limited nature of zoster necessitates only **symptomatic treatment** with analgesics. However, as mentioned previously, more aggressive treatment will not only give better pain relief but also accelerate healing and, more importantly, may decrease the incidence of postherpetic neuralgia.

2. **Antiviral drugs** including adenine arabinoside[3] (10 mg/kg over 12 h daily for 5 days) and acyclovir[4] (500 mg/m^2 tid for 7 days) have been shown to accelerate healing of vesicles and provide faster pain relief. There is also a suggestion that antiviral therapy will decrease the incidence of postherpetic neuralgia. This effect is most marked when antiviral therapy is begun as early as possible in the course of the illness.

3. There is considerable reason to believe **sympathetic blockade** will act synergistically with antiviral chemotherapy to accelerate healing and provide complete pain relief, while reducing the likelihood of the development of postherpetic neuralgia. The best results are obtained when blockade is performed within several days of the initial symptoms, preferably before vesicles develop. Bonica and Buckley recommend performing blocks on a daily basis for 5 to 7 days, and then 3 times weekly until pain relief persists.[5] It appears that paravertebral sympathetic block and epidural block are equally effective, although placement of an epidural catheter allows maintenance of sympathetic block over an extended period of time.

4. The use of **systemic corticosteroids** may also accelerate healing and decreases postherpetic neuralgia. One dosage schedule consists of prednisone 60 mg daily for 1 week, tapered to 30 mg in the second week, and 15 mg daily in the third week.[6]

5. Subcutaneous injection of **local anesthetic and steroid mixtures** has also been used effectively in herpes zoster. Mayne et al. recommend the use of 0.2% triamcinolone in 0.25% bupivacaine, injected throughout the affected area, 2 or 3 times weekly until improvement is seen, at which time treatments are decreased to once weekly until resolution.[6]

III. Postherpetic neuralgia

A. Incidence

1. When healing of the vesicular eruption is followed by **persistent pain in a dermatomal distribution,** the diagnosis of postherpetic neuralgia can be made.

2. The incidence of postherpetic neuralgia is **age-related.** Its incidence may be greater than 50% in patients over age 60. In addition, the duration of postherpetic neuralgia is much more likely to be prolonged in the elderly.

3. **Diabetes mellitus** reportedly **increases the risk** of postherpetic neuralgia.

4. Postherpetic neuralgia is more commonly seen **after ophthalmic herpes zoster.**

B. Pathophysiology

1. Numerous theories have been proposed to explain the development of postherpetic neuralgia. Most authorities feel that this disorder represents **deafferentation pain,** which is perpetuated at a central level.

2. This **central mechanism** is supported by the general lack of response to section of peripheral nerves. It is also supported by the better success rate seen with centrally acting drugs such as antidepressants (see section **III.D.2.b**).

C. Clinical presentations

1. Postherpetic neuralgia is characterized by a **constant burning, aching pain,** often with a superimposed shooting component. The afflicted area can be hypoesthetic or hyperesthetic. Dysesthesias such as formication (the sensation of ants crawling on the skin) are not uncommon.

2. Although other conditions may mimic postherpetic neuralgia, the development of **pain in a dermatomal distribution** after a previous vesicular eruption is pathognomonic of postherpetic neuralgia.

D. Treatment of postherpetic neuralgia

1. Numerous pharmacologic, regional anesthetic, and surgical therapies have been used in an attempt to relieve postherpetic neuralgia. Unfortunately, many of these therapies are of doubtful efficacy, and none is completely effective. As stated above, the most effective strategy appears to be one of preventing the development of postherpetic neuralgia through the **aggressive treatment of herpes zoster** in its earliest stages.

2. **Pharmacologic therapy**

   a. **Narcotic analgesics should be used with great care** in patients with postherpetic neuralgia. Effective analgesia occurs at narcotic levels that are close to toxic. Because of the chronic nature of the disorder, development of drug dependence is a very real risk. However, short-term use of narcotics may be needed while evaluating other long-term therapies.

b. **Tricyclic antidepressants** have been used in a number of studies with encouraging results. Although many patients with postherpetic neuralgia are depressed, these drugs can be effective even in the absence of depression. There is some evidence that the addition of a phenothiazine may improve pain relief. Loeser suggests a single bedtime dose of amitriptyline 25 mg, increased to 75 mg over a period of 10 days, combined with fluphenazine 1 mg q6h.[1] Several authors have postulated that a therapeutic window exists with the tricyclic antidepressants and that high doses may not be as effective as lower doses.[7] It is important to note that phenothiazines may have exaggerated side effects in the elderly, and their use in this group should be carefully monitored.[2]

c. **Anticonvulsants** have been utilized in the treatment of postherpetic neuralgia. They are generally used in combination with an antidepressant. Their addition to an antidepressant regimen appears to be particularly effective when there is a significant lancinating component to the pain. **Carbamazepine** is most commonly used (100 mg bid titrated slowly upward until relief is obtained or blood levels are in the anticonvulsant range) although **valproic acid** and **phenytoin** (Dilantin) are also reported to be effective. Their dosage should also be increased in a stepwise fashion until relief or anticonvulsant blood levels are achieved.

d. **Capsaicin** is thought to selectively stimulate and then block small-diameter afferent nociceptive transmission by depleting neurotransmitter peptides such as substance P. Capsaicin has also been used for other chronic pains of peripheral origin and limited spatial extent such as diabetic neuropathy, ischemic neuropathy, contact dermatitis, and reflex sympathetic dystrophy. Guidelines in the use of capsaicin require supervision and patient education. They include the following:

(1) Application should be 4–5 times per day for at least 4 weeks. The onset and best response may be delayed until that time. Less frequent use may be ineffective.

(2) Patients should wash their hands after each application to prevent inadvertent contact with the eye.

(3) Patients should be seen weekly or bimonthly to encourage continued use and to deal with burning after capsaicin administration. This will become more bearable after the first week and can be tolerated if there is pretreatment with topical lidocaine (5%).

(4) At the end of 4 weeks, treatment should be withdrawn and reinstituted if there is the recurrence of pain.

3. **Regional block therapy**

a. **Local anesthetic blockade** of either somatic or sympathetic nerves has been reported to give good immediate relief. Over time, however, pain tends to recur. The best results are obtained when blocks are initiated soon after the development of neuralgia. Bonica and Buckley point out that although neural blockade provides inconsistent relief, the procedure is benign enough that it is worth a trial in patients with postherpetic neuralgia, especially in view of the lack of success of other therapies. They recommend a series of blocks done every other day, until a total of 7 to 10 is reached. Lack of success indicates that further blocks are unlikely to provide significant relief.[5]

b. **Neurolytic blockade** can be quite effective in providing short-term pain relief. Persistent anesthesia in the blocked area, however, can become as distressing to the patient as was the original pain.

4. **Ablative surgical therapy**

a. An impressive array of surgical treatments of postherpetic neuralgia have been attempted. These include peripheral nerve section, undermining of the affected skin, rhizotomy, thalamotomy, and lobotomy. None of these treatments has been shown to be consistently successful.

b. Friedman and Bullitt have reported their experience with **dorsal root entry zone (DREZ)** lesions: 91% of their patients had immediate relief, yet this dropped to 53% at 6 months and 25% at 18 months and beyond. In addition, a significant number of patients (22 of 32) developed postoperative lower extremity weakness.[8]

    c. This **lack of consistent success** under the best of circumstances points up the need to investigate all other avenues before performing an invasive and destructive procedure.

5. Electrical stimulation

    a. Transcutaneous electrical nerve stimulation (TENS) has been used with some success. The most important characteristics in its favor are its low cost and its lack of side effects. **Acupuncture,** like TENS, is more effective than the conventional technique.[9]

    b. Dorsal column stimulation shares with TENS the advantage of being only minimally invasive. Patients who obtain good relief from a trial can undergo internalization of the system.

    c. Intracerebral stimulation of the ventral posteromedial nucleus of the thalamus has been reported to provide long-term pain relief in one third of patients.[10] This procedure is maximally invasive, so it is **reserved for patients with disabling pain.**

6. The unfortunate truth remains that **no treatment** of postherpetic neuralgia **is consistently effective.** Because of the low probability of long-term success, any treatment regimen contemplated should also have a low probability of producing patient injury.

References

1. Loeser JD. Herpes zoster and post-herpetic neuralgia. In Bonica JJ (ed.), *The Management of Pain* (2nd ed.). Philadelphia: Lea & Febiger, 1990.
2. Portenoy RK, Duma C, Foley KM. Acute herpetic and post-herpetic neuralgia: clinical review and current management. *Ann Neurol* 20:651, 1986.
3. Whitley RJ, Chien LT, Dolin R, et al. Adenine arabinoside therapy of herpes zoster in the immunosuppressed. NIAID Collaborative Antiviral Study. *N Engl J Med* 294:1193, 1976.
4. Balfour HH, Bean B, Laskin OL, et al. Acyclovir halts progression of herpes zoster in immunocompromised patients. *N Engl J Med 308:1448, 1983.*
5. Bonica JJ, Buckley FP. Regional analgesia with local anesthetics. In Bonica JJ (ed.), *The Management of Pain* (2nd ed.). Philadelphia: Lea & Febiger, 1990.
6. Mayne GE, Brown M, Arnold P, Moya F. Pain of herpes zoster and post-herpetic neuralgia. In Raj PP (ed.), *Practical Management of Pain.* Chicago: Year Book Medical Publishers, 1986.
7. Watson CPN. Therapeutic window for amitriphyline analgesia. *Can Med Assoc J* 130:105, 1984.
8. Friedman AH, Bullitt E. Dorsal root entry zone lesions in the treatment of pain following brachial plexus avulsion, spinal cord injury and herpes zoster. *Appl Neurophysiol* 51:164, 1988.
9. Sjolund BH, Eriksson M, Loeser JD. Transcutaneous and implanted electric stimulation of peripheral nerves. In Bonica JJ (ed.), *The Management of Pain* (2nd ed.). Philadelphia: Lea & Febiger, 1990.
10. Siegfried J. Monopolar electrical stimulation of nucleus ventroposter-omedialis thalami for post-herpetic facial pain. *Appl Neurophysiol* 45:179, 1982.

Index

The letter *t* following a page number denotes a table, and *f* denotes a figure.